Cardiovascular Magnetic Resonance

Editor

SUBHA V. RAMAN

HEART FAILURE CLINICS

www.heartfailure.theclinics.com

Consulting Editor
EDUARDO BOSSONE

Founding Editor
JAGAT NARULA

January 2021 • Volume 17 • Number 1

ELSEVIER

1600 John F. Kennedy Boulevard • Suite 1800 • Philadelphia, Pennsylvania, 19103-2899

http://www.theclinics.com

HEART FAILURE CLINICS Volume 17, Number 1
January 2021 ISSN 1551-7136, ISBN-13: 978-0-323-71175-3

Editor: Joanna Collett
Developmental Editor: Laura Fisher

Heart Failure Clinics (ISSN 1551-7136) is published quarterly by Elsevier Inc., 360 Park Avenue South, New York, NY 10010-1710. Months of publication are January, April, July, and October. Business and editorial offices: 1600 John F. Kennedy Boulevard, Suite 1800, Philadelphia, PA 19103-2899. Periodicals postage paid at New York, NY, and additional mailing offices. Subscription prices are USD 277.00 per year for US individuals, USD 661.00 per year for US institutions, USD 100.00 per year for US students and residents, USD 300.00 per year for Canadian individuals, USD 684.00 per year for Canadian institutions, USD 315.00 per year for international individuals, USD 684.00 per year for international institutions, and USD 100.00 per year for Canadian and foreign students/residents. To receive student and resident rate, orders must be accompanied by name of affiliated institution, date of term, and the *signature* of program/residency coordinator on institution letterhead. Orders will be billed at individual rate until proof of status is received. Foreign air speed delivery is included in all *Clinics* subscription prices. All prices are subject to change without notice. **POSTMASTER:** Send address changes to *Heart Failure Clinics*, Elsevier Health Sciences Division, Subscription Customer Service, 3251 Riverport Lane, Maryland Heights, MO 63043. **Customer Service: 1-800-654-2452 (US and Canada). From outside of the US and Canada, call 314-447-8871. Fax: 314-447-8029. For print support, E-mail: JournalsCustomerService-usa@elsevier.com. For online support, E-mail: JournalsOnlineSupport-usa@elsevier.com.**

Reprints. For copies of 100 or more of articles in this publication, please contact the Commercial Reprints Department, Elsevier Inc., 360 Park Avenue South, New York, NY 10010-1710. Tel.: 212-633-3874; Fax: 212-633-3820; E-mail: reprints@elsevier.com.

Heart Failure Clinics is covered in *MEDLINE/PubMed (Index Medicus).*

Contributors

CONSULTING EDITOR

EDUARDO BOSSONE, MD, PhD, FCCP, FESC, FACC
Division of Cardiology, AORN Antonio
Cardarelli Hospital, Naples, Italy

EDITOR

SUBHA V. RAMAN, MD
Professor and Chief, Krannert Institute of
Cardiology, Indiana University School of
Medicine, Indianapolis, Indiana, USA

AUTHORS

ASHISH ANEJA, MD, FACC, FSCMR, FASE
Associate Professor, Department of
Cardiovascular Diseases, Case Western
Reserve University, MetroHealth Medical
Center, Cleveland, Ohio, USA

ANNA BARITUSSIO, MD, PhD
Department of Cardiac, Thoracic, Vascular
Sciences and Public Health, University
Hospital Padua, Padua, Italy

WENDY BOTTINOR, MD, MSCI
Department of Internal Medicine, Division of
Cardiovascular Medicine, Pauley Heart Center,
Virginia Commonwealth University, Division of
Cardiovascular Medicine, Department of
Medicine, Vanderbilt University School of
Medicine, Nashville, Tennessee, USA

CHIARA BUCCIARELLI-DUCCI, MD, PhD
Department of Cardiology, Bristol Heart
Institute, University Hospitals Bristol and
Weston NHS Foundation Trust, Bristol Medical
School, Translational Health Sciences,
University of Bristol, Bristol National Institute of
Health Research (NIHR) Centre University of
Bristol and University Hospitals Bristol NHS
Foundation Trust, Bristol, United Kingdom

FRANCESCO CAPUANO, PhD
Department of Industrial Engineering, Federico
II University of Naples, Naples, Italy

ROSANGELA COCCHIA, MD
Cardiology Division, A Cardarelli Hospital,
Naples, Italy

CARLA CONTALDI, MD, PhD
Department of Cardiology, University Hospital
of Salerno, Salerno, Italy

ESTEFANIA De GARATE, MD
Department of Cardiology, Bristol Heart
Institute, University Hospitals Bristol and
Weston NHS Foundation Trust, Bristol Medical
School, Translational Health Sciences,
University of Bristol, Bristol, United Kingdom

SANTO DELLEGROTTAGLIE, MD, PhD
Cardiovascular Magnetic Resonance
Laboratory, Hospital Villa dei Fiori, Naples, Italy

ANEESH S. DHORE-PATIL, MD
Cardiology Fellow, Tulane University Heart and
Vascular Center, Tulane University, New
Orleans, Louisiana, USA

MOHAMMED S.M. ELBAZ, PhD
Department of Radiology, Feinberg School of
Medicine, Northwestern University, Chicago,
Illinois, USA

FRANCESCO FERRARA, MD, PhD
Department of Cardiology, University Hospital
of Salerno, Salerno, Italy

J. PAUL FINN, MD
Diagnostic Cardiovascular Imaging Research
Laboratory, Department of Radiology, David
Geffen School of Medicine at UCLA, Physics
and Biology in Medicine Graduate Program,
University of California, Los Angeles, Los
Angeles, California, USA

AAKASH N. GUPTA, BS
Department of Radiology, Feinberg School of
Medicine, Northwestern University, Chicago,
Illinois, USA

BRIAN P. HALLIDAY, PhD
National Heart and Lung Institute, Imperial
College, CMR Unit, Royal Brompton Hospital,
London, United Kingdom

DANIEL J. HAMMERSLEY, MBBS
National Heart and Lung Institute, Imperial
College, CMR Unit, Royal Brompton Hospital,
London, United Kingdom

KATE HANNEMAN, MD, MPH, FRCPC
Department of Medical Imaging, University
Health Network, University of Toronto, Division
of Radiology, Toronto General Hospital,
Toronto, Ontario, Canada

IWAN HARRIES, MBBCh, BSc
Department of Cardiology, Bristol Heart
Institute, University Hospitals Bristol and
Weston NHS Foundation Trust, Bristol Medical
School, Translational Health Sciences,
University of Bristol, Bristol, United Kingdom

NATALIE HO, MD
Division of Cardiology, Scarborough Health
Network, Scarborough General Hospital,
Toronto, Ontario, Canada

PENG HU, PhD
Diagnostic Cardiovascular Imaging Research
Laboratory, Department of Radiology, David
Geffen School of Medicine at UCLA, Physics
and Biology in Medicine Graduate Program,
University of California, Los Angeles, Los
Angeles, California, USA

W. GREGORY HUNDLEY, MD
Department of Internal Medicine, Division of
Cardiovascular Medicine, Pauley Heart Center,
Virginia Commonwealth University, Richmond,
Virginia, USA

CHRISTOPHER JANISH, MD
Cardiology Fellow, Division of Cardiology,
Krannert Institute of Cardiology at Indiana
University School of Medicine, Indianapolis,
Indiana, USA

OMAR JAWAID, MD
Cardiology Fellow, Division of Cardiology,
Krannert Institute of Cardiology at Indiana
University School of Medicine, Indianapolis,
Indiana, USA

RICHARD E. JONES, MBChB
National Heart and Lung Institute, Imperial
College, CMR Unit, Royal Brompton Hospital,
London, United Kingdom

SABRA C. LEWSEY, MD MPH
Division of Cardiology, Department of
Medicine, Johns Hopkins School of Medicine,
Johns Hopkins Hospital, Baltimore, Maryland,
USA

KATE LIANG, MBBCh
Department of Cardiology, Bristol Heart
Institute, University Hospitals Bristol and
Weston NHS Foundation Trust, Bristol Medical
School, Translational Health Sciences,
University of Bristol, Bristol, United Kingdom

LUKAS MACH, MD
National Heart and Lung Institute, Imperial
College, CMR Unit, Royal Brompton Hospital,
London, United Kingdom

MICHAEL MARKL, PhD
Department of Radiology, Feinberg School of
Medicine, Department of Biomedical
Engineering, McCormick School of
Engineering, Northwestern University,
Evanston, Illinois, USA

GAETANO MIRTO
Engineer, Clinical Engineering Division, A
Cardarelli Hospital, Naples, Italy

VIVEK MUTHURANGU, MD(res)
Professor of Cardiovascular Imaging and
Physics, Institute of Cardiovascular Science,
University College London, London, United
Kingdom

GILLIAN NESBITT, MD
Division of Cardiology, Mount Sinai Hospital,
Toronto, Ontario, Canada

KIM-LIEN NGUYEN, MD
Division of Cardiology, David Geffen School of
Medicine at UCLA, VA Greater Los Angeles
Healthcare System, Diagnostic Cardiovascular
Imaging Research Laboratory, Department of
Radiology, David Geffen School of Medicine at
UCLA, Physics and Biology in Medicine
Graduate Program, University of California, Los
Angeles, Los Angeles, California, USA

ROBERT O. BONOW, MD, FAHA, FESC
Department of Medicine-Cardiology,
Northwestern University Feinberg School of
Medicine, Chicago, Illinois, USA

**EDUARDO BOSSONE, MD, PhD, FCCP,
FESC, FACC**
Division of Cardiology, AORN Antonio
Cardarelli Hospital, Naples, Italy

ELLEN OSTENFIELD, MD, PhD
Department of Medical Imaging and
Physiology, Cardiac Imaging, Skåne University
Hospital, Lund, Sweden

ALBERTO PALAZZUOLI, MD, PhD
Cardiovascular Diseases Unit, Department of
Internal Medicine, Le Scotte Hospital,
University of Siena, Siena, Italy

SANJAY K. PRASAD, MD
National Heart and Lung Institute, Imperial
College, CMR Unit, Royal Brompton Hospital,
London, United Kingdom

SUBHA V. RAMAN, MD
Professor and Chief, Krannert Institute of
Cardiology, Indiana University School of
Medicine, Indianapolis, Indiana, USA

BRIGIDA RANIERI, PhD
IRCCS SDN, Naples, Italy

ROOPA A. RAO, MBBS
Assistant Professor of Clinical Medicine,
Division of Cardiology, Krannert Institute of
Cardiology at Indiana University School of
Medicine, Indianapolis, Indiana, USA

SALVATORE REGA
Medical School, Federico II University of
Naples, Naples, Italy

LUIGIA ROMANO, MD
General and Emergency Radiology Division, A
Cardarelli Hospital, Naples, Italy

MICHAEL SCHÄR, PhD
Division of Magnetic Resonance Research,
Department of Radiology, Johns Hopkins
School of Medicine, Johns Hopkins Hospital,
Baltimore, Maryland, USA

DAVID E. SOSNOVIK, MD
Cardiology Division, Cardiovascular Research
Center, Department of Radiology, Athinoula A.
Martinos Center for Biomedical Imaging,
Massachusetts General Hospital, Harvard
Medical School, Boston, Massachusetts, USA;
Division of Health Sciences and Technology,
Harvard Medical School and Massachusetts
Institute of Technology, Cambridge,
Massachusetts, USA

JOEVIN SOURDON, PhD
Aix-Marseille Université, CNRS, CRMBM,
Faculté de Médecine, Marseille, France;
Division of Cardiology, Department of
Medicine, Johns Hopkins School of Medicine,
Baltimore, Maryland, USA

ANNA AGNESE STANZIOLA, MD
Department of Respiratory Diseases, Monaldi
Hospital, University "Federico II," Naples, Italy

**PAALADINESH THAVENDIRANATHAN, MD,
SM, FRCPC, FASE**
Department of Medical Imaging, University
Health Network, University of Toronto, Division
of Cardiology, Peter Munk Cardiac Centre,
Division of Cardiology, Toronto General
Hospital, Toronto, Ontario, Canada

CORY R. TRANKLE, MD
Department of Internal Medicine, Division of
Cardiovascular Medicine, Pauley Heart Center,

Virginia Commonwealth University, Richmond, Virginia, USA

SETH URETSKY, MD, FACC
Medical Director of Cardiovascular Imaging, Assistant Director, Cardiology Fellowship Program, Department of Cardiovascular Medicine, Gagnon Administration, Meade B, Morristown Medical Center/Atlantic Health System, Morristown, New Jersey, USA

ROBERT G. WEISS, MD
Division of Cardiology, Department of Medicine, Johns Hopkins School of Medicine, Baltimore, Maryland, USA

MATTHEW WILLIAMS, MBChB, BSc
Department of Cardiology, Bristol Heart Institute, University Hospitals Bristol and Weston NHS Foundation Trust, Bristol Medical School, Translational Health Sciences, University of Bristol, Bristol, United Kingdom

STEVEN WOLFF, MD, PhD, FACR
Owner, NeoSoft, LLC, Pewaukee, Wisconsin, USA

Contents

Use of cardiac magnetic resonance (CMR) to aid in diagnosis, management, and prognosis of ischemic and nonischemic cardiomyopathy has advanced tremendously in the past several decades. These advances have expanded our understanding of both ischemic and nonischemic cardiomyopathies while also allowing for new avenues of diagnosis and treatment. This review summarizes key concepts of CMR technology and CMR use in the diagnosis and prognosis in ischemic, infiltrative, inflammatory, and other nonischemic cardiomyopathies and discusses the use of CMR in the patient presenting with ventricular arrhythmia with unclear diagnosis and advances in CMR in the management cardiomyopathy.

 Video content accompanies this article at http://www.heartfailure.theclinics.com.

Classification of heart failure is based on the left ventricular ejection fraction (EF): preserved EF, midrange EF, and reduced EF. There remains an unmet need for further heart failure phenotyping of ventricular structure-function relationships. Because of high spatiotemporal resolution, cardiac magnetic resonance (CMR) remains the reference modality for quantification of ventricular contractile function. The authors aim to highlight novel frameworks, including theranostic use of ferumoxytol, to enable more efficient evaluation of ventricular function in heart failure patients who are also frequently anemic, and to discuss emerging quantitative CMR approaches for evaluation of ventricular structure-function relationships in heart failure.

Cardiovascular magnetic resonance represents the imaging modality of choice for the investigation of patients with heritable cardiomyopathies. The combination of gold-standard volumetric analysis with tissue characterization can deliver precise phenotypic evaluation of both cardiac morphology and the underlying myocardial substrate. Cardiovascular magnetic resonance additionally has an established role in risk-stratifying patients with heritable cardiomyopathy and an emerging role in guiding therapies. This article explores the application and utility of cardiovascular magnetic resonance techniques with specific focus on the major heritable cardiomyopathies.

> Ischemic heart disease is the most common cause of cardiovascular morbidity and mortality. Cardiac magnetic resonance (CMR) improves on other noninvasive modalities in detection, assessment, and prognostication of ischemic heart disease. The incorporation of CMR in clinical trials allows for smaller patient samples without the sacrifice of power needed to demonstrate clinical efficacy. CMR can accurately quantify infarct acuity, size, and complications; guide therapy; and prognosticate recovery. Timing of revascularization remains the holy grail of ischemic heart disease, and viability assessment using CMR may be the missing link needed to help reduce morbidity and mortality associated with the disease

> Right heart and pulmonary circulation disorders are generally caused by right ventricle (RV) pressure overload, volume overload, and cardiomyopathy, and they are associated with distinct clinical courses and therapeutic approaches, although they often may coexist. Cardiac magnetic resonance (CMR) provides a noninvasive accurate and reproducible multiplanar anatomic and functional assessment, tissue characterization, and blood flow evaluation of the right heart and pulmonary circulation. This article reviews the current status of the CMR, the most recent techniques, the new parameters and their clinical utility in diagnosis, prognosis, and therapeutic management in the right heart and pulmonary circulation disorders.

> Cardiac magnetic resonance (CMR) imaging is a unique imaging modality, which provides accurate noninvasive tissue characterization. Various CMR sequences can be utilized to identify and quantify patterns of myocardial edema, fibrosis, and infiltrates, which are important determinants for diagnosis and prognostication of heart failure. This article describes available methods of tissue characterization imaging applied in CMR. The presence and patterns of abnormal tissue characterization are related to common etiologies of heart failure and the techniques employed to demonstrate this. CMR provides the opportunity to identify the etiology of heart failure based on the recognition of different patterns of myocardial abnormalities.

> Advances in technology have made it possible to image the microstructure of the heart with diffusion-weighted magnetic resonance. The technique provides unique insights into the cellular architecture of the myocardium and how this is perturbed in a range of disease contexts. In this review, the physical basis of diffusion MRI and the challenges of implementing it in the beating heart are discussed. Cutting edge acquisition and analysis techniques, as well as the results of initial clinical studies, are reported.

The heart has the highest energy demands per gram of any organ in the body and energy metabolism fuels normal contractile function. Metabolic inflexibility and impairment of myocardial energetics occur with several common cardiac diseases, including ischemia and heart failure. This review explores several decades of innovations in cardiac magnetic resonance spectroscopy modalities and their use to noninvasively identify and quantify metabolic derangements in the normal, failing, and diseased heart. The implications of this noninvasive modality for predicting significant clinical outcomes and guiding future investigation and therapies to improve patient care are discussed.

Over the past decade, cardiovascular magnetic resonance (CMR) has become a mainstream noninvasive imaging tool for assessment of adult and pediatric patients with congenital heart disease. It provides comprehensive anatomic and hemodynamic information that echocardiography and catheterization alone do not provide. Extracardiac anatomy can be delineated with high spatial resolution, intracardiac anatomy can be imaged in multiple planes, and functional assessment can be made accurately and with high reproducibility. In patients with heart failure, CMR provides not only reference standard evaluation of ventricular volumes and function but also information about the possible causes of dysfunction.

HEART FAILURE CLINICS

SERIES OF RELATED INTEREST

Cardiology Clinics
http://www.cardiology.theclinics.com/
Cardiac Electrophysiology Clinics
https://www.cardiacep.theclinics.com/
Interventional Cardiology Clinics
https://www.interventional.theclinics.com/

THE CLINICS ARE AVAILABLE ONLINE!
Access your subscription at:
www.theclinics.com

Preface
Cardiovascular Magnetic Resonance in Heart Failure

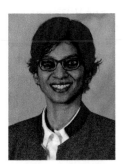

Subha V. Raman, MD
Editor

Failure is not fatal, but failure to change might be.[1]

The burden of heart failure (HF) on individuals, families, clinicians, and society cannot be overstated.[2] Upon hearing the diagnosis, patients may feel particularly oppressed by the term "failure"—a weight added to life-altering symptoms that brought them to the attention of clinical practitioners, scientists, and trainees. Those affected in the modern era, both patients and caregivers, may come across bleak statistics regarding HF-associated morbidity and mortality on their inevitable quest for information to find a way forward.

What does hope look like for someone receiving a new diagnosis of HF? Hope is the promise of better days, when a precise diagnosis points to effective treatments that restore one to the cherished activities of life curtailed by illness. Hope is also precision in prognosis, without which it is difficult to engage in shared decision making about potentially life-altering interventions. And, finally, hope is a lifeline to possibilities as yet undefined. It is the possibility of benefit, if not for oneself, then for a broader community, conveyed in investigations that leverage precision in diagnosis and prognosis to do even better than what we offer today.

Cardiovascular magnetic resonance (CMR) offers hope across the entire spectrum of HF. As the renowned authors in this issue of *Heart Failure Clinics* detail, CMR often holds the key to accurate diagnosis when traditional approaches have proved unrevealing, or when therapies instituted based on previously assumed diagnoses have been ineffective. CMR is most helpful when initiated by and interpreted with appropriate clinical acumen. As with any test, one's direct assessment of the patient helps guide the CMR examination and, in turn, consideration of treatment options based on the results. For instance, a patient presenting with HF found to have multivessel obstructive coronary artery disease and left ventricular systolic dysfunction may be referred for CMR-based viability assessment. Accurate quantification of concomitant significant mitral regurgitation with the detection of viable myocardium may favor surgical revascularization with mitral valve repair over multivessel percutaneous intervention.[3]

Heart Failure Clin 17 (2021) xiii–xiv
https://doi.org/10.1016/j.hfc.2020.10.001
1551-7136/21/© 2020 Published by Elsevier Inc.

heartfailure.theclinics.com

Prognosis is a particularly important measure in HF.[4] Guidelines advocate titration of medical therapy as tolerated; however, if there is extensive myocardial scar by late gadolinium enhancement CMR suggesting poor prognosis with medical therapy alone, discussions regarding advanced HF interventions such as device placement or cardiac transplantation could be initiated in a more timely manner. Prognosis may change, too, if one's initial assumptions need to be revised after CMR-based biomarkers indicate a myocardial disease that was not previously suspected. Consider, for instance, the patient thought to have "idiopathic" HF with preserved ejection fraction who undergoes CMR that reveals an infiltrative process amenable to disease-specific therapy.

Thousands of patients with HF are to be thanked for helping establish the evidence presented in this compendium that CMR can favorably impact HF outcomes. As the technology continues to advance toward noninvasive visualization and quantitation of mechanistically based disease features, CMR will be central in trials of novel therapies for HF. Alterations in myocardial energetics and myofiber architecture are both early mechanisms on the road to functional cardiac impairment and adverse cardiac remodeling. Both are well within the crosshairs of future trials using mechanistically informed CMR biomarkers to better diagnose and treat individuals at risk and further reduce the downstream burden of an HF diagnosis. Such a reduction can only be delivered through active partnerships between HF clinicians and CMR collaborators, with the publications in this issue of *Heart Failure Clinics* as a set of guideposts to achieve patient benefit via coordinated research and clinical care.

Subha V. Raman, MD
Krannert Institute of Cardiology
Indiana University School of Medicine
1800 North Capital Avenue
Indianapolis, IN 46202, USA

E-mail address:
suraman@iu.edu

REFERENCES

1. Wooden J. They Call Me Coach. New York: McGraw-Hill Education; 2004.
2. Virani SS, Alonso A, Benjamin EJ, et al. American Heart Association Council on E, Prevention Statistics C and Stroke Statistics S. Heart Disease and Stroke Statistics—2020 Update: a report from the American Heart Association. Circulation 2020;141:e139–596.
3. Uretsky S, Argulian E, Narula J, et al. Use of cardiac magnetic resonance imaging in assessing mitral regurgitation: current evidence. J Am Coll Cardiol 2018;71:547–63.
4. Gulati A, Japp AG, Raza S, et al. Absence of myocardial fibrosis predicts favorable long-term survival in new-onset heart failure. Circ Cardiovasc Imaging 2018;11:e007722.

When to Use Cardiovascular Magnetic Resonance in Patients with Heart Failure

Roopa A. Rao, MBBS[a],*, Omar Jawaid, MD[b], Christopher Janish, MD[b], Subha V. Raman, MD[c]

KEYWORDS

- Cardiac magnetic resonance • Heart failure • Late gadolinium enhancement

KEY POINTS

- Cardiac magnetic resonance (CMR) is comprehensive and accurate in determining the cause of cardiomyopathy or heart failure (HF) of unknown cause.
- Tissue characterization with qualitative late gadolinium enhancement as well as quantitative T1, T2, and T2* mapping afford detailed assessment of the myocardium.
- CMR is the gold standard to noninvasively quantify biventricular size and function, regional morphology, and tissue composition, all key to making the right diagnosis and selecting optimal therapies for cardiomyopathy/HF.
- Across a broad range of acquired and heritable cardiomyopathies, CMR provides specific biomarkers of disease that also have utility in establishing prognosis and tracking treatment response.

INTRODUCTION

Imaging in cardiovascular medicine has seen tremendous innovation in the past decade. Advances in echocardiography, cardiac computed tomography, cardiac magnetic resonance (CMR), and nuclear imaging have expanded the repertoire of diagnostic testing for the practicing clinician. This has been driven by patients' increasing complexity in an aging population. In particular, the rising burden of cardiomyopathies, both ischemic and nonischemic, has brought CMR to the forefront. CMR can assess scar burden, ventricular tachycardia substrate, and myocardial viability in ischemic cardiomyopathies, while also providing diagnostic clarity when applied to patients with nonischemic cardiomyopathy. In this review, the use of CMR is discussed with respect to both ischemic and nonischemic cardiomyopathy, its utility in diagnosis of the cause, prognostication, and treatment modifications.

COMMON CARDIAC MAGNETIC RESONANCE TERMINOLOGY SIMPLIFIED FOR THE CLINICIAN

One of the strengths of CMR is the ability to customize the examination through utilization of specific sequence to answer clinical questions. Multidimensional myocardial characterization, unique to CMR among various diagnostic tools, affords for many conditions noninvasive microscopic examination of the myocardium. In-depth discussion of the specifics of these sequences is

[a] Division of Cardiology, Krannert Institute of Cardiology at Indiana University School of Medicine, 1701, Senate Boulevard, MPC II, Suite 2000, Indianapolis, IN 46202, USA; [b] Division of Cardiology, Krannert Institute of Cardiology at Indiana University School of Medicine, 1800 North Capital Avenue, Indianapolis, IN 46202, USA; [c] Krannert Institute of Cardiology, Indiana University School of Medicine, 1800 North Capital Avenue, Indianapolis, IN 46202, USA
* Corresponding author.
E-mail address: rrao@iuhealth.org

Heart Failure Clin 17 (2021) 1–8
https://doi.org/10.1016/j.hfc.2020.09.001

beyond the scope of this review, but a brief understanding should be beneficial to the clinician.

1. Late gadolinium enhancement (LGE): indicates myocardial damage. Typical gadolinium-based contrast agents should be eliminated from intact myocardium after 10 to 15 minutes; persistence in the myocardium is visualized as enhancement after a delay using LGE imaging techniques. The pattern of LGE indicates mechanism of damage (eg, subendocardial = ischemic, midwall = nonischemic, epicardial = inflammatory).
2. T1—longitudinal relaxation: T1-weighted imaging or quantitative T1 mapping can be performed without contrast (eg, "native T1") as well as postcontrast. Native T1 values may indicate fat or iron infiltrate if significantly decreased or extracellular expansion by edema, infiltrate, or fibrosis if significantly elevated.
3. T2—transverse relaxation: T2-weighted imaging or quantitative T2 mapping is typically performed before contrast administration. Myocardial T2 that is elevated may indicate inflammation and/or edema. "T2-star" (T2*) is shortened by local iron deposition.
4. Myocardial extracellular volume fraction (ECV): computed from pre- and postcontrast T1 maps in conjunction with hematocrit. ECV elevation indicates myocardial interstitial expansion.

WHEN TO USE CARDIAC MAGNETIC RESONANCE IN NONISCHEMIC CARDIOMYOPATHY?

CMR increases the diagnostic yield in patients routinely labeled as idiopathic cardiomyopathy. In a study of 500 patients with nonischemic cardiomyopathy, CMR identified specific cause of heart failure in 36% of patients versus 20% by using echocardiography.[1] Ischemic type of scar is seen in about 13% of patients thought to have nonischemic cardiomyopathy. LGE is seen in about 10% to 30% of patients with nonischemic cardiomyopathy. The nonischemic pattern of LGE is usually midmyocardial linear striae, not following any vascular territory. The presence of midwall fibrosis by LGE portends worse prognosis, with increase in mortality and arrhythmic events.[2] LGE in the septum is associated with large increase in the risk of death and sudden cardiac death (SCD) even if the extent is small.[3]

Use of CMR, as with any diagnostic test, should be directed by clinical acumen. It's utility is greatest when the differential diagnosis of a condition, could be more effectively narrowed down with

CMR and can also modulate treatment. Routine CMR in all comers with nonischemic heart failure was shown in the OUTSMART-HF study to be no better than selective CMR for identifying specific heart failure causes.[1] This concept is still evolving, and future studies will shed more light into this.

In the next section the authors discuss some of the common causes of nonischemic cardiomyopathy and how CMR helps in overall care of the patient.

MYOCARDITIS

Myocarditis, often viral in cause, is the inflammation of the myocardium with varying clinical presentations from asymptomatic to fulminant heart failure. Clinical course is heterogeneous with full recovery or progression to end-stage heart failure or SCD. About 10% to 20% of chronic myocarditis can progress to dilated cardiomyopathy.

CMR helps in identifying different features of myocarditis such as edema, hyperemia and capillary leak, myocardial necrosis, and scar. Newer parametric CMR techniques such as T1 mapping, ECV fraction, and T2 mapping have evolved in the last decade to improve diagnostic accuracy in acute[4] and chronic myocarditis. CMR-based Lake Louis Criteria for diagnosis of myocarditis, originally developed in 2009 and modified in 2018,[5] has increased the diagnostic accuracy.

Endomyocardial biopsy is limited to fulminant myocarditis or myocarditis presenting with advanced heart block and life-threatening ventricular arrhythmias; although historically the gold standard, it is limited by sampling a few regions of the endocardium of the right ventricle. CMR can help in identifying the site of myocardial biopsy to improve the yield. There is good correlation between LGE seen on CMR and myocarditis features on biopsy. However, in most cases, CMR findings have abated the need for biopsy.

The LGE is usually seen in the free lateral myocardial wall. Endocardium is usually spared, which distinguishes this from ischemic cause. The lateral free-wall LGE is usually seen in parvovirus B19 infection, and human herpesvirus 6 mainly affects ventricular septum. Recent studies have shown association of location of LGE to prognosis in myocarditis. In ITAMY registry, LGE in anteroseptal wall had increased cardiac death, implantable cardiac defibrillator (ICD) firing, cardiac arrest, and hospitalization for heart failure.[6] Ventricular septal LGE can also be a predictor of chronic ventricular dysfunction, as well as ventricular dilatation at follow-up. Presence of LGE at 6-months CMR is associated with worse prognosis particularly with LGE midwall septal pattern.[7] SCD is unlikely with no LGE.

IRON OVERLOAD CARDIOMYOPATHY

Abnormal deposition of iron in myocardial tissue can lead to restrictive cardiomyopathy or dilated cardiomyopathy. Accumulation of toxic iron radicals can damage the myocardium. The accumulation in the conduction system can cause complete heart block, bradycardia, and atrial fibrillation. Primary iron overload can happen from hereditary hemochromatosis or secondary from multiple blood transfusions from various hematological disorders such as thalassemia and myelodysplastic syndrome.

CMR plays a key role in diagnosis and management of IOC and can be used as screening tool.[8] Serum ferritin level or hepatic iron cannot predict myocardial iron content. Myocardial uptake is lower than liver, hence cardiac findings lag liver manifestations. MRI-derived T2* relaxation time can assess the amount of iron in the myocardium. Normal T2* value at 1.5 T is greater than or equal to 20 msec. Iron-overloaded myocardium has shorter relaxation time, value less than 10 msec indicating severe and 10 to 20 msec indicating moderate to severe disease.

T2* value is associated with heart failure and risk of arrhythmias. Anderson and colleagues[9] initially validated T2* relaxometry and showed that as myocardial iron load increased, there was progressive decline in ejection fraction. In a prospective study of 652 patients with thalassemia major, the occurrence of heart failure within 1 year was 47%, 21%, and 0.2% in patients with T2* less than 6 ms, 6 to 10 ms, and greater than 10 ms, respectively. Arrhythmias occurred in 19% of patients with T2* less than 6 ms, 18% of those with T2* 6 to 10 ms, and 4% of those with T2* greater than 10 ms.[10]

Chelation therapy is the treatment of choice for IOC from blood transfusion and is heavily guided by the amount of iron in the myocardium. In no or mild myocardial involvement, a single-drug regimen is used to keep the T2* time greater than 20 msec. In moderate to severe disease 2 drug combinations or intravenous infusion is used to increase the T2* to greater than 20 msec.[8] The overall survival of patients with thalassemia has improved, and this has been partly attributed to better treatment based on MRI findings.

AMYLOIDOSIS

Amyloidosis is a systemic disease with deposition of fibrillatory protein amyloid in the extracellular tissue. There are more than 30 different types of amyloid protein with most common being light chain and transthyretin amyloid.

Unexplained left ventricular hypertrophy (LVH) evaluation is challenging, as it could be subtle and initial clue to the infiltrative disease (**Fig. 1**).

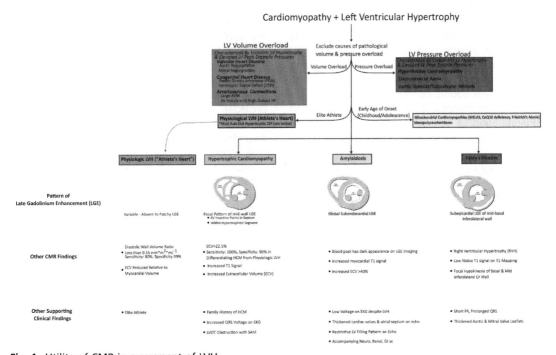

Fig. 1. Utility of CMR in assessment of LVH.

In light-chain amyloidosis CMR has high sensitivity and specificity. CMR should be considered early to evaluate cardiac involvement, as this can detect disease when echocardiogram can only have subtle features. In transthyretin amyloidosis either CMR or pyrophosphate scan can be used for diagnosis. CMR can help in assessing the myocardial thickness, assess the size of the atria, pericardial effusion, right heart involvement with thickening, and atrial dilatation.

Amyloid infiltration expands the extracellular space, and gadolinium is chelated into this space giving the characteristic appearance of diffuse subendocardial or transmural LGE. Subendocardial disease is usually seen during the early phase of the disease. Transmural LGE is usually seen more in transthyretin than light-chain amyloidosis.

In LGE imaging, blood usually seems bright. However, in amyloidosis, gadolinium binds to amyloid protein and is extracted relatively quickly giving blood a dark appearance (fast first-pass metabolism and high extraction from tissue uptake). This characteristic appearance of diffuse subendocardial enhancement along with dark blood appearance helps in differentiating it from other diseases with LVH.

Disease burden of amyloid in cardiac tissue can be quantitated by T1 mapping and ECV fraction. Both these techniques can be an early marker of disease. It has been shown to be present before the onset of LVH/LGE/biomarker elevation.[11] T1 mapping value has linear relationship, being high in advanced disease. Intramyocardial T1 gradient also has shown survival benefit, with 85% accuracy.[12] ECV values greater than 40% suggest amyloidosis. Hence both T1 mapping and ECV assessment provide prognostic utility and help in diagnosing the disease. T1 mapping can be useful when contrast agents cannot be given.

As in other disease states, CMR has helped in understanding of the histopathological changes and has reduced the need for cardiac biopsy.

FABRY DISEASE

Fabry disease is a X-linked disorder due to deficiency of the lysosomal enzyme alpha-galactosidase A, leading to accumulation of glycosphingolipids in the various organs. Myocardial involvement is the common cause of mortality and morbidity in Fabry disease. It causes ventricular arrhythmias, severe conduction disturbances, heart failure, and SCD. Accumulation of glycosphingolipids causes inflammation, LVH, and ultimately fibrosis. Unexplained LVH in relatively young patients can be misdiagnosed as hypertrophic cardiomyopathy (HCM), as 1% of such patients are found to have Fabry disease.[13] CMR along with echo helps in diagnosing the disease and monitoring the therapy.

LGE has a characteristic appearance and is typically seen as midwall enhancement in basal inferolateral wall for unknown reasons and often occurring on a nonhypertrophied segment. In most patients subendocardium is spared, distinguishing it from ischemic disease.

T1 relaxation time is reduced (as in IOC), and this can be seen in subclinical cases with marginal LVH. T1 relaxation can be used to detect early disease even when LVH is not apparent. In a study by Sado and colleagues,[14] low T1 value was observed in 40% patients with Fabry disease without LVH and in greater than 90% of patients with LVH. However, T1 relaxation time can be pseudonormal if relaxation time coexists with fibrosis.

In a recent large retrospective study of 90 patients with 4 years of follow-up, LGE was linked to increased cardiac events such as ventricular arrhythmias, bradycardia requiring pacemaker placement, severe heart failure, and SCD. As in HCM, LGE involving greater than 15% of LV mass was associated with the highest risk for cardiac event.[15]

HYPERTROPHIC CARDIOMYOPATHY

The diagnosis of HCM heavily relies on the noninvasive assessment of the LV wall thickness. However, echocardiography can be inconclusive due to poor acoustic windows or poor assessment of echo-blind areas such as the posterior part of the septum, apex, and anterolateral wall, where HCM features could be seen. CMR has better spatial resolution and provides sharp contrast between blood and myocardium aiding in the accurate assessment of the wall thickness. CMR provides a complete tomographic view of the myocardium, better evaluation of aneurysms and thrombus. When HCM diagnosis was inconclusive, about 6% of pts were identified by CMR compared with echo.[16] CMR can also assess the mitral valve structure and can give accurate assessment of mitral valve regurgitation and outflow tract.

Up to 50% to 70% of all patients with HCM have some evidence of LGE, which is mostly evident in the hypertrophied segment. LGE can also be seen in different locations and pattern.[16] Presence of LGE has been linked to LV dysfunction and occurrence of heart failure symptoms as well as greater disease expression.[17] In a study by Maron and colleagues[18] of 202 patients, 53% of patients with preserved ejection fraction had LGE and all patients with ejection fraction less than 50% had LGE.

One of the dreaded complications in HCM is SCD. Presence of LGE has been associated with 7-fold increase in nonsustained ventricular tachycardia and with SCD. Chan and colleagues[19] found that compared with patients without LGE, SCD risk increased substantially across the range of LGE. LGE greater than or equal to 15% of the LV mass conferred a greater than >2-fold risk in patients otherwise considered low risk.[17] Each 10% increase in LGE was associated with 40% relative risk increase in SCD. They also found that patients with increased LGE were at an increased risk of progression of heart failure and future heart transplantation. They proposed consideration of ICD for primary prevention in patients with LGE greater than 15% of LV mass.

Decisions regarding ICD implantation can be clinically very challenging despite clear-cut guidelines. Shared decision-making is often practiced and extent of LGE can be used as a diagnostic tool (Recommendation from ACC/AHA Class II b indication [level of evidence: C]).

In HCM at tissue level, there is myocardial disarray, microvascular disease, and myocardial fibrosis. Although myocardial fibrosis is assessed by LGE (regional scar), interstitial fibrosis is assessed by T1 mapping. Studies have shown increased T1, T2, and ECV values, even in patients with normal LV thickness and without LGE, indicating early remodeling before morphologic expression of the disease.[20]

UTILITY OF CARDIAC MAGNETIC RESONANCE IN PATIENTS PRESENTING WITH HEART FAILURE AND VENTRICULAR ARRHYTHMIAS

Ventricular tachycardia is an uncommon but serious first presentation of nonischemic cardiomyopathy, fulminant myocarditis, or a complication of known ischemic cardiomyopathy. CMR can offer rapid diagnosis with high sensitivity and specificity in a multitude of cardiomyopathies. Presence of full-thickness or endocardial LGE can hint toward undiagnosed coronary artery disease. In this section, arrhythmogenic right ventricular cardiomyopathy, cardiac sarcoidosis, and giant cell myocarditis are discussed.

ARRHYTHMOGENIC RIGHT VENTRICULAR CARDIOMYOPATHY

Arrhythmogenic right ventricular cardiomyopathy is a rare genetic cardiomyopathy characterized by mostly autosomal dominant inheritance; the most common genes being affected are those related to cardiac desmosomes and gap junctions. The 2019 consensus guidelines revised the diagnostic criteria to include CMR features.[21] The hallmark of this disease is fatty infiltrate predominantly of the right ventricle resulting in progressive right ventricular dysfunction as well as ventricular arrhythmias. Surface echocardiogram may demonstrate right ventricular dysfunction; however, overall sensitivity is low, ranging from 60% to 80% in studied populations.[21]

In contrast to echocardiography, CMR offers more detailed and accurate measurements of the right ventricle. When this disease is suspected, CMR has diagnostic sensitivity and specificity ranging 68% to 89% and 85% to 97%, respectively. Characteristic findings on CMR include fatty infiltrate of the right and rarely LV, aneurysmal changes and dilatation with reduced right ventricular function, right ventricular wall motion abnormalities, right ventricular hypertrophy, trabecular disarray, and free-wall thinning.[22,23] Increasingly, LV dysfunction with fatty infiltrate and abnormal strain have been characterized in these patients, with up to 76% of patients demonstrating LV involvement, these findings indicating more advanced, high-risk disease. LGE can help identify patients at higher risk of ventricular arrhythmias as well as aid in mapping ventricular tachycardia reentry circuits for possible endocardial or epicardial ablation.[21,22]

CARDIAC SARCOIDOSIS

Cardiac sarcoidosis is a rare inflammatory, infiltrative cardiomyopathy characterized by granulomatous invasion of the myocardium. Patients often present with ventricular arrhythmias, conduction abnormalities as well as LV dysfunction. Although echocardiography can be useful as an initial screening modality, CMR is far more sensitive. Echocardiography can demonstrate basal thinning of the interventricular septum; however, this finding is only found in 25% of patients with confirmed cardiac disease; overall, echocardiographic findings are abnormal in 14% to 46% of patients.[24]

In contrast, CMR can provide diagnostic clarity as well as risk stratify patients.[5,6] Sarcoidosis can be diagnosed by CMR, with near 100% sensitivity and 78% specificity in patients suspected of cardiac sarcoidosis.[24] Follow-up confirmatory testing with either cardiac PET or endomyocardial biopsy can be pursued. CMR typically demonstrates patchy wall thinning, aneurysmal changes, as well as multifocal LGE in the basal anteroseptum, inferoseptum, subepicardium, and right ventricle. In addition, T2 weighting demonstrating myocardial edema can identify areas of active inflammation.[24,25] Thus, appropriate CMR use can act as gatekeeper for further advanced or invasive diagnostics.

GIANT CELL MYOCARDITIS

Giant cell myocarditis is an extremely rare, but highly lethal, inflammatory, infiltrative cardiomyopathy. There is debate on whether cardiac sarcoidosis and giant cell myocarditis are the same disease entity with a spectrum of disease severity.

It is often seen in the context of a fulminant myocarditis in a young patient, often younger than 40 years. The gold standard remains endomyocardial biopsy; however, sensitivity ranges from 68% to 93%.[26] Echocardiography remains the initial diagnostic test given ease of use and widespread availability; however, no constellation of findings are predictive.[26,27] CMR offers some diagnostic clarity, with similar findings to cardiac sarcoidosis with patchy midmyocardial and epicardial inflammatory infiltrates, increased myocardial edema with T2 weighting, and diffuse LGE with often subendocardial sparing.[26,27]

CARDIAC MAGNETIC RESONANCE IN ISCHEMIC CARDIOMYOPATHY—REVASCULARIZE OR NOT TO REVASCULARIZE?

Patients with coronary artery disease and LV dysfunction have a substantial chance at improvement if viable segments are revascularized. Kim, and colleagues[28] in a landmark study showed that with no LGE, 78% had improvement in contractility, while with greater than 50% transmural LGE, 90% did not show benefit from revascularization. Also, there are reports of benefit from revascularization if end diastolic diameter less than 5.5 cm if there is no transmural scar. Low-dose dobutamine CMR has been shown to have improved predictive accuracy for recovery postrevascularization with LGE less than 75%. However, randomized controlled trials have not shown elusive benefit in viability assessment. Even though jury is not out, limiting viability to high-risk patients (older age, ejection fraction <40%, significant cocomorbidities) seems reasonable.[29]

OTHER UTILITIES OF CARDIAC MAGNETIC RESONANCE IN CARDIOMYOPATHY

Electrocardiogram-gated cine imaging is the gold standard for assessment of LV and right ventricular systolic and diastolic volumes as well as regional and global LV and right ventricular systolic function with high reproducibility and low interobserver variability.

In patients undergoing placement of LV lead for cardiac resynchronization therapy in ischemic or

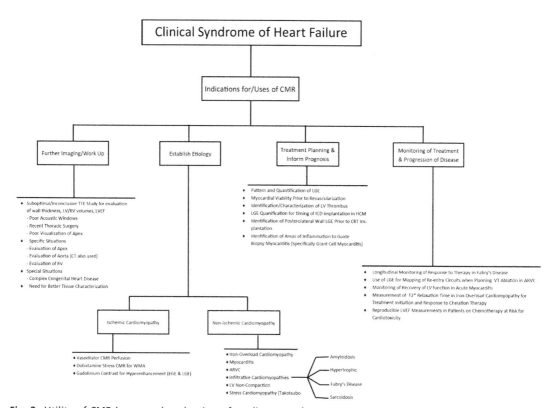

Fig. 2. Utility of CMR in general evaluation of cardiomyopathy.

nonischemic cardiomyopathy, degree of LGE has been associated with decreased responsiveness to resynchronization therapy. LV lead deployment away from scarred myocardium can result in a better clinical outcome.[30]

Accruing evidence supports the CMR technique of T1 mapping for noninvasive monitoring of heart transplant rejection to prevent unnecessary biopsy.

SUMMARY

CMR has evolved over the years to be in the forefront of diagnosing and managing myocardial disease (**Fig. 2**). It provides a platform for better understanding of the disease process underlying heart failure and cardiomyopathy, establishing diagnosis, and predicting treatment effectiveness. The clinical decision-making can be individualized. CMR has become an integral part in the care of patients with heart failure.

ACKNOWLEDGMENTS

Omar Jawaid MD and Christopher Janish have contributed equally to the article.

DISCLOSURE

The authors have nothing to disclose.

REFERENCES

1. Ian Paterson D, Wells George, Erthal Fernanda, et al. A randomized controlled trial of routine versus selective cardiac magnetic resonance for patients with nonischemic heart failure (IMAGE-HF 1B). Circulation 2020;141:818–27.
2. Halliday BP, Cleland JGF, Goldberger JJ, et al. Personalizing risk stratification for sudden death in dilated cardiomyopathy: the past, present, and future. Circulation 2017;136:215–31.
3. Halliday Brian P, John Baksi A, Gulati Ankur, et al. Outcome in dilated cardiomyopathy related to the extent, location, and pattern of late gadolinium enhancement. JACC Cardiovasc Imaging 2019; 12(Issue 8 Part 2):1645–55.
4. Kotanidis CP, Bazmpani MA, Haidich AB, et al. Diagnostic accuracy of cardiovascular magnetic resonance in acute myocarditis: a systematic review and meta-analysis. JACC Cardiovasc Imaging 2018;11(11):1583–90 [Epub 2018 Feb 14].
5. Ferreira VM, Schulz-Menger J, Holmvang G, et al. Cardiovascular magnetic resonance in nonischemic myocardial inflammation.expert recommendations. J Am Coll Cardiol 2018;72(24):3158–76.
6. Aquaro GD, Perfetti M, Camastra G, et al. Cardiac MR with late gadolinium enhancement in acute myocarditis with preserved systolic function: ITAMY study.cardiac magnetic resonance working group of the Italian society of cardiology. J Am Coll Cardiol 2017;70(16):1977–87.
7. Giovanni DA, Yacob GH, Giovanni Camastra J, et al. Prognostic value of repeating cardiac magnetic resonance in patients with acute myocarditis. J Am Coll Cardiol 2019;74(20):2439–48.
8. Dimitrios T. Kremastinos and dimitrios farmakis. iron overload cardiomyopathy in clinical practice. Circulation 2011;124:2253–63.
9. Anderson LJ, Holden S, Davis B, et al. Cardiovascular T2-star (T2*) magnetic resonance for the early diagnosis of myocardial iron overload. Eur Heart J 2001;22:2171–9.
10. Kirk P, Roughton M, Porter JB, et al. Cardiac T2* magnetic resonance for prediction of cardiac complications in thalassemia major. Circulation 2009; 120:1961–8.
11. Marianna F, Ćorović A, Paul S, et al. Myocardial amyloidosis: the exemplar interstitial disease. JACC Cardiovasc Imaging 2019;12(11 Pt 2): 2345–56.
12. Maceira AM, Joshi J, Prasad SK, et al. Cardiovascular magnetic resonance in cardiac amyloidosis. Circulation 2005;111:186–93.
13. Hagège A, Réant P, Habib G, et al. Fabry disease in cardiology practice: literature review and expert point of view. Arch Cardiovasc Dis 2019;112(4): 278–87.
14. Sado DM, White SK, Piechnik, et al. Indentification and assessment of Anderson- Fabry disease by cardiovascular magnetic resonance non contrast myocardial T1 mapping. Circ Cardiovasc Imaging 2013;6:392–8.
15. Hanneman K, Karur GR, Wasim S, et al. Left ventricular hypertrophy and late gadolinium enhancement at cardiac MRI are associated with adverse cardiac events in fabry disease. Radiology 2020;294:42–9.
16. Gersh BJ, Maron BJ, Bonow RO, et al. 2011 ACCF/ AHA guideline for the diagnosis and treatment of hypertrophic cardiomyopathy. Circulation 2011;124: e783–831.
17. Dumonta CA, Monserrata L, Soler R, et al. Clinical significance of late gadolinium enhancement on cardiovascular magnetic resonance in patients with hypertrophic cardiomyopathy. Rev Esp Cardiol 2007; 60(1):15–23.
18. Maron MS, Appelbaum E, HarriganIn CJ, et al. Clinical profile and significance of delayed enhancement in hypertrophic cardiomyopathy. Circ Heart Fail 2008;1:184–91.
19. Chan RH, Maron BJ, Olivotto I, et al. Prognostic value of quantitative contrast-enhanced cardiovascular magnetic resonance for the evaluation of sudden death risk in patients with hypertrophic cardiomyopathy. Circulation 2014;130:484–95.

20. Weng Z, Yao J, Chan RH, et al. Prognostic value of LGE-CMR in HCM: a meta-analysis. JACC Cardiovasc Imaging 2016;9(12):1392–402.

21. Towbin JA, McKenna WJ, Abrams DJ, et al. 2019 HRS expert consensus statement on evaluation, risk stratification, and management of arrhythmogenic cardiomyopathy. Heart Rhythm 2019;16(11): e301–72.

22. te Riele AS, Tandri H, Bluemke DA. Arrhythmogenic right ventricular cardiomyopathy (ARVC): cardiovascular magnetic resonance update. J Cardiovasc Magn Reson 2014;16:50. https://doi.org/10.1186/s12968-014-0050-8. Available at:.

23. Jain A, Tandri H, Calkins H, et al. Role of cardiovascular magnetic resonance imaging in arrhythmogenic right ventricular dysplasia. J Cardiovasc Magn Reson 2008;10:32.

24. Blankstein R, Waller AH. Evaluation of known or suspected cardiac sarcoidosis. Circ Cardiovasc Imaging 2016;9(3):e000867.

25. Hulten E, Aslam S, Osborne M, et al. Cardiac sarcoidosis-state of the art review. Cardiovasc Diagn Ther 2016;6(1):50–63.

26. Kandolin R, Lehtonen J, Salmenkivi K, et al. Diagnosis, treatment, and outcome of giant-cell myocarditis in the era of combined immunosuppression. Circ Heart Fail 2013;6(1):15–22.

27. Ghaly M, Schiliro D, Stepczynski J. Giant cell myocarditis: a time sensitive distant diagnosis. Cureus 2020;12(1):e6712.

28. Kim RJ, Wu E, Rafael A, et al. The use of contrast-enhanced magnetic resonance imaging to identify reversible myocardial dysfunction. N Engl J Med 2000;343:1445–53.

29. Bock A, Estep JD. Myocardial viability: heart failure perspective.Ashley Bock 1, Jerry D Estep. Curr Opin Cardiol 2019;34(5):459–65.

30. Leyva F. The role of cardiovascular magnetic resonance in cardiac resynchronization therapy. Heart Failure Clin 2017;13(1):63–77.

Cardiac Magnetic Resonance Quantification of Structure-Function Relationships in Heart Failure

Kim-Lien Nguyen, MD[a,b,c],*, Peng Hu, PhD[b,c], J. Paul Finn, MD[b,c]

KEYWORDS

- Heart failure • Cardiovascular magnetic resonance • Strain • Diffusion tensor • 4D flow
- Cardiac function and morphology • Myocardial microstructure • Ferumoxytol

KEY POINTS

- Novel cardiovascular magnetic resonance (CMR) approaches enable characterization of ventricular structure-function relationships in heart failure patients beyond the ventricular ejection fraction.
- Ferumoxytol may improve CMR imaging by facilitating steady-state contrast-enhanced image acquisition.
- Technical developments for functional imaging include a shift from 2-dimensional multislice cine acquisition to 5-dimensional imaging, which may enable simultaneous evaluation of cardiopulmonary physiology.
- Tissue motion mapping using feature tracking CMR has emerged as a clinically useful tool for myocardial strain quantification and has gained traction beyond conventional myocardial tagging and tissue velocity mapping methods.
- Diffusion tensor and intracardiac 4-dimensional flow mapping are promising techniques for characterization of tissue microstructure and evaluation of intracardiac blood flow's impact on ventricular morphology.

 Video content accompanies this article at http://www.heartfailure.theclinics.com.

INTRODUCTION

Heart failure (HF) affects approximately 6.5 million adults in the United States and is expected to increase in prevalence because of an aging population and cardiometabolic disorders.[1] Although imperfect, the left ventricular ejection fraction (LVEF) serves as a surrogate marker for combined left ventricular (LV) function and structural phenotyping of HF. Current classification of HF is based solely on the ejection fraction (EF) and can be divided into the following: (1) HF with preserved EF (HFpEF, LVEF $\geq$50%), (2) reduced EF (HFrEF, LVEF <40%), and (3) midrange EF (HFmrEF, LVEF 40%–49%). Echocardiography is the mainstay of initial LVEF assessment in patients who

Funding: The authors acknowledge grant support from the American Heart Association (18TPA34170049), the National Institutes of Health (R01HL127153, R01HL148182), and the Veterans Health Administration (I01-CX001901).
[a] Division of Cardiology, David Geffen School of Medicine at UCLA, VA Greater Los Angeles Healthcare System, Los Angeles, CA, USA; [b] Diagnostic Cardiovascular Imaging Research Laboratory, Department of Radiology, David Geffen School of Medicine at UCLA, Los Angeles, CA, USA; [c] Physics & Biology in Medicine Graduate Program, University of California, Los Angeles, Los Angeles, CA, USA
* Corresponding author. 300 Medical Plaza, Los Angeles, CA 90095.
E-mail address: klnguyen@ucla.edu

present with signs and symptoms of HF. However, cardiovascular magnetic resonance (CMR) imaging serves as the standard reference modality for quantification of ventricular volume, global and regional contractile function, and ventricular mass because of its high spatiotemporal resolution. In the past decade, however, advances in CMR have shifted the paradigm beyond quantification of ventricular EF to provide other quantitative signatures of ventricular function.

Most recently, the use of LVEF to categorize cardiomyopathies and to serve as a proxy for contractility in the failing heart has been called into question because of dependency of LVEF on load and heart rate as well as interobserver variability when derived from 2-dimensional (2D) cardiac ultrasound.[2] Historically, the concept of ventricular EF arose from development of angiographic techniques to reliably measure stroke volume. Kennedy and colleagues[3] first defined the EF as the stroke volume divided by end-diastolic volume (EDV; or the ejected ventricular volume). Sonnenblick[4] later demonstrated EF to be related to sarcomere shortening. Together, these findings serve as the basis for historical and current use of LVEF as a measurement of contractile function. As a measure for diagnosis, prognosis, treatment, and development of new therapeutics, the LVEF has stood the test of time through its strong inverse association with mortality and its prediction of both clinical outcomes and therapeutic response across a wide range of patients and disease states.

One unmet area in HF phenomapping whereby CMR stands to fill a large gap is HFpEF and HFmrEF. Beyond ventricular function, volume, and mass, CMR can provide additional information on tissue characteristics, perfusion, myocardial mechanics, tissue microarchitecture, and intraventricular blood flow patterns. Excellent, detailed discussions of technical CMR principles[5,6] and imaging protocols[7,8] are available in the published literature. In this work, the authors provide a summary of technical advances in novel CMR methods to improve quantitative assessment of ventricular contractile structure-function relationships.

VENTRICULAR STRUCTURE-FUNCTION RELATIONSHIP

The relationship between myocardial architecture and ventricular function is complex. Myocardial deformation, microstructural orientation, and LV shape contribute to the overall EF. Ventricular contraction occurs along the longitudinal axis with circumferential shortening and radial thickening. From the LV apex to base, cardiomyocytes have a left-handed helical course at the epicardium, transitioning to circumferential arrangements at the midmyocardium, and turning toward a right-handed helical pattern at the endocardium.[9] The helical arrangement contributes to myocardial rotation and torsion during contraction. Cardiomyocytes serve as fundamental contractile elements and only shorten by ~15% and thicken by ~8% during systole. Secondary organization of myocytes consist of laminar structures (~5–10 cardiomyocytes thick) termed sheets[10] or sheetlets that are surrounded by collagen and multiple other local subpopulations of countersloping sheetlets (shear layers).[11] Together, the reorientation of the sheetlets and shear layer slippage serves as the main contributors to LV wall thickening and base-to-apex systolic shortening.

THERANOSTIC USE OF FERUMOXYTOL IN HEART FAILURE

Thirty percent to 50% of HF patients have anemia of chronic disease.[12] Guidelines[13] and expert opinions[14] recommend intravenous rather than oral iron repletion because supplementation has been shown to improve exercise capacity, HF symptoms, and health-related quality of life; yet, not all patients are adequately treated. Many HF patients also have concomitant cardiorenal disease, which limits the use of gadolinium-based magnetic resonance (MR) contrast agents. Even in the absence of renal dysfunction, data have emerged to support accumulation of gadolinium in brain and other tissues.[15,16] CMR with cine imaging is typically performed without contrast agents. However, some techniques to further characterize ventricular function may benefit from contrast enhancement. Contrast agents with paramagnetic properties are used in CMR imaging to modify the T1, T2, and T2* relaxation times of local tissues, and the relative effects are visualized as tissue contrast using different CMR pulse sequences. In the context of HF whereby patients have anemia and renal dysfunction, ferumoxytol (Feraheme; AMAG Pharmaceuticals, Waltham, MA, USA) may be used on-label for therapeutic (treatment of anemia)[14,17] and off-label for diagnostic purposes.[18–21] Ferumoxytol is an intravenous iron-oxide nanoparticle that has been approved by the Food and Drug Administration (FDA) for treatment of iron-deficiency anemia and was originally developed as an MR contrast agent,[22,23] but manufacturers eventually pursued a therapeutic indication. As an ultrasmall, superparamagnetic, iron-oxide nanoparticle with an intravascular half-life of 14 to 15 hours and a high r_1 of 15 L mmol^{-1}s^{-1}, ferumoxytol is predominantly an intravascular contrast agent, but its biodistribution and metabolism by the reticuloendothelial system can be leveraged for a variety of imaging indications[18–21,24] beyond the current capabilities of commercially available gadolinium-based contrast agents (**Fig. 1**). The long half-life enables a long temporal window for high-resolution, high signal-to-noise (SNR) vascular imaging,[20,21] whereas delayed imaging at later time points (1–10 days after injection) enables tracking of macrophage activity.[25–27] Despite its promising applications, ferumoxytol received an FDA black-box warning for potential anaphylactic allergic reactions related to its postmarketing therapeutic use.[28] With vigilant monitoring of vital signs, dilution, and slow infusion, no further reports of fatal anaphylaxis allergic reactions have been reported. In contrast, the diagnostic use of ferumoxytol has shown favorable safety profile in both single-center[29–32] and multicenter reports.[33] The total amount of ferumoxytol used for diagnostic purposes is typically less than half the therapeutic dose. Several caveats merit mention: (1) high ferumoxytol concentration may be associated with susceptibility artifacts, (2) effects may be present on MRIs for up to 6 months, and (3) dilution factor and short echo time must be carefully chosen for specific indications.

VENTRICULAR EJECTION FRACTION, VOLUME, AND MASS
Two-Dimensional Imaging

Conventional quantification of ventricular volume, EF, and mass is derived from a stack of breath-held, 2D multislice, short-axis, cine MRIs acquired from the ventricular base to apex. Each 2D slice is 6–8 mm in thickness, and the interslice gap is 2–4 mm. The segmented raw image data are acquired for each cardiac phase of every cardiac cycle and takes a total of 6 to 7 minutes if acceleration approaches are used. Images are typically acquired at end-expiration to ensure consistent cardiac positioning within the thoracic cavity. The data are then averaged to generate a movie (typically 25–30 frames; see **Fig. 1**). Acquisition of cine images can be performed using spoiled-gradient echo fast low-angle shot (FLASH)[34] or balanced steady-state free precession (bSSFP)[35,36] pulse sequences. FLASH relies on blood inflow to generate blood-myocardial contrast and has low contrast-to-noise ratio (CNR), especially at short repetition times (TR) and with low flow rates. bSSFP is based on steady-state signal (T2 to T1 ratio) and remains the cornerstone for cine MRIs. Relative to FLASH, bSSFP has higher in-plane resolution with shorter acquisition time and better overall image quality. Shorter TR is possible with SSFP while maintaining consistent high blood-myocardial contrast.

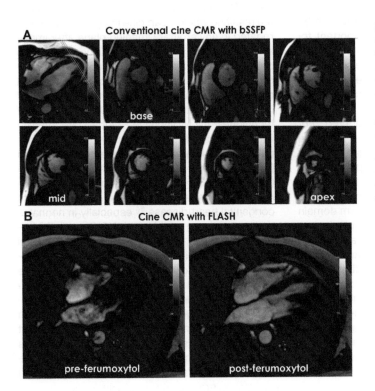

A Conventional cine CMR with bSSFP

base

mid

apex

B Cine CMR with FLASH

pre-ferumoxytol   post-ferumoxytol

Fig. 1. Quantification of LVEF, volume, and mass can be accomplished with noncontrast cine CMR using a bSSFP pulse sequence (*A*) or from a fast low-angle single-shot (FLASH) (*B*) sequence. Using a long-axis image (*A, upper left panel*), multislice 2D short-axis images from base to apex are acquired perpendicular to the long-axis and then segmented offline to derive measures of LV function (EF, volume, mass). Relative to noncontrast cine CMR images obtained from FLASH (*B, left panel*), ferumoxytol-enhanced cine FLASH CMR images (*B, right panel*) have improved image quality with less artifacts and more homogenous bloodpool.

However, SSFP tends to yield slightly higher LV EDV (13.3 ± 11.6 mL, P<.0001) and end-systolic volume (ESV; 12.2 ± 11.7 mL, P<.0001) with lower ventricular mass (21.5 ± 10.1 g, P<.0001).[37,38] LVEF by SSFP is slightly lower relative to LVEF by gradient echo (3.8 ± 4.6%, P<.0001); differences in LV stroke volume is negligible (0.7 ± 11.6 mL, P = .69).

Image Acceleration

To improve overall scan time, several acceleration strategies[39–41] may be used to speed up image acquisition and reduce the acquisition time of each 2D cine slice to 4 to 5 seconds. These approaches all involve some form of data undersampling and can be classified as parallel imaging, prior-knowledge-driven imaging including several k-t methods,[42] and compressed sensing. Of these approaches, parallel imaging is most widely used, and 2 variants are commercially available: sensitivity encoding (SENSE) and GeneRalized Autocalibrating Partially Parallel Acquisitions (GRAPPA). SENSE formulates the image reconstruction problem as an inverse problem and leverages intrinsic redundancies in multicoil image encoding to recover the image from undersampled k-space data. Although parallel imaging along with improved coil arrays can reduce scan time by 3- to 4-fold, prior-knowledge-driven approaches or the combination of prior-knowledge-driven and parallel imaging can achieve higher acceleration relative to parallel imaging alone. The latter combination of approaches is especially important for dynamic imaging, such as cardiac cine imaging, because these methods leverage close correlation between dynamic frames to achieve greater k-space undersampling. With acceleration, however, tradeoffs between acceleration and occurrence of artifacts need to be considered. For parallel imaging, SNR and CNR used in image quality comparisons may require consideration of spatially varying noise, whereas temporal fidelity of images reconstructed from certain knowledge-driven methods need further validation.

In compressed sensing,[43] the transform domain L1-norm minimization using nonlinear optimization methods is applied at the time of image reconstruction to take advantage of the intrinsic data sparsity of medical images in a predefined transform domain, such as wavelet. Compressed sensing theory does not require multicoil MRI data. However, practical implementations of compressed sensing sometimes combines the L1-norm minimization with a k-space data consistency measure based on multicoil data and its associated data redundancy.[44] Whole-heart, cine

CMR with compressed sensing is commercially available on more recent state-of-the-art scanners and can be completed in a single breath-hold.[45] Relative to conventional multislice breath-held SSFP, whole-heart, single breath-held SSFP using compressed sensing yields an LVEF mean difference of 1.3 ± 4.3% (P = .11), LV ESV mean difference of 2.0 ± 11.7 mL (P = .24), LV EDV mean difference of 9.9 ± 10.2 mL (P = .0009), LV stroke volume mean difference of 8.8 ± 12.8 mL (P = .11), and LV mass mean difference of −2.5 ± 9.6 g (P = .18).[45] With compressed sensing and incorporation of machine-learning methods, including deep neural networks, further efficiency may be achieved.[41]

Three-Dimensional and Four-Dimensional Imaging

Potential gains from 3-dimensional (3D) imaging with wider field of view have led to increased interest in 4-dimensional (4D; 3D + cardiac phase-resolved) CMR techniques.[46–60] For conventional CMR scans, multiple additional 2D breath-held slices are acquired in customized imaging planes to answer specific clinical questions in addition to a stack of 2D short-axis cine images. Isotropic, non-angulated 3D CMR acquisitions with parallel and undersampling reconstruction and respiratory gating have been incorporated into several strategies of 2D and 3D sequences[61–63] to create whole-heart 3D imaging. With newer 4D CMR techniques, the resulting whole-heart cine images can be interrogated in any arbitrary imaging plane after image acquisition and inline reconstruction. Although promising, these approaches are not yet commercially available because vendors have not perceived demand by users, and insufficient cost-benefit analyses are available. One set of techniques, 4D MUltiphase Steady-state Imaging with Contrast (MUSIC),[52] and its sister, self-gated 4D MUltiphase Steady-state Imaging with Contrast Using ROtating Cartesian K-space (ROCK-MUSIC),[53,55,64] has demonstrated technical feasibility and early value in patients with congenital heart disease,[54] especially in neonates and very young children. MUSIC and ROCK-MUSIC leverage the off-label use of ferumoxytol contrast to achieve submillimeter isotropic in-plane spatial resolution (**Fig. 2**). MUSIC uses the ventilator signal for gating, whereas ROCK-MUSIC is a free-breathing imaging technique. Both are effective for generating high-resolution 4D cine images inclusive of both the beating heart and relevant pulsatile thoracoabdominal vessels within 5 to 10 minutes, which depends on the required temporal resolution. Availability of 3D

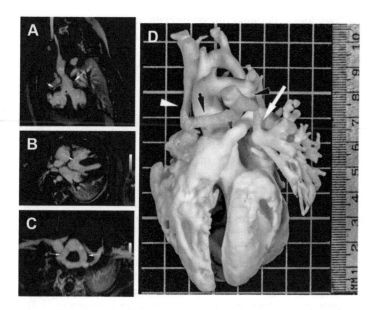

Fig. 2. Ferumoxytol-enhanced 4D MUSIC CMR. Multiplanar reformats of 4D MUSIC in a 3-month-old girl (7.7 kg) with tetralogy of Fallot (ToF) and a double aortic arch. (*A*) Characteristic features of ToF including right ventricular (RV) hypertrophy with dynamic RV outflow tract obstruction, an overriding aorta (Ao), and a perimembranous ventricular septal defect (*asterisk*) are clearly visualized on dynamic review (Video 1). Both proximal courses of the left and right coronary arteries (*A, white arrow*) are also well visualized; the distal right coronary artery can also be seen coursing along the right ventricle. (*B*) The large ventricular septal defect (*B, white arrow*) and the double aortic arch forming a complete vascular ring (*C*) are clearly delineated, without dynamic compression of the trachea (Video 2). (*D*) 3D print shows anomalous pulmonary venous drainage with the left innominate vein (*D, black arrow*) dipping inferiorly before joining the right innominate vein (*D, white arrowhead*) to form a right-sided superior vena cava. The left superior vertical vein (*D, black arrowhead*) joins the low bridging left innominate vein (*D, black arrow*) and the left superior pulmonary vein (*D, white arrow*), which forms the confluence of the superior pulmonary venous trunk (see Video 1). (*From* Nguyen KL, Han F, Zhou Z et al. 4D MUSIC CMR: Value-based imaging of neonates and infants with congenital heart disease. J Cardiovasc Magn Reson. 2017;19:40.)

and 4D datasets of ventricular function has paved the way for image-based computational models of cardiac structure and function in several disease states through advanced applications, such as statistical shape modeling.[65,66]

Five-Dimensional Imaging

Most recently, a framework for free-breathing MRI was developed that may offer simultaneous evaluation of cardiopulmonary physiology: eXtra-Dimensional Golden-angle RAdial Sparse Parallel (XD-GRASP) imaging.[67] XD-GRASP builds on iterative GRASP[68] whereby continuous multidimensional data are acquired and then sorted into undersampled datasets with distinct motion-states. Compressed sensing is used to reconstruct the motion-sorted datasets from radial k-space data. The extra dimensions may provide additional physiologic information, which can be extracted during reconstruction. Based on a 5-dimensional (5D) whole-heart sparse imaging framework,[69] simultaneous evaluation of myocardial motion and high-resolution cardiac and respiratory motion-resolved acquisitions can be achieved in a single continuous noncontrast examination. These techniques were applied to a 4D flow sequence (XD flow) for simultaneous

assessment of cardiopulmonary physiology and where information about ventricular function can be extracted from the anatomic images.[70]

Real-Time Imaging

Patients with HF frequently have irregular heart rhythms or difficulty with breath-holding; in these cases, real-time cine CMR may be used. Feasibility of real-time CMR[71,72] can be facilitated by exploitation of nonlinear algorithms, and has progressed to encompass modified use of radial sampling,[73] parallel imaging,[74,75] sparse sampling with iterative reconstruction,[76–79] compressed sensing,[80,81] and unsupervised motion-corrected reconstruction (MOCO-RT).[82] Real-time cine CMR uses a fast low-angle single-shot acquisition approach,[71,72] but more recently has transitioned to bSSFP[79,82] to improve the SNR as well as spatiotemporal characteristics. The MOCO-RT technique relies on bSSFP, free-breathing, Cartesian, real-time cine acquisition with GRAPPA, and inline unsupervised motion correction. Relative to conventional segmented 2D bSSFP cine, MOCO-RT yields an LVEF mean difference of 1.9% (95% confidence interval [CI] −1.9%–5.6%), LV ESV mean difference of −4.9 mL (95% CI −15.6–5.8 mL), LV EDV mean difference of −5.8 mL (95% CI −26.7–

15.0 mL). Compared with other approaches for real-time cine imaging, the MOCO-RT technique's inline reconstruction makes it a more clinically relevant technique with potential for widespread adoption.

Postprocessing of Cine Images

Commercially available software can be used to segment and quantify ventricular volume, EF, and mass from multislice 2D cine images. The routine use of commercial software to analyze 4D datasets remains in the research realm. Potential sources for variability in ventricular volumes merit consideration. The most common error for variability in volumes is selection of the basal short-axis slice, which is defined as the most basal slice whereby 50% of the slice's circumference consists of myocardium. This error is offset by using a combination of long-axis and short-axis images when selecting the most basal short-axis slice. Other sources of error include endocardial and epicardial contouring, inexperienced operators, and lack of standardization within an imaging laboratory. More recent iterations of commercially available CMR processing software have incorporated artificial intelligence into segmentation algorithms to further reduce variability and sources of error. Postprocessing of 4D and 5D datasets relies on in-house methods, and there are a limited number of commercially available software that

currently accommodate these data for clinical workflow.

GLOBAL AND REGIONAL MYOCARDIAL MECHANICS

Ventricular structure and function relationships can also be further characterized by quantifying myocardial strain and tissue velocities from myocardial tagging, tissue displacement, and tissue phase mapping techniques.[83] Global and regional myocardial contractility can be described through measures of longitudinal, circumferential, and radial strain and strain rate as well as rotational mechanics, including torsion and twist using tagging or tissue displacement imaging. Myocardial tagging[84,85] involves labeling segments of the ventricular myocardium with dark bands that are perpendicular to the imaging planes to create grid or linear patterns (**Fig. 3**). Tagging can be done in Cartesian or in polar coordinates.[86] The latter is better for the ventricular shape and enables higher density of tag lines that are in either the circular or radial direction. The evolution of tagging CMR pulse sequences is nicely outlined by Ibrahim.[85] "Tags" are applied at the onset of the R wave, deform throughout the cardiac cycle, and enable both visualization and quantification of global and regional strain and strain rate. One drawback is fading of the tags as magnetization recovers toward equilibrium because of spin-lattice relaxation throughout the cardiac cycle,

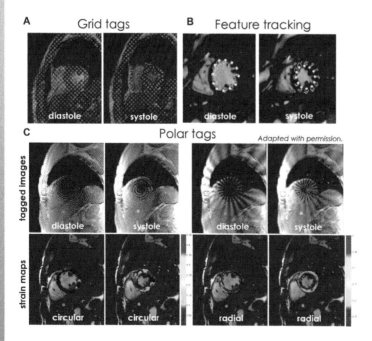

Fig. 3. Myocardial mechanics can be quantified using rectilinear grid tags (*A*), feature tracking (*B*), or polar tags (*C*) in the circular and radial directions. Global and regional strain curves can be used to derive longitudinal, circumferential, and radial strain and strain rate. Rotational mechanics (torsion) is quantified using short-axis images. ([C] *Adapted from* Nasiraei-Moghaddam A, Finn JP. Tagging of cardiac magnetic resonance images in the polar coordinate system: physical principles and practical implementation. Magn Reson Med. 2014;71:1755; with permission. (Figure 6 in original).)

especially near end-diastole. Binomial rectilinear grid tags are limited by spatial limits between the tag lines. Other challenges include lack of widely affordable and available commercial software for analyzing specific types of tag lines for strain measurements. Although 3D tagging is possible as a research tool, most clinical CMR workflow relies on 2D myocardial tagging.

Tissue displacement techniques,[85] such as displacement encoding with simulated echoes (DENSE), strain encoding (SENC), or feature tracking,[87,88] can also be used for derivation of global and regional strain. DENSE displays tissue motion information at the pixel level: the vector orientation and length reflect direction and magnitude, respectively. Unlike DENSE, SENC, or tagging, feature tracking is a postprocessing technique that is applied retrospectively to routinely acquired cine images for derivation of strain measurements (see Fig. 3). Feature tracking software tracks endocardial features after user-defined epicardial and endocardial borders are delineated. Global longitudinal strain is derived from 3 long-axis cine images, whereas global circumferential and radial strain are derived from short-axis cine images. Relative to conventional tagging or other tissue displacement techniques, feature tracking has been more widely incorporated into routine clinical CMR workflow because of its simplicity, and postprocessing is possible with several commercially available CMR quantification software. Limitations of feature tracking include pixel size (displacement smaller than the pixel size may not be detected), artifacts from through plane motion, and 2D tracking. Global strain values are more reproducible than regional strain with the most consistent parameter being global longitudinal strain. Global circumferential and longitudinal strain values less negative than -17% or -20%, respectively, are considered pathologic. In patients with HFpEF (n = 206), feature tracking-derived global longitudinal strain was associated with HF hospitalizations and cardiovascular death (hazard ratio 1.06% per 1% strain increase, 95% CI 1.01–1.11, $P = .03$).[89] These findings are consistent with a larger, multicenter study (n = 1274) showing global longitudinal strain derived from feature tracking is an independent predictor of all-cause mortality in patients with HFpEF; each 1% worsening in global longitudinal strain was associated with a 22.8% increased risk of death after adjusting for clinical and other imaging factors.[90] The impact of using feature tracking-derived global longitudinal strain extends to stress testing. In patients with known or suspected coronary artery disease, blunted global longitudinal strain at peak vasodilator stress perfusion CMR independently predicted major adverse cardiovascular events (death, nonfatal myocardial infarction, HF hospitalization, sustained ventricular tachycardia, and late revascularization).[91]

DIFFUSION TENSOR FOR TISSUE MICROSTRUCTURE

Myocardial microstructure is crucial to ventricular architecture, shape, and overall contractile function.[92,93] Until diffusion tensor (DT) CMR was available, in vivo dynamic evaluation of cardiac microstructure in the mammalian heart was not possible. Developments in DT MR have been most robust in neuroimaging, but Edelman and colleagues,[94] in 1994, were able to overcome cardiac bulk motion using a stimulated echo acquisition mode (STEAM) technique to capture the first in vivo diffusion cardiac images. Both diffusion-weighted (DW) and DT-CMR take advantage of the Brownian motion of water molecules in myocardial tissue (cardiomyocytes and extracellular matrix) to provide measurements about the myocardial tissue's underlying microstructural organization.[95]

DT-CMR relies on information obtained from DW images. By using strong bipolar gradients (diffusion gradients) to sensitize the MR signal to the diffusivity of water molecules, DW imaging generates several images with different degrees of diffusion weighing based on the b-values (units of seconds per square millimeter). Typical b-values range from 450 to 600 s/mm^2 and reflect the gradient amplitude, duration, and temporal separation between the gradient pulses. The water diffusivity along a particular spatial direction can be calculated by performing an exponential fit on the signal intensities from the DW images. For DT-CMR, the 3D DT is calculated from DW images with multidirectional diffusion encoding gradients. DT-CMR in vivo data can be acquired using (1) cardiac and respiratory dual-gated stimulated echo pulse sequences, such as STEAM,[94,96] (2) velocity-compensated (M1 gradient moment nulled) and/or acceleration-compensated (M2 gradient moment nulled) spin echo (SE) echo-planar imaging (EPI) sequences,[97–100] or (3) SE-EPI techniques with postprocessing using principal component analysis for motion filtering.[101] M1/M2-nulled approaches use motion-compensated diffusion encoding gradients to reduce signal phase errors and signal void caused by cardiac motion; these techniques, however, inevitably increase the echo time and further reduce the SNR. STEAM does not require high-performance gradients because a significant contribution to the b-value comes from the long mixing time in STEAM rather than from the strong bipolar gradients in conventional SE-EPI approaches.[95] STEAM, however, can be sensitive to relative motion that occurs between the time of the stimulated echo encoding and the time of the diffusion readout, which happens one heartbeat later. Therefore, it is crucial to ensure that the heart is in the same breathing position and at the same time point within the cardiac cycle between these 2 successive heartbeats. Reliable cardiac position and timing within the cardiac cycle may be achieved using electrocardiogram-gating and navigator-based respiratory gating, respectively.[96] In a typical STEAM scan, for every 2D slice, 8 breath-held images are acquired over ~18 heartbeats and averaged. The images are postprocessed using proprietary software algorithms to generate 3D DT maps that reflect different components of myocyte organization and behavior. Several recent clinical research studies[102–105] conducted in small groups of normal volunteers and patients have relied on STEAM. Pathologic conditions included hypertrophic cardiomyopathy, dilated cardiomyopathy, myocardial infarction, congenital heart disease, and amyloidosis.[95,105] Because of the intrinsic 50% SNR loss when stimulated echoes are acquired, STEAM has relatively lower SNR than single-shot SE-EPI acquisitions using similar pulse sequence parameters, which may be compensated by incorporating larger voxel sizes (eg, $2.8 \times 2.8 \times 8$ mm^2).[104] Moreover, STEAM is dependent on 2 regular R-R intervals, is less applicable to patients with dysrhythmia, and is susceptible to confounding effects of myocardial deformation because of the long diffusion time.

Several quantitative DT-CMR parameters merit discussion because of their physiologic and clinical implications in structure-function relationships. DT-CMR relies on a 3D eigensystem whereby the *eigenvalues* (λ_1, λ_2, λ_3) describe the magnitude of directional diffusivity, and the *eigenvectors* (E1, E2, E3) describe the direction (**Fig. 4**). E1 is the principal eigenvector and corresponds to the average intravoxel cardiomyocyte orientation, whereas E2 reflects the predominant sheetlet orientation and E3 reflects the normal sheetlet orientation.[106–109] The average eigenvector is represented by each imaging voxel, and 3D diffusion maps convey pixelwise information. *Mean diffusivity* (MD) is similar to mean apparent diffusion coefficient from DW imaging and reflects the average of the eigenvalues. MD represents the packing of myocytes; low values indicate tight packing, and higher values indicate greater interstitial pathologic condition. *Fractional anisotropy* (FA) values

parallel changes in tissue organization; a low FA may indicate greater myocyte disarray. Using DT-CMR, MD and FA values can differentiate between cardiac amyloidosis and hypertrophic cardiomyopathy.[105] MD and FA are scalar diffusivity parameters and are reported as global values across the midventricle in healthy volunteers; they can vary depending on the pulse sequence, cardiac phase, and b-values used during the image acquisition. Cardiomyocyte orientation is described using the *helix angle* (HA, E1A), which is the angulation created by E1 and the circumferential direction (see **Fig. 4**). Sheetlet orientation is described by E2A, which is the angulation between E2 projected onto the cross-myocyte plane. In healthy myocardium, FA is highest in the mid-myocardium (0.46 ± 0.04) relative to the endocardium (0.40 ± 0.04) and epicardium (0.39 ± 0.004).[103] MD exhibits a transmural gradient that increases from epicardium ($0.87 \pm 0.07 \times 10^{-3}$ mm^2/s) to endocardium ($0.91 \pm 0.08 \times 10^{-3}$ mm^2/s).[110] Transmural gradient of the HA reflecting cardiomyocyte orientation is small (transverse angle is between $-20°$ and $+20°$).[109] Sheetlet orientation (E2A), however, varies throughout the cardiac cycle and is likely due to radial strain. Biphasic E2A variation is present using STEAM[111]: $26 \pm 6°$ in diastole, $54 \pm 6°$ in systole. Together, measures of diffusivity, cardiomyocyte orientation, and sheetlet orientation can characterize dynamic microstructural alterations that affect the overall ventricular geometry and function (**Fig. 5**).

FOUR-DIMENSIONAL INTRACARDIAC BLOOD FLOW

Ventricular geometry or shape is influenced by the impact of intracardiac blood flow over time. To preserve energy during the cardiac cycle, blood flow through the ventricle generates vortices. These intraventricular blood flow vortices are affected by changes in ventricular geometry and have different formation time, size, shape, strength, depth, and direction based on cardiac structure and function. In HF patients, the intracardiac blood flow pattern is altered and has been shown to be associated with decreased preservation of LV inflow kinetic energy. These parameters lend insight about the impact of intracardiac blood flow on LV remodeling and overall function.

Recent advances in MR hardware and in image reconstruction and acceleration have enabled the clinical use of 4D flow CMR for visualization and quantification of vascular[112] and intracardiac blood flow and energy distribution.[113,114] 4D flow phase contrast pulse sequences are typically

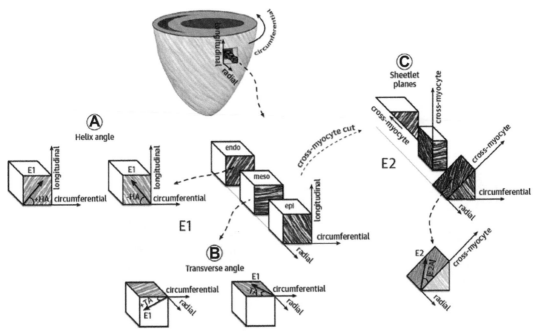

Fig. 4. Eigenvectors projected onto cardiac plane. The primary eigenvector (E1) is projected on the circumferential-longitudinal plane giving rise to the HA (*A*). E1 is projected on the circumferential-radial plane giving rise to the transverse angle (*B*). The voxels are cut in a cross-myocyte direction, showing the plane perpendicular to E1 (*C*). Projecting the second eigenvector (E2) onto the sheetlet plane gives E2A. endo, endocardium; meso, mesocardium; epi, epicardium; TA, transverse angle. (*From* Khalique Z, Ferreira PF, Scott AD et al. Diffusion tensor cardiovascular magnetic resonance imaging: a clinical perspective. JACC Cardiovasc. Imaging. 2020;13(5):1244; with permission.)

non-breath-held because of long acquisition time (10–25 minutes). Several image acceleration techniques are used to reduce acquisition time, and a variety of respiratory motion compensation or self-gating strategies are used to cope with the additional time window required for adequate spatial and temporal resolution. A spatial resolution of less than $3.0 \times 3.0 \times 3.0$ mm^3 with high temporal resolution is necessary for quantification of intracardiac blood flow. The maximum flow velocity (or the velocity encoding sensitivity [VENC]) is typically set at 10% higher than the maximal expected velocity to avoid velocity aliasing. If the VENC is set too high, an increase in velocity noise may occur. To include both early and late diastolic filling, retrospective cardiac gating is used. Because several sources of error can lead to large discrepancies in 4D flow data, careful preprocessing may be needed. Major sources of error include eddy current effects, concomitant Maxwell field effects, gradient nonlinearity, and phase wraps. Many of these errors are corrected inline by the reconstruction algorithms on the scanner software. If velocity aliasing occurs, however, additional phase-unwrapping steps may be necessary. For quality control, quantitative

verification based on the conservation of mass principle is also used. A useful check is the consistency in net aortic and pulmonary artery outflow, which should be equal in the absence of intracardiac shunts. Another internal check of the acquired data is verification of 4D flow with a validated 2D phase-contrast scan.

Once acquired, 4D flow datasets can be reformatted to user-defined 2D views, and blood flow information (velocity direction and magnitude, kinetic energy, and vorticity) is color coded using commercially available software. Data can be presented as 2D velocity vector or 2D streamline displays to reflect velocity direction. 3D visualization of intracardiac flow is also possible. Three emerging quantitative parameters of relevance for structure-function relationships include (1) particle tracing quantification to evaluate blood volume transportation efficiency,[115,116] (2) intracardiac kinetic energy quantification ($E = (1/2)mv^2$, where m = mass, v = velocity) for HF classification,[117–119] and (3) vortical flow[120–122] as an indicator of maladaptive ventricular shape. The interplay among intracardiac blood volume transport efficiency, kinetic energy, and altered vortical flow is grounded in the physics of fluid dynamics

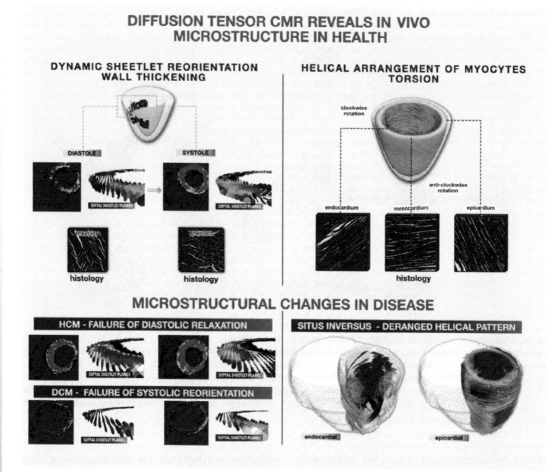

Fig. 5. DT-CMR in health and in disease states. In healthy left ventricles (LV), DT-CMR demonstrates reorientation of cardiomyocyte sheetlets from "wall-parallel" in diastole to "wall-perpendicular" in systole to cause LV wall thickening responsible for the predominant contraction (*upper left panel*). Sheetlets in hypertrophic cardiomyopathy (HCM) fail to relax to the expected diastolic position, whereas in dilated cardiomyopathy (DCM), sheetlets fail to rotate to the expected systolic position (*lower left panel*). DT-CMR demonstrates the helical arrangement of cardiomyocytes, with a right-handed helix in the endocardium, circumferential in the mesocardium, and left-handed helix in the epicardium (*upper right panel*). Contraction drives clockwise rotation basally and anti-clockwise rotation apically, resulting in LV torsion. In patients with situs inversus, torsion is impaired (*lower right panel*). (*From* Khalique Z, Ferreira PF, Scott AD et al. Diffusion tensor cardiovascular magnetic resonance imaging: a clinical perspective. JACC Cardiovasc. Imaging. 2020;13(5):1237; with permission.)

and can be related to the mechanical function of the ventricle. Relative to patients with normal LV function, patients with impaired LV function have persistence of vortical flow (vortex formation) in both diastole and systole (**Fig. 6**).[123] Because particle tracing enables tracking of the 3D trajectory of blood volume (equal to the voxel size) over the entire cardiac cycle, blood flow components in healthy and pathologic states can be classified into direct flow, retained flow, delayed ejection, or residual volume. A higher percentage of direct flow is assumed to be associated with more efficient transport of intracardiac blood volume. In

HF patients (n = 34 dilated cardiomyopathy, n = 30 ischemic cardiomyopathy, n = 36 healthy volunteers), direct-flow average intracardiac kinetic energy had an independent predictive relationship with 6-minute walk distance (a prognostic measure of functional capacity, $\beta = 0.280$, $P = .035$; model R^2 0.466, $P = .002$), but neither EF nor LV volumes were independently predictive.[124] In Fontan patients, both intracardiac kinetic energy and vortical flow are altered,[125,126] and in patients with total cavopulmonary connections, exercise capacity has been linked to energy loss.[127] With dobutamine-induced stress in Fontan

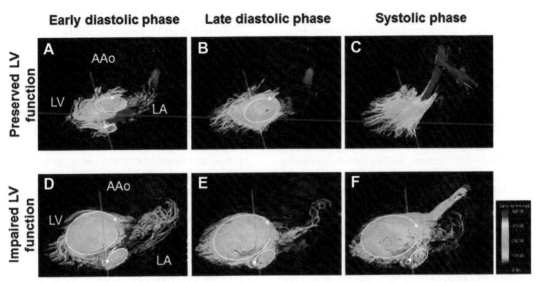

Fig. 6. Color-rendered streamline 4D flow CMR images with intraventricular vortex patterns. Relative to a patient with normal LV function (*upper panel, A-C*), the patient with reduced LV function (*lower panel, D-F*) has altered vortical flow (*white circular arrows*) throughout of the cardiac cycle (early diastole, late diastole, and during systole). Note the absence of vortex formation during systole in the setting of normal LV function and persistence of vortex formation during systole in the setting of impaired LV function. AAo, ascending aorta; LA, left atrium; LV, left ventricle. (*From* Suwa K, Saitoh T, Takehara Y, et al. Intra-left ventricular flow dynamics in patients with preserved and impaired left ventricular function: Analysis with 3D cine phase contrast MRI (4D-Flow). J Magn Reson Imaging. 2016;44(6):1493-1503.; with permission.)

patients, kinetic energy, viscous energy loss, and vorticity increases and percent change between rest-stress have negative correlation with Vo_{2max} (kinetic energy, r = −0.83, P = .003; energy loss, r = −0.80, P = .006; vorticity volume, r = −0.64, P = .047).[127]

SUMMARY

Diagnosis, prognosis, treatment, and development of new therapeutics require reliable imaging biomarkers of contractile function beyond the EF. With robust computational power, the development of image-based, multidimensional, patient-specific HF models that incorporate myocardial deformation, tissue microstructure, and intracardiac flow data to provide structure-function relationships is on the horizon. New CMR methods have potential to facilitate HF phenotyping by enabling more granular characterization of ventricular structure-function relationships. Although exciting, a major limitation to widespread translation of CMR techniques is vendor adoption and commercialization. Until demand for such techniques follows market metrics and comparative-effectiveness studies with clinical outcomes data are available, many of the described developments will remain in the research realm, and access will be limited to the few patients at medical centers with active technical CMR research and industry relationships.

DISCLOSURE

The authors have nothing to disclose.

SUPPLEMENTARY DATA

Supplementary data related to this article can be found online at https://doi.org/10.1016/j.hfc.2020.08.001.

REFERENCES

1. Benjamin EJ, Blaha MJ, Chiuve SE, et al. Heart disease and stroke statistics-2017 update: a report from the American Heart Association. Circulation 2017;135:e146–603.
2. Konstam MA, Abboud FM. Ejection fraction: misunderstood and overrated (changing the paradigm in categorizing heart failure). Circulation 2017;135:717–9.
3. Kennedy JW, Baxley WA, Figley MM, et al. Quantitative angiocardiography. I. The normal left ventricle in man. Circulation 1966;34:272–8.
4. Sonnenblick EH. Correlation of myocardial ultrastructure and function. Circulation 1968;38:29–44.

5. Ridgway JP. Cardiovascular magnetic resonance physics for clinicians: part I. J Cardiovasc Magn Reson 2010;12:71.

6. Biglands JD, Radjenovic A, Ridgway JP. Cardiovascular magnetic resonance physics for clinicians: part II. J Cardiovasc Magn Reson 2012;14:66.

7. Schulz-Menger J, Bluemke DA, Bremerich J, et al. Standardized image interpretation and post-processing in cardiovascular magnetic resonance - 2020 update : Society for Cardiovascular Magnetic Resonance (SCMR): Board of Trustees Task Force on Standardized Post-Processing. J Cardiovasc Magn Reson 2020;22:19.

8. Kramer CM, Barkhausen J, Bucciarelli-Ducci C, et al. Standardized cardiovascular magnetic resonance imaging (CMR) protocols: 2020 update. J Cardiovasc Magn Reson 2020;22:17.

9. Streeter DD Jr, Spotnitz HM, Patel DP, et al. Fiber orientation in the canine left ventricle during diastole and systole. Circ Res 1969;24:339–47.

10. LeGrice IJ, Smaill BH, Chai LZ, et al. Laminar structure of the heart: ventricular myocyte arrangement and connective tissue architecture in the dog. Am J Physiol 1995;269:H571–82.

11. Kung GL, Nguyen TC, Itoh A, et al. The presence of two local myocardial sheet populations confirmed by diffusion tensor MRI and histological validation. J Magn Reson Imaging 2011;34:1080–91.

12. Rocha BML, Cunha GJL, Menezes Falcão LF. The burden of iron deficiency in heart failure: therapeutic approach. J Am Coll Cardiol 2018;71:782–93.

13. Ponikowski P, Voors AA, Anker SD, et al. 2016 ESC Guidelines for the diagnosis and treatment of acute and chronic heart failure: the Task Force for the diagnosis and treatment of acute and chronic heart failure of the European Society of Cardiology (ESC) Developed with the special contribution of the Heart Failure Association (HFA) of the ESC. Eur Heart J 2016;37:2129–200.

14. Auerbach M, Gafter-Gvili A, Macdougall IC. Intravenous iron: a framework for changing the management of iron deficiency. Lancet Haematol 2020;7:e342–50.

15. Huckle JE, Altun E, Jay M, et al. Gadolinium deposition in humans: when did we learn that gadolinium was deposited in vivo? Invest Radiol 2016;51:236–40.

16. McDonald RJ, Levine D, Weinreb J, et al. Gadolinium retention: a research roadmap from the 2018 NIH/ACR/RSNA workshop on gadolinium chelates. Radiology 2018;289(2):517–34.

17. Auerbach M, Chertow GM, Rosner M. Ferumoxytol for the treatment of iron deficiency anemia. Expert Rev Hematol 2018;11(10):829–34.

18. Neuwelt EA, Hamilton BE, Varallyay CG, et al. Ultrasmall superparamagnetic iron oxides (USPIOs): a future alternative magnetic resonance (MR) contrast agent for patients at risk for nephrogenic systemic fibrosis (NSF)? Kidney Int 2009;75:465–74.

19. Bashir MR, Bhatti L, Marin D, et al. Emerging applications for ferumoxytol as a contrast agent in MRI. J Magn Reson Imaging 2015;41:884–98.

20. Finn JP, Nguyen KL, Han F, et al. Cardiovascular MRI with ferumoxytol. Clin Radiol 2016;71:796–806.

21. Toth GB, Varallyay CG, Horvath A, et al. Current and potential imaging applications of ferumoxytol for magnetic resonance imaging. Kidney Int 2017;92(1):47–66.

22. Anzai Y, Prince MR, Chenevert TL, et al. MR angiography with an ultrasmall superparamagnetic iron oxide blood pool agent. J Magn Reson Imaging 1997;7:209–14.

23. Prince MR, Zhang HL, Chabra SG, et al. A pilot investigation of new superparamagnetic iron oxide (ferumoxytol) as a contrast agent for cardiovascular MRI. J Xray Sci Technol 2003;11:231–40.

24. Nguyen KL, Shao J, Ghodrati VK, et al. Ferumoxytol-enhanced CMR for vasodilator stress testing: a feasibility study. JACC Cardiovasc Imaging 2019;12(8 Pt 1):1582–4.

25. Alam SR, Shah AS, Richards J, et al. Ultrasmall superparamagnetic particles of iron oxide in patients with acute myocardial infarction: early clinical experience. Circ Cardiovasc Imaging 2012;5:559–65.

26. Alam SR, Stirrat C, Richards J, et al. Vascular and plaque imaging with ultrasmall superparamagnetic particles of iron oxide. J Cardiovasc Magn Reson 2015;17:83.

27. Stirrat CG, Alam SR, MacGillivray TJ, et al. Ferumoxytol-enhanced magnetic resonance imaging assessing inflammation after myocardial infarction. Heart 2017;103:1528–35.

28. U.S. Food and Drug Administration. FDA Drug Safety Communication: FDA strengthens warnings and changes prescribing instructions to decrease the risk of serious allergic reactions with anemia drug Feraheme (ferumoxytol). 2015. Available at: http://www.fda.gov/Drugs/DrugSafety/ucm440138.htm. Accessed March 30, 2015.

29. Ning P, Zucker EJ, Wong P, et al. Hemodynamic safety and efficacy of ferumoxytol as an intravenous contrast agents in pediatric patients and young adults. Magn Reson Imaging 2016;34:152–8.

30. Muehe AM, Feng D, von Eyben R, et al. Safety report of ferumoxytol for magnetic resonance imaging in children and young adults. Invest Radiol 2016;51:221–7.

31. Nguyen KL, Yoshida T, Han F, et al. MRI with ferumoxytol: a single center experience of safety

across the age spectrum. J Magn Reson Imaging 2017 Mar;45(3):804–12.

32. Varallyay CG, Toth GB, Fu R, et al. What does the boxed warning tell us? Safe practice of using ferumoxytol as an MRI contrast agent. AJNR Am J Neuroradiol 2017;38(7):1297–302.

33. Nguyen KL, Yoshida T, Kathuria-Prakash N, et al. Multicenter safety and practice for off-label diagnostic use of ferumoxytol in MRI. Radiology 2019; 293:554–64.

34. Atkinson DJ, Edelman RR. Cineangiography of the heart in a single breath hold with a segmented turboFLASH sequence. Radiology 1991;178:357–60.

35. Carr JC, Simonetti O, Bundy J, et al. Cine MR angiography of the heart with segmented true fast imaging with steady-state precession. Radiology 2001;219:828–34.

36. Miller S, Simonetti OP, Carr J, et al. MR imaging of the heart with cine true fast imaging with steady-state precession: influence of spatial and temporal resolutions on left ventricular functional parameters. Radiology 2002;223:263–9.

37. Moon JC, Lorenz CH, Francis JM, et al. Breath-hold FLASH and FISP cardiovascular MR imaging: left ventricular volume differences and reproducibility. Radiology 2002;223:789–97.

38. Plein S, Bloomer TN, Ridgway JP, et al. Steady-state free precession magnetic resonance imaging of the heart: comparison with segmented k-space gradient-echo imaging. J Magn Reson Imaging 2001;14:230–6.

39. Kozerke S, Plein S. Accelerated CMR using zonal, parallel and prior knowledge driven imaging methods. J Cardiovasc Magn Reson 2008;10:29.

40. Yang AC, Kretzler M, Sudarski S, et al. Sparse reconstruction techniques in magnetic resonance imaging: methods, applications, and challenges to clinical adoption. Invest Radiol 2016;51:349–64.

41. Bustin A, Fuin N, Botnar RM, et al. From compressed-sensing to artificial intelligence-based cardiac MRI reconstruction. Front Cardiovasc Med 2020;7:17.

42. Tsao J, Boesiger P, Pruessmann KP. k-t BLAST and k-t SENSE: dynamic MRI with high frame rate exploiting spatiotemporal correlations. Magn Reson Med 2003;50:1031–42.

43. Lustig M, Donoho D, Pauly JM. Sparse MRI: the application of compressed sensing for rapid MR imaging. Magn Reson Med 2007;58:1182–95.

44. Uecker M, Lai P, Murphy MJ, et al. ESPIRiT–an eigenvalue approach to autocalibrating parallel MRI: where SENSE meets GRAPPA. Magn Reson Med 2014;71:990–1001.

45. Vincenti G, Monney P, Chaptinel J, et al. Compressed sensing single-breath-hold CMR for fast quantification of LV function, volumes, and mass. JACC Cardiovasc Imaging 2014;7:882–92.

46. Park J, Larson AC, Zhang Q, et al. 4D radial coronary artery imaging within a single breath-hold: cine angiography with phase-sensitive fat suppression (CAPS). Magn Reson Med 2005;54: 833–40.

47. Kressler B, Spincemaille P, Nguyen TD, et al. Three-dimensional cine imaging using variable-density spiral trajectories and SSFP with application to coronary artery angiography. Magn Reson Med 2007;58:535–43.

48. Lai P, Larson AC, Park J, et al. Respiratory self-gated four-dimensional coronary MR angiography: a feasibility study. Magn Reson Med 2008;59: 1378–85.

49. Liu J, Spincemaille P, Codella NC, et al. Respiratory and cardiac self-gated free-breathing cardiac CINE imaging with multiecho 3D hybrid radial SSFP acquisition. Magn Reson Med 2010;63:1230–7.

50. Liu J, Nguyen TD, Zhu Y, et al. Self-gated free-breathing 3D coronary CINE imaging with simultaneous water and fat visualization. PLoS One 2014; 9:e89315.

51. Coppo S, Piccini D, Bonanno G, et al. Free-running 4D whole-heart self-navigated golden angle MRI: Initial results. Magn Reson Med 2015;74:1306–16.

52. Han F, Rapacchi S, Khan S, et al. Four-dimensional, multiphase, steady-state imaging with contrast enhancement (MUSIC) in the heart: a feasibility study in children. Magn Reson Med 2015;74: 1042–9.

53. Han F, Zhou Z, Han E, et al. Self-gated 4D multiphase, steady-state imaging with contrast enhancement (MUSIC) using rotating cartesian K-space (ROCK): validation in children with congenital heart disease. Magn Reson Med 2016; 78(2):472–83.

54. Nguyen KL, Han F, Zhou Z, et al. 4D MUSIC CMR: value-based imaging of neonates and infants with congenital heart disease. J Cardiovasc Magn Reson 2017;19:40.

55. Zhou Z, Han F, Rapacchi S, et al. Accelerated ferumoxytol-enhanced 4D multiphase, steady-state imaging with contrast enhancement (MUSIC) cardiovascular MRI: validation in pediatric congenital heart disease. NMR Biomed 2017;30. https:// doi.org/10.1002/nbm.3663.

56. Moghari MH, Barthur A, Amaral ME, et al. Free-breathing whole-heart 3D cine magnetic resonance imaging with prospective respiratory motion compensation. Magn Reson Med 2018;80:181–9.

57. Moghari MH, Uecker M, Roujol S, et al. Accelerated whole-heart MR angiography using a variable-density poisson-disc undersampling pattern and compressed sensing reconstruction. Magn Reson Med 2018;79:761–9.

58. Bustin A, Ginami G, Cruz G, et al. Five-minute whole-heart coronary MRA with sub-millimeter

isotropic resolution, 100% respiratory scan efficiency, and 3D-PROST reconstruction. Magn Reson Med 2019;81:102–15.

59. Usman M, Ruijsink B, Nazir MS, et al. Free breathing whole-heart 3D CINE MRI with self-gated Cartesian trajectory. Magn Reson Imaging 2017;38: 129–37.

60. Cheng JY, Hanneman K, Zhang T, et al. Comprehensive motion-compensated highly accelerated 4D flow MRI with ferumoxytol enhancement for pediatric congenital heart disease. J Magn Reson Imaging 2015;43(6):1355–68.

61. Larson AC, Kellman P, Arai A, et al. Preliminary investigation of respiratory self-gating for free-breathing segmented cine MRI. Magn Reson Med 2005;53:159–68.

62. Larson AC, White RD, Laub G, et al. Self-gated cardiac cine MRI. Magn Reson Med 2004;51:93–102.

63. Uribe S, Muthurangu V, Boubertakh R, et al. Whole-heart cine MRI using real-time respiratory self-gating. Magn Reson Med 2007;57:606–13.

64. Zhou Z, Han F, Yoshida T, et al. Improved 4D cardiac functional assessment for pediatric patients using motion-weighted image reconstruction. MAGMA 2018;31:747–56.

65. Fonseca CG, Backhaus M, Bluemke DA, et al. The Cardiac Atlas Project–an imaging database for computational modeling and statistical atlases of the heart. Bioinformatics 2011;27:2288–95.

66. Medrano-Gracia P, Cowan BR, Ambale-Venkatesh B, et al. Left ventricular shape variation in asymptomatic populations: the Multi-Ethnic Study of Atherosclerosis. J Cardiovasc Magn Reson 2014;16:56.

67. Feng L, Axel L, Chandarana H, et al. XD-GRASP: golden-angle radial MRI with reconstruction of extra motion-state dimensions using compressed sensing. Magn Reson Med 2016;75:775–88.

68. Feng L, Grimm R, Block KT, et al. Golden-angle radial sparse parallel MRI: combination of compressed sensing, parallel imaging, and golden-angle radial sampling for fast and flexible dynamic volumetric MRI. Magn Reson Med 2014;72: 707–17.

69. Feng L, Coppo S, Piccini D, et al. 5D whole-heart sparse MRI. Magn Reson Med 2018;79:826–38.

70. Cheng JY, Zhang T, Alley MT, et al. Comprehensive multi-dimensional MRI for the simultaneous assessment of cardiopulmonary anatomy and physiology. Sci Rep 2017;7:5330.

71. Zhang S, Uecker M, Voit D, et al. Real-time cardiovascular magnetic resonance at high temporal resolution: radial FLASH with nonlinear inverse reconstruction. J Cardiovasc Magn Reson 2010; 12:39.

72. Uecker M, Zhang S, Frahm J. Nonlinear inverse reconstruction for real-time MRI of the human heart using undersampled radial FLASH. Magn Reson Med 2010;63:1456–62.

73. Frahm J, Haase A, Matthaei D. Rapid NMR imaging of dynamic processes using the FLASH technique. Magn Reson Med 1986;3:321–7.

74. Breuer FA, Kellman P, Griswold MA, et al. Dynamic autocalibrated parallel imaging using temporal GRAPPA (TGRAPPA). Magn Reson Med 2005;53:981–5.

75. Feng L, Srichai MB, Lim RP, et al. Highly accelerated real-time cardiac cine MRI using k-t SPARSE-SENSE. Magn Reson Med 2013;70: 64–74.

76. Kellman P, Chefd'hotel C, Lorenz CH, et al. High spatial and temporal resolution cardiac cine MRI from retrospective reconstruction of data acquired in real time using motion correction and resorting. Magn Reson Med 2009;62:1557–64.

77. Hansen MS, Sørensen TS, Arai AE, et al. Retrospective reconstruction of high temporal resolution cine images from real-time MRI using iterative motion correction. Magn Reson Med 2012;68:741–50.

78. Xue H, Kellman P, Larocca G, et al. High spatial and temporal resolution retrospective cine cardiovascular magnetic resonance from shortened free breathing real-time acquisitions. J Cardiovasc Magn Reson 2013;15:102.

79. Camargo GC, Erthal F, Sabioni L, et al. Real-time cardiac magnetic resonance cine imaging with sparse sampling and iterative reconstruction for left-ventricular measures: comparison with gold-standard segmented steady-state free precession. Magn Reson Imaging 2017;38:138–44.

80. Usman M, Atkinson D, Odille F, et al. Motion corrected compressed sensing for free-breathing dynamic cardiac MRI. Magn Reson Med 2013;70: 504–16.

81. Kido T, Kido T, Nakamura M, et al. Compressed sensing real-time cine cardiovascular magnetic resonance: accurate assessment of left ventricular function in a single-breath-hold. J Cardiovasc Magn Reson 2016;18:50.

82. Rahsepar AA, Saybasili H, Ghasemiesfe A, et al. Motion-corrected real-time cine magnetic resonance imaging of the heart: initial clinical experience. Invest Radiol 2018;53:35–44.

83. Scatteia A, Baritussio A, Bucciarelli-Ducci C. Strain imaging using cardiac magnetic resonance. Heart Fail Rev 2017;22:465–76.

84. Zerhouni EA, Parish DM, Rogers WJ, et al. Human heart: tagging with MR imaging–a method for noninvasive assessment of myocardial motion. Radiology 1988;169:59–63.

85. Ibrahim el SH. Myocardial tagging by cardiovascular magnetic resonance: evolution of techniques–pulse sequences, analysis algorithms, and applications. J Cardiovasc Magn Reson 2011;13:36.

86. Nasiraei-Moghaddam A, Finn JP. Tagging of cardiac magnetic resonance images in the polar coordinate system: physical principles and practical implementation. Magn Reson Med 2014;71(5):1750–9.

87. Hor KN, Gottliebson WM, Carson C, et al. Comparison of magnetic resonance feature tracking for strain calculation with harmonic phase imaging analysis. JACC Cardiovasc Imaging 2010;3:144–51.

88. Hor KN, Baumann R, Pedrizzetti G, et al. Magnetic resonance derived myocardial strain assessment using feature tracking. J Vis Exp 2011;12(48):2356.

89. Kammerlander AA, Donà C, Nitsche C, et al. Feature tracking of global longitudinal strain by using cardiovascular MRI improves risk stratification in heart failure with preserved ejection fraction. Radiology 2020;296(2):290–8.

90. Romano S, Judd RM, Kim RJ, et al. Feature-tracking global longitudinal strain predicts mortality in patients with preserved ejection fraction: a multicenter study. JACC Cardiovasc Imaging 2020;13:940–7.

91. Romano S, Romer B, Evans K, et al. Prognostic implications of blunted feature-tracking global longitudinal strain during vasodilator cardiovascular magnetic resonance stress imaging. JACC Cardiovasc Imaging 2020;13:58–65.

92. Udelson JE. Left ventricular shape: the forgotten stepchild of remodeling parameters. JACC Heart Fail 2017;5:179–81.

93. Udelson JE, Konstam MA. Relation between left ventricular remodeling and clinical outcomes in heart failure patients with left ventricular systolic dysfunction. J Card Fail 2002;8:S465–71.

94. Edelman RR, Gaa J, Wedeen VJ, et al. In vivo measurement of water diffusion in the human heart. Magn Reson Med 1994;32:423–8.

95. Nielles-Vallespin S, Scott A, Ferreira P, et al. Cardiac diffusion: technique and practical applications. J Magn Reson Imaging 2020;52(2):348–68.

96. Nielles-Vallespin S, Mekkaoui C, Gatehouse P, et al. In vivo diffusion tensor MRI of the human heart: reproducibility of breath-hold and navigator-based approaches. Magn Reson Med 2013;70:454–65.

97. Nguyen C, Fan Z, Sharif B, et al. In vivo three-dimensional high resolution cardiac diffusion-weighted MRI: a motion compensated diffusion-prepared balanced steady-state free precession approach. Magn Reson Med 2014;72:1257–67.

98. Welsh CL, DiBella EV, Hsu EW. Higher-order motion-compensation for in vivo cardiac diffusion tensor imaging in rats. IEEE Trans Med Imaging 2015;34:1843–53.

99. Stoeck CT, von Deuster C, Genet M, et al. Second-order motion-compensated spin echo diffusion tensor imaging of the human heart. Magn Reson Med 2016;75:1669–76.

100. Aliotta E, Wu HH, Ennis DB. Convex optimized diffusion encoding (CODE) gradient waveforms for minimum echo time and bulk motion-compensated diffusion-weighted MRI. Magn Reson Med 2017;77:717–29.

101. Delattre BM, Viallon M, Wei H, et al. In vivo cardiac diffusion-weighted magnetic resonance imaging: quantification of normal perfusion and diffusion coefficients with intravoxel incoherent motion imaging. Invest Radiol 2012;47:662–70.

102. Ferreira PF, Kilner PJ, McGill LA, et al. In vivo cardiovascular magnetic resonance diffusion tensor imaging shows evidence of abnormal myocardial laminar orientations and mobility in hypertrophic cardiomyopathy. J Cardiovasc Magn Reson 2014;16:87.

103. McGill LA, Scott AD, Ferreira PF, et al. Heterogeneity of fractional anisotropy and mean diffusivity measurements by in vivo diffusion tensor imaging in normal human hearts. PLoS One 2015;10:e0132360.

104. Nielles-Vallespin S, Khalique Z, Ferreira PF, et al. Assessment of myocardial microstructural dynamics by in vivo diffusion tensor cardiac magnetic resonance. J Am Coll Cardiol 2017;69:661–76.

105. Khalique Z, Ferreira PF, Scott AD, et al. Diffusion tensor cardiovascular magnetic resonance in cardiac amyloidosis. Circ Cardiovasc Imaging 2020;13:e009901.

106. Hsu EW, Muzikant AL, Matulevicius SA, et al. Magnetic resonance myocardial fiber-orientation mapping with direct histological correlation. Am J Physiol 1998;274:H1627–34.

107. Scollan DF, Holmes A, Winslow R, et al. Histological validation of myocardial microstructure obtained from diffusion tensor magnetic resonance imaging. Am J Physiol 1998;275:H2308–18.

108. Tseng WY, Wedeen VJ, Reese TG, et al. Diffusion tensor MRI of myocardial fibers and sheets: correspondence with visible cut-face texture. J Magn Reson Imaging 2003;17:31–42.

109. Chen J, Liu W, Zhang H, et al. Regional ventricular wall thickening reflects changes in cardiac fiber and sheet structure during contraction: quantification with diffusion tensor MRI. Am J Physiol Heart Circ Physiol 2005;289:H1898–907.

110. Pope AJ, Sands GB, Smaill BH, et al. Three-dimensional transmural organization of perimysial collagen in the heart. Am J Physiol Heart Circ Physiol 2008;295:H1243–52.

111. McGill LA, Ferreira PF, Scott AD, et al. Relationship between cardiac diffusion tensor imaging

parameters and anthropometrics in healthy volunteers. J Cardiovasc Magn Reson 2016;18:2.

112. Dyverfeldt P, Bissell M, Barker AJ, et al. 4D flow cardiovascular magnetic resonance consensus statement. J Cardiovasc Magn Reson 2015;17:72.

113. Crandon S, Elbaz MSM, Westenberg JJM, et al. Clinical applications of intra-cardiac four-dimensional flow cardiovascular magnetic resonance: a systematic review. Int J Cardiol 2017;249:486–93.

114. Zhong L, Schrauben EM, Garcia J, et al. Intracardiac 4D flow MRI in congenital heart disease: recommendations on behalf of the ISMRM Flow & Motion Study Group. J Magn Reson Imaging 2019;50:677–81.

115. Bolger AF, Heiberg E, Karlsson M, et al. Transit of blood flow through the human left ventricle mapped by cardiovascular magnetic resonance. J Cardiovasc Magn Reson 2007;9:741–7.

116. Wigström L, Ebbers T, Fyrenius A, et al. Particle trace visualization of intracardiac flow using time-resolved 3D phase contrast MRI. Magn Reson Med 1999;41:793–9.

117. Carlsson M, Heiberg E, Toger J, et al. Quantification of left and right ventricular kinetic energy using four-dimensional intracardiac magnetic resonance imaging flow measurements. Am J Physiol Heart Circ Physiol 2012;302:H893–900.

118. Kanski M, Arvidsson PM, Töger J, et al. Left ventricular fluid kinetic energy time curves in heart failure from cardiovascular magnetic resonance 4D flow data. J Cardiovasc Magn Reson 2015;17:111.

119. Wong J, Chabiniok R, deVecchi A, et al. Age-related changes in intraventricular kinetic energy: a physiological or pathological adaptation? Am J Physiol Heart Circ Physiol 2016;310:H747–55.

120. Töger J, Kanski M, Arvidsson PM, et al. Vortex-ring mixing as a measure of diastolic function of the human heart: phantom validation and initial observations in healthy volunteers and patients with heart failure. J Magn Reson Imaging 2016;43:1386–97.

121. Töger J, Kanski M, Carlsson M, et al. Vortex ring formation in the left ventricle of the heart: analysis by 4D flow MRI and Lagrangian coherent structures. Ann Biomed Eng 2012;40:2652–62.

122. Elbaz MS, Calkoen EE, Westenberg JJ, et al. Vortex flow during early and late left ventricular filling in normal subjects: quantitative characterization using retrospectively-gated 4D flow cardiovascular magnetic resonance and three-dimensional vortex core analysis. J Cardiovasc Magn Reson 2014;16:78.

123. Suwa K, Saitoh T, Takehara Y, et al. Intra-left ventricular flow dynamics in patients with preserved and impaired left ventricular function: analysis with 3D cine phase contrast MRI (4D-Flow). J Magn Reson Imaging 2016;44:1493–503.

124. Stoll VM, Hess AT, Rodgers CT, et al. Left ventricular flow analysis. Circ Cardiovasc Imaging 2019;12:e008130.

125. Sjöberg P, Heiberg E, Wingren P, et al. Decreased diastolic ventricular kinetic energy in young patients with Fontan circulation demonstrated by four-dimensional cardiac magnetic resonance imaging. Pediatr Cardiol 2017;38:669–80.

126. Kamphuis VP, Elbaz MSM, van den Boogaard PJ, et al. Disproportionate intraventricular viscous energy loss in Fontan patients: analysis by 4D flow MRI. Eur Heart J Cardiovasc Imaging 2019;20:323–33.

127. Kamphuis VP, Elbaz MSM, van den Boogaard PJ, et al. Stress increases intracardiac 4D flow cardiovascular magnetic resonance-derived energetics and vorticity and relates to VO(2)max in Fontan patients. J Cardiovasc Magn Reson 2019;21:43.

Cardiovascular Magnetic Resonance in Heritable Cardiomyopathies

Daniel J. Hammersley, MBBS[a,b], Richard E. Jones, MBChB[a,b],
Lukas Mach, MD[a,b], Brian P. Halliday, PhD[a,b], Sanjay K. Prasad, MD[a,b],*

KEYWORDS

- Cardiomyopathy • Heritable • Inherited • Cardiovascular magnetic resonance

KEY POINTS

- Cardiovascular magnetic resonance (CMR) is the imaging modality of choice for many heritable cardiomyopathies because it affords gold-standard evaluation of cardiac morphology in tandem with tissue characterization of the underlying myocardial substrate.
- CMR additionally has an important role in risk stratification of patients with heritable cardiomyopathies.
- There is now an emerging role for CMR in guiding therapies and evaluating treatment response for patients with heritable cardiomyopathies.

INTRODUCTION

Cardiomyopathy is an umbrella term that describes a heterogeneous group of disorders characterized by structural and functional abnormalities of the myocardium in the absence of significant coronary artery disease, hypertension, primary valvular disease, or congenital heart disease.[1] In many cases cardiomyopathies have an underlying genetic basis and are termed heritable or inherited cardiomyopathies. Cardiomyopathy is associated with a significant global health burden, driven principally by heart failure (HF) or arrhythmic sequelae including sudden cardiac death. Amid aspirations to transition toward more personalized therapies, there is a pressing need for precision phenotypic evaluation to optimize diagnostic accuracy and characterize risk. In this article the utility, recent advances, and future horizons of cardiovascular magnetic resonance (CMR) in heritable cardiomyopathies is outlined and explored.

CLASSIFYING THE ROLES OF CARDIOVASCULAR MAGNETIC RESONANCE IN HERITABLE CARDIOMYOPATHIES

The principal utility of cardiovascular imaging in patients with cardiomyopathies can broadly be divided into 3 domains:

1. Establishing the underlying diagnosis and identifying disease etiology
2. Informing risk stratification and prognosis
3. Guiding clinical management and evaluating treatment response

CARDIOVASCULAR MAGNETIC RESONANCE TECHNIQUES USED IN HERITABLE CARDIOMYOPATHIES

Several different CMR-based sequences and techniques contribute to the evaluation of heritable cardiomyopathies.

Funding: The authors acknowledge support from the NHLI Foundation, the Royal Brompton Cardiovascular Research Centre, Elliot's Touch, the British Heart Foundation, Cardiomyopathy UK, and the Alexander Jansons Fund.
 a National Heart & Lung Institute, Imperial College, London SW3 6LY, UK; b CMR Unit, The Royal Brompton Hospital, Sydney Street, London SW3 6NP, UK
* Corresponding author. CMR Unit, The Royal Brompton Hospital, Sydney Street, London SW3 6NP, UK.
E-mail address: s.prasad@rbht.nhs.uk

Heart Failure Clin 17 (2021) 25–39
https://doi.org/10.1016/j.hfc.2020.08.004
1551-7136/21/© 2020 Elsevier Inc. All rights reserved.

Cine-Cardiovascular Magnetic Resonance

Through the acquisition of high-spatial-resolution cine images with clear blood–endocardial border delineation, CMR represents the gold-standard imaging modality for quantification of cardiac chamber volumes and myocardial mass.[2,3] Cine-CMR is subject to less operator dependence and intraobserver and interobserver variability than other imaging modalities.[4]

Late Gadolinium Enhancement Cardiovascular Magnetic Resonance

Late gadolinium enhancement (LGE)-CMR is an important technique for myocardial tissue characterization. This technique uses the intrinsic properties of gadolinium based extracellular contrast agents to shorten the T1 recovery time. In normal myocardium, myocytes are densely packed and the volume of distribution of gadolinium is small, precluding hyperenhancement on T1-weighted imaging. Expansion of the myocardial extracellular space results in gadolinium accumulation and delayed clearance, which in turn causes hyperenhancement on T1-weighted images.[5] In patients with cardiomyopathy, the most common cause of LGE is myocardial replacement fibrosis. Correlation between LGE and histologic replacement fibrosis is well described across numerous nonischemic cardiomyopathies.[6–8] The prevalence, typical patterns, and extent of LGE vary between different cardiomyopathies, offering diagnostic utility. LGE observed in cardiomyopathy can typically be distinguished from LGE secondary to myocardial infarction, owing to sparing of the subendocardium (**Fig. 1**).[9] One important consideration with LGE-CMR imaging relates to the requirement to null signal to a reference normal myocardial region, which can result in underestimation in conditions characterized by a more diffuse fibrosis.[10]

Parametric Mapping

Parametric mapping is an alternative tissue characterization technique based on mapping the magnetic relaxation properties (T1, T2, and T2* relaxation time) of each voxel within an image.[11] Precontrast and postcontrast T1 mapping can be used in conjunction with hematocrit to calculate extracellular volume (ECV) by estimating the concentration of contrast in the extracellular space relative to the blood pool at steady state.[12] Histologic validation studies have demonstrated that both native T1 (precontrast) and ECV correlate with diffuse interstitial fibrosis across a range of cardiovascular conditions, including cardiomyopathies.[8,12–15] T2 mapping is used to evaluate myocardial edema. T2* mapping is a technique used to assess for myocardial iron overload.

Cardiovascular Magnetic Resonance Feature Tracking

Myocardial strain measures the degree of myocardial deformation from a fixed point throughout the cardiac cycle and can be evaluated using either transthoracic echocardiography (TTE) or CMR-based techniques.[16] CMR feature tracking (CMR-FT) is a technique used to evaluate myocardial strain by tracking individual anatomic features.[17] Left ventricular (LV) global longitudinal strain (GLS) offers a reproducible alternative measure of LV contractile performance to LV ejection fraction (LVEF) that is less affected by geometric confounders such as cavity size. Although CMR-FT is currently not routinely used for clinical purposes, LV GLS may be more sensitive to subtle systolic

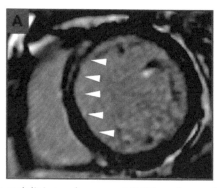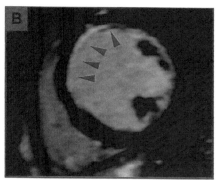

Fig. 1. Late gadolinium enhancement (LGE) cardiovascular magnetic resonance (CMR) in a patient with nonischemic dilated cardiomyopathy (DCM) demonstrating midwall LGE of the basal septum (*A; white arrowheads* indicate myocardial regions with midwall LGE); and in a patient with ischemic heart disease demonstrating subendocardial LGE of the midventricular anteroseptal and anterior segments caused by myocardial infarction (*B; red arrowheads* indicate regions of subendocardial infarction).

dysfunction than standard volumetric analysis, which may be of particular utility in the diagnosis of early-stage cardiomyopathies.[18]

DILATED CARDIOMYOPATHY

Nonischemic dilated cardiomyopathy (DCM) is a primary disease of the myocardium characterized by LV dilatation with systolic impairment in the absence of obstructive coronary artery disease or adverse loading conditions.[19] DCM represents a common morphologic phenotype expressed among a highly heterogeneous component group of patients. The adoption of a disease definition based on cardiac morphology results in the inclusion of extensively varied pathology under a single moniker. Although historically cases of DCM were attributed to a single overarching etiology, it has become clear that many cases result from the complex interaction between genetic susceptibility and environmental triggers, including pregnancy, myocarditis, endocrinopathy, toxin exposure (alcohol and chemotherapy), and chronic tachycardia.[2,20,21] Familial disease is defined by the presence of confirmed DCM in 2 or more family members[19] and occurs in 20% to 30% of cases.[22] In approximately 40% of these cases, a pathogenic or likely pathogenic molecular genetic cause can be identified.[23] DCM is the most common cardiomyopathy worldwide, with an estimated population prevalence of 1 in 250.[24] Despite refinement in therapies, DCM remains the leading indication for heart transplantation globally.[24] The 5-year mortality is 20%, driven principally by HF and sudden cardiac death (SCD).[24] Current selection criteria for primary prevention implantable cardioverter defibrillator (ICD) therapy for patients with DCM are based on a single measure of left ventricular ejection fraction (LVEF); this is widely regarded as an inadequate determinant of ICD candidacy. The DANISH (Defibrillator Implantation in Patients with Nonischemic Systolic Heart Failure) study reported that primary-prevention ICD therapy for such patients did not improve all-cause mortality, despite reducing SCD, supporting the view that current ICD selection criteria are failing to identify those most likely to benefit.[25] There is therefore an important unmet need to refine these selection criteria and a long-standing interest in the integration of CMR to optimize this process.

Cardiovascular Magnetic Resonance in the Diagnosis of Dilated Cardiomyopathy

Morphological and function
The morphologic diagnostic criteria for DCM include LV dilatation and systolic impairment. As the gold-standard imaging modality for volumetric analysis, CMR is optimally placed to detect even marginal degrees of ventricular dilatation or systolic impairment, and this may be important in identifying early DCM. The European Society of Cardiology Working Group on myocardial and pericardial disease recently released a position statement that acknowledged a spectrum of mild disease often identified in a preclinical form in asymptomatic family members, including isolated LV dilatation and hypokinetic nondilated cardiomyopathy.[19]

Exclusion of coronary artery disease
A further diagnostic criterion for DCM is the absence of significant flow-limiting coronary artery disease. Most patients with DCM undergo an anatomic coronary evaluation with either invasive coronary angiography or a computed tomography coronary angiogram at the point of initial diagnostic workup. In some cases it may be feasible to exclude significant coronary disease by combining a CMR-based functional test, such as a stress-perfusion study, with LGE-CMR to exclude myocardial infarction. Such an approach may be adopted in patients considered to be at low risk of coronary artery disease because of their young age and absence of conventional risk factors. Coronary artery recanalization, spasm, or coronary embolism may cause myocardial infarction in the absence of angiographic obstructive coronary disease, and can result in LV systolic dysfunction (LVSD) being incorrectly attributed to DCM. One study demonstrated that 13% of patients diagnosed with DCM on the basis of coronary angiography in fact had evidence of infarction on LGE-CMR that was indistinguishable from patients with established ischemic heart disease.[9] CMR is thus a powerful discriminator of the etiology of LVSD and is particularly important in distinguishing ischemic from nonischemic pathologic features. A further study demonstrated that the use of LGE-CMR alone in patients with new-onset HF resulted in accurate identification of the underlying etiology with 100% sensitivity, 96% specificity, and 95% diagnostic accuracy.[26]

Exclusion of differential diagnoses
Myocarditis is an inflammatory disease of the myocardium and, although a distinct clinical entity from DCM, may show overlapping clinical features in the acute setting. CMR can be used to distinguish between DCM and acute myocarditis (**Fig. 2**). Making this distinction is important because it has implications for the timeline of future investigations, clinical follow-up, family screening and prognosis. Three hallmark features

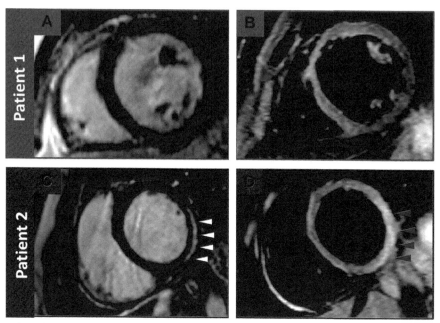

Fig. 2. The utility of CMR to distinguish dilated cardiomyopathy from acute myocarditis. Patient 1 has dilated cardiomyopathy with subtle midwall LGE in the interventricular septum (A) and no areas of increased myocardial signal on T2 short-tau inversion recovery (T2 STIR) imaging (B). Patient 2 has acute myocarditis with subepicardial LGE in the basal inferior/inferolateral segments (C; *white arrowheads* indicate LGE) with corresponding high myocardial signal on T2 STIR imaging (D; *red arrowheads* indicate area of high signal).

are recognized in the CMR Lake Louise diagnostic criteria for myocarditis: (1) myocardial edema on T2-weighted imaging; (2) myocardial hyperemia and capillary leak on early gadolinium enhancement; (3) necrosis and fibrosis on LGE. Presence of 2 of the 3 criteria has a diagnostic accuracy of 78%.[27] Several LGE patterns are described, the most common of which is subepicardial LGE in the lateral wall.[27] Through T2 parametric mapping, focal regions of interest can be analyzed with a quantitative readout of corresponding T2 relaxation time. The gold-standard investigation for myocarditis is endomyocardial biopsy, although its clinical application is limited by its invasive nature, the risk of complications, and the potential for sampling error.

Cardiac sarcoidosis is another condition that can mimic DCM and is thus an important disorder to exclude in the initial DCM diagnostic workup. In most cases the LVEF is preserved, whereas a smaller proportion of patients are associated with LV dilatation and systolic impairment, and such cases may exhibit a number of features common also to DCM. The Heart Rhythm Society have produced expert consensus diagnostic criteria,[28] although this leans heavily on requirements for histologic evidence of extracardiac or cardiac sarcoidosis; in practice up to 65% of patients with cardiac sarcoidosis have no extracardiac disease, and access to cardiac biopsy may be limited.[29] Numerous CMR features may favor a diagnosis of cardiac sarcoidosis over DCM. These include evidence of myocardial edema on T2-weighted imaging, an LGE pattern that is atypical for DCM, and extracardiac features of sarcoidosis identified on the scan (eg, hilar lymphadenopathy). Cardiac sarcoidosis is associated with highly variable patterns of LGE, which may be subepicardial, midwall, subendocardial, or transmural.[30]

Iron overload cardiomyopathy, also termed cardiac hemosiderosis, is an infiltrative cardiomyopathy caused by accumulation of iron in the myocardium. The most common cause globally is long-term blood transfusion therapy, although it can represent a cardiac manifestation of the inherited systemic disease hereditary hemochromatosis. The cardiac phenotype may mimic DCM in cases of heavy iron overload. CMR is the only imaging modality capable of noninvasively measuring cardiac iron load using T2* techniques. Importantly, iron overload cardiomyopathy is treatable and potentially reversible[31]; it should be considered as a potential alternative diagnosis in patients with underlying risk factors presenting with LVSD.[32] CMR has been successfully used to risk stratify and guide therapy in patients with iron overload cardiomyopathy.[33,34]

The Contributory Role of Late Gadolinium Enhancement Cardiovascular Magnetic Resonance in Identifying the Etiology of Dilated Cardiomyopathy

Approximately 30% to 40% of patients with DCM demonstrate LGE on CMR as a result of myocardial replacement fibrosis. The most commonly encountered pattern is linear midwall enhancement of the septum.[6] In some cases, the pattern of LGE may provide a clue as to the underlying etiology, although it is important to emphasize that etiology cannot be accurately determined by LGE characteristics alone. A study of 89 patients with DCM-associated genetic mutations identified distinct phenotypic features on LGE-CMR that distinguished disease caused by desmoplakin (*DSP*) and filamin C (*FLNC*) mutations from other disease-causing variants.[35] LGE in subjects with *DSP/FLNC* mutations was typically found in the basal lateral segment with a subepicardial ring-like pattern (**Fig. 3**A, B).[35] Truncating variants to the sarcomeric protein titan (TTNtv) represents the most common genetic cause of DCM. In contrast to the findings with *DSP/FLNC*, the largest study of 716 patients (83 with TTNtv) did not identify a characteristic LGE signature associated with TTNtv-DCM.[36] DCM caused by pathogenic mutations to *LMNA*, the gene that encodes the Lamin A and C proteins, is associated with a highly malignant disease characterized by high penetrance, prevalent ventricular arrhythmia, atrioventricular block, and progression to advanced HF. Large CMR-based studies of patients with laminopathy are restricted by early ICD implantation and high rates of SCD. Existing small series indicate that DCM caused by pathogenic *LMNA* mutation is associated with a high prevalence of septal midwall LGE, often observed early in the disease course and frequently preceding significant LV dilatation or systolic impairment (**Fig. 3**C).[37–39]

The Role of Cardiovascular Magnetic Resonance in the Risk Stratification of Patients with Dilated Cardiomyopathy

Late gadolinium enhancement cardiovascular magnetic resonance

The association between the presence of LGE and SCD has been established in numerous studies.[6,40–43] In a large prospective study of 472 patients with DCM, LGE was strongly associated with a composite arrhythmic end point (SCD or aborted SCD) even after adjustment for LVEF, with a significant but less powerful association found with all-cause mortality and a composite HF end point.[6] These findings have recently been replicated in a multicenter study of 12 institutions across 4 countries.[44] There does not appear to be a linear dose-response effect observed with increasing LGE mass in patients with DCM; LGE presence alone appears to be a better predictor of risk.[45] LGE-CMR also is a powerful predictor of life-threatening arrhythmia in patients with mild to moderate DCM, with one single-center study demonstrating that LGE was strongly associated with SCD or aborted SCD in patients with DCM and LVEF greater than 40% and no pre-existing ICD indication.[46] Importantly these patients would generally not be eligible for ICD implantation under current guidelines.

T1 Mapping

A multicenter study has demonstrated that native T1 is predictive of both all-cause mortality and a composite HF end point (HF death or hospitalization) in patients with DCM.[47] A smaller single-center study has additionally demonstrated an association between native T1 and appropriate ICD

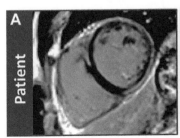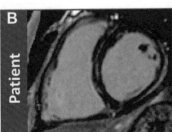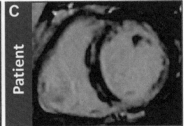

Fig. 3. The contributory role of LGE-CMR in identifying underlying etiology in patients with genetic DCM. Patient A has DCM associated with a pathogenic *DSP* variant, with extensive subepicardial LGE in the basal inferior, lateral, and anterior walls. Patient B has DCM caused by a pathogenic nonsense variant to *FLNC*, with extensive subepicardial LGE of the basal inferior, lateral, and anterior walls with midwall extension into the basal septum. Patient C has DCM associated with a pathogenic missense variant to *LMNA*, with prominent midwall LGE of the basal septum.

therapy or sustained ventricular arrhythmia, although larger multicenter studies are required to validate this arrhythmic association.[48]

Cardiovascular magnetic resonance feature tracking

A large multicenter study of 1012 patients with LVEF less than 50% (49.9% nonischemic DCM) demonstrated an association between CMR-FT LV GLS and all-cause mortality, finding that each 1% worsening in GLS was associated with an 89.1% increased risk of death after adjustment for clinical and imaging variables, including LVEF and LGE, in both ischemic and nonischemic pathology.[49] Studies evaluating the relationship between CMR-FT LV GLS and adverse outcomes with greater granularity are indicated to identify whether this association was principally driven by HF or arrhythmic death.

Cardiovascular Magnetic Resonance in the Clinical Management and Evaluation of Therapy Response in Dilated Cardiomyopathy

Current treatments for patients with DCM are centered around neurohumoral blockade and device therapy (ICDs for prevention of SCD and/or cardiac resynchronization therapy [CRT]).[50] One area of particular interest is in the ability of CMR to guide CRT implantation based on selective deployment of pacing leads to areas of nonscarred myocardium. In a study of 559 patients with both DCM and ischemic HF, CMR-guided

CRT resulted in improvement in symptoms and a reduction in adverse outcomes. Of particular note, pacing areas of scarred myocardium was associated with both SCD and adverse HF events.[51] CMR may offer additional utility in predicting which patients will undergo LV reverse remodeling. Several studies have found that the presence of LGE is associated with failure to reverse remodel.[52–54] It is thus feasible that CMR may be able to identify patients likely to benefit from early referral for advanced therapies because of limited capacity for improvement with pharmacotherapy; larger multicenter studies are warranted to validate these early findings and test this hypothesis.

Follow-up CMR scans may be of particular value in 2 different clinical circumstances for patients with DCM. The first is to evaluate both cardiac structure and function and to assess for development or progression of fibrosis following clinical deterioration. The second circumstance is in the evaluation of therapy response, with particular emphasis on the detection of LV reverse remodeling, especially in patients being considered for device therapy. The utility of CMR in the diagnosis, risk stratification, and management of patients with DCM is summarized in **Fig. 4**.

HYPERTROPHIC CARDIOMYOPATHY

Hypertrophic cardiomyopathy (HCM) is a heritable cardiomyopathy defined by the presence of

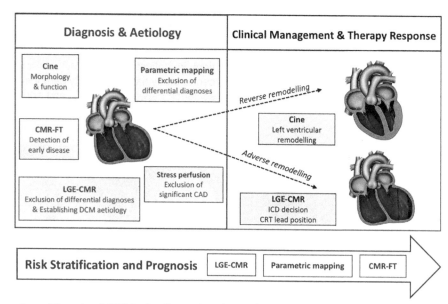

Fig. 4. Overview of the role of CMR in the diagnosis, risk stratification, and clinical management of patients with dilated cardiomyopathy. CAD, coronary artery disease; CMR-FT, cardiovascular magnetic resonance feature tracking; CRT, cardiac resynchronization therapy; DCM, dilated cardiomyopathy; ICD, implantable cardiac defibrillator; LGE-CMR, late gadolinium enhancement cardiovascular magnetic resonance.

increased LV wall thickness that cannot be explained by abnormal loading conditions.[55] Approximately 40% to 70% of patients have obstructive HCM, defined by the presence of an LV intracavity gradient of $\geq$30 mm Hg at rest or during exercise.[56] Historical data have suggested an HCM population prevalence of 1 in 500, although more contemporaneous measures indicate that this may be an underestimate.[57,58] Sarcomeric mutations are found in 60% of cases. A smaller proportion (5%–10%) is caused by other etiologies (including neuromuscular disease, hereditary syndromes, and storage disorders). In the remainder of cases, the etiology remains unknown; some of these cases may relate to undiscovered genetic causes.[56] Established sequelae of HCM include progression to HF, atrial fibrillation, and SCD. Advances in treatment and risk stratification have resulted in significant improvement in clinical outcomes, with contemporary disease-related mortality rates estimated at less than 0.5% per year.[59,60]

Cardiovascular Magnetic Resonance in the Diagnosis of Hypertrophic Cardiomyopathy

Cardiovascular magnetic resonance in the evaluation of the extent of left ventricular hypertrophy

The diagnosis of HCM in adults is made on the basis of LV wall thickness $\geq$15 mm in $\geq$1 myocardial segments in the absence of adverse loading conditions.[55] CMR offers incremental diagnostic value over alternative modalities in several specific circumstances. Establishing a diagnosis in patients for whom echocardiographic imaging is technically suboptimal because of poor acoustic windows is one such circumstance.[61] CMR is also more sensitive than TTE in the detection of regional mild LV hypertrophy (LVH), with one study finding that CMR identified mild focal LVH in 10% of sarcomeric mutation carriers reported to have normal wall thickness on TTE.[62] An additional study found that CMR offered greater precision for identifying regional LVH in the anterolateral LV wall.[63] CMR is also the gold-standard imaging modality for evaluating LV mass.[64] Although the most common pattern of hypertrophy observed in HCM is asymmetric basal septal hypertrophy, morphologic variants exist (**Fig. 5**). CMR is the imaging modality of choice in apical and midcavity HCM and is superior to TTE for identifying associated apical aneurysms.[65] In a study of 1299 patients with HCM, only 16 of 28 patients (57%) with apical aneurysms were identified by TTE, whereas all cases were identified by CMR.[66]

Cardiovascular magnetic resonance in the evaluation of left ventricular outflow tract gradients

Left ventricular outflow tract (LVOT) obstruction has implications for the management, natural history, and prognosis of HCM.[61] Although CMR is capable of measuring LVOT and intracavity gradients using velocity encoded imaging, continuous-wave Doppler echocardiography remains the first-line investigation for this purpose and can be readily used with exercise stress protocols. This exemplifies the importance of a multimodality imaging approach in patients with HCM; such a strategy is recommended in a recent European Association of Cardiovascular Imaging expert consensus document.[67]

Exclusion of alternative causes of left ventricular hypertrophy

LGE is found in up to 70% of patients with HCM. The distribution of LGE is most commonly patchy and located in the midwall of the most hypertrophied segments and at the right ventricular (RV) insertion points.[68] Several studies have demonstrated increased native T1 and ECV levels in HCM, reflecting more diffuse fibrosis.[69,70] Integrating LGE-CMR with parametric mapping is of incremental value in determining pathologic LVH etiology (**Fig. 6**). The storage disorder Anderson-Fabry disease is an import differential diagnosis and can be distinguished from HCM by low native T1 values and characteristic midwall LGE in the basal inferolateral wall.[71,72] HCM phenocopies also include those associated with PRKAG2 mutation, and low native T1 may also help to distinguish these cases during the early stages of disease.[73] Cardiac amyloid is a rare infiltrative cardiomyopathy associated with concentric LVH, preserved systolic function, restrictive physiology, and significant biatrial dilatation. The hallmark CMR features of cardiac amyloidosis include markedly increased native T1 and ECV values and diffuse circumferential subendocardial LGE with abnormal LGE kinetics.[74] A further important clinical distinction is between HCM and hypertensive heart disease, especially in patients with intermediate control of blood pressure. CMR features that favor a diagnosis of HCM over hypertensive heart disease include normal rather than hyperdynamic LVEF, absence of LGE, and less extensive hypertrophy; however, such findings should be interpreted in the broader clinical context with specific focus on control of blood pressure and family history.

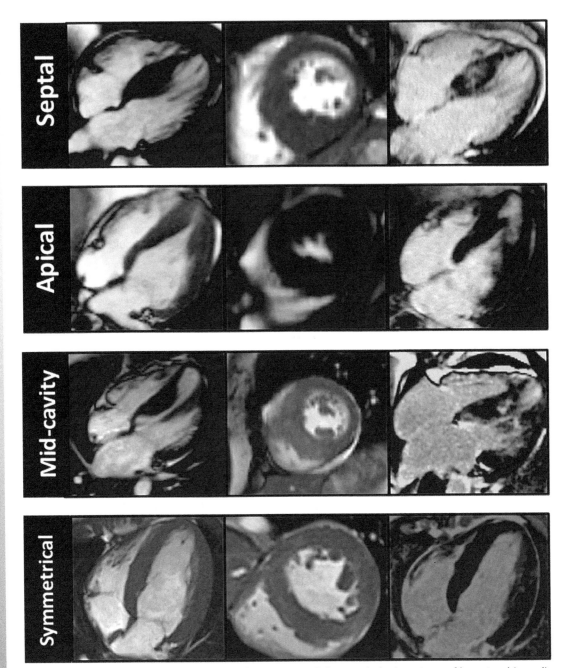

Fig. 5. CMR horizontal long axis, short axis, and LGE images of the morphologic variants of hypertrophic cardiomyopathy: septal, apical, midcavity, and symmetrical.

The Role of Cardiovascular Magnetic Resonance in the Risk Stratification of Patients with Hypertrophic Cardiomyopathy

LGE-CMR also has a role in risk-stratifying patients with HCM. A meta-analysis of 5 studies, including 2993 patients with HCM, showed that LGE was associated with a 3.4-fold increase in the risk of SCD, a 2.9-fold increase in the risk of cardiovascular death, and a 1.8-fold increase in all-cause mortality.[75] Of note, the extent of LGE was also associated with SCD risk after adjusting for baseline characteristics, which is an important finding given the high prevalence of LGE in patients with HCM.[75] LGE ≥15% of LV myocardial mass was associated with a 2-fold increase in SCD risk in one large multicenter study and has

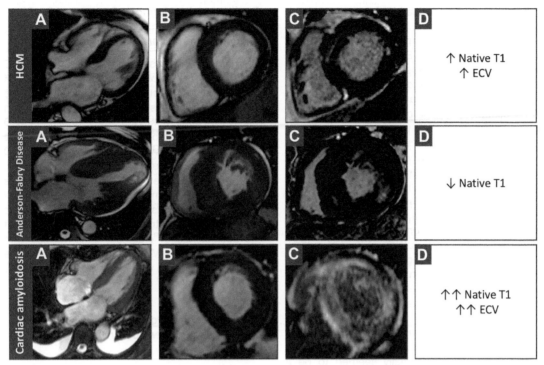

Fig. 6. The utility of CMR to distinguish the etiology of pathologic left ventricular hypertrophy using LGE-CMR with parametric mapping. (*A*) Horizontal long axis; (*B*) short axis; (*C*) LGE; (*D*) T1-mapping summary. ECV, extracellular volume; HCM, hypertrophic cardiomyopathy.

been proposed as a potentially useful threshold value.[76] A recent study has also found that progression of LGE on serial CMRs was associated with a composite end point of HF progression, cardiac hospitalization, and ventricular tachycardia.[77] The role of parametric mapping in risk stratification is currently unclear, and the results of the Hypertrophic Cardiomyopathy Registry are eagerly awaited to explore this further.[78]

Cardiovascular Magnetic Resonance in the Clinical Management and Evaluation of Therapy Response in Hypertrophic Cardiomyopathy

As the gold-standard imaging modality for LV mass, CMR may play a role in serial imaging of patients with HCM to assess for disease progression, although this depends on local service availability. Another important role is in surgical planning in patients referred for septal myomectomy, especially those with complex multilevel obstruction and those with RV outflow tract obstruction.[55] CMR also plays a role in evaluating hypertrophy regression and myocardial scar after septal reduction therapy with either myomectomy or alcohol septal ablation.[79,80]

ARRHYTHMOGENIC CARDIOMYOPATHIES

Arrhythmogenic cardiomyopathy (ACM) is an arrhythmogenic disorder of the myocardium that is not caused by ischemic, hypertensive, or valvular heart disease.[81] This group of conditions incorporates the autosomal dominant cardiomyopathies arrhythmogenic RV cardiomyopathy (ARVC) and arrhythmogenic LV cardiomyopathy (ALVC).[81] ARVC is the best studied of the ACMs, characterized by fibrofatty replacement of the RV myocardium, with additional features that may include RV dilatation with wall motion abnormalities, ventricular arrhythmia, ECG abnormalities, and a family history.[82] The diagnosis is typically made using the revised 2010 Task Force Criteria (TFC).[82] ALVC describes ACM of LV origin and may have considerable phenotypic overlap with DCM.[81] The revised TFC are not applicable to ALVC, and the diagnostic criteria, including the CMR characteristics, require further consensus and refinement.

Cardiovascular Magnetic Resonance in the Diagnosis of Arrhythmogenic Cardiomyopathy

Right ventricular morphology and function
It must be emphasized that ARVC is not a diagnosis that can be made on the basis of cardiac

imaging alone. The revised TFC integrate histology, ECG abnormalities, arrhythmia, and family history in addition to morphologic cardiac abnormalities assessed by TTE, CMR, or RV angiography.[82] CMR is considered the gold-standard modality for the evaluation of the right ventricle and is more sensitive than TTE for the detection of RV dilatation, systolic dysfunction, wall motion abnormalities, and wall thinning. In a study of 102 patients with confirmed ARVC, a significant proportion of patients who met CMR-based TFC did not fulfill echocardiographic criteria, indicating that these imaging modalities should not be used interchangeably in the assessment of suspected cases.[83] A CMR-based study has additionally identified the "Accordion Sign," describing an extended area of focal bulging of the RV outflow tract and subtricuspid regions, observed in 60% of asymptomatic mutation carriers, thereby potentially acting as a novel CMR-based imaging biomarker of early disease.[84]

Detection of fibrofatty infiltration

Although the ability of fast spin-echo sequences to detect fatty infiltration initially seemed to be a promising potential adjunct in establishing a diagnosis of ARVC, the technique has been hampered by low sensitivity and findings that RV fat deposition occurs in numerous other pathological and physiological states.[85]

Late gadolinium enhancement cardiovascular magnetic resonance

LGE of the right ventricle is observed in some patients with ARVC,[86] although such findings were not recognized in the revised TFC, principally because of the notable limitation resulting from the RV wall thinning in ARVC, making this a less sensitive technique than LGE-CMR imaging of the left ventricle. Discerning fibrosis from fat additionally remains challenging.

Cardiovascular magnetic resonance to exclude arrhythmogenic right ventricular cardiomyopathy mimics

Numerous alternative conditions are associated with morphological abnormalities of the right ventricle, including pectus excavatum, ischemic heart disease, cardiac sarcoidosis, myocarditis, and conditions associated with RV overload (intracardiac shunts, anomalous pulmonary venous drainage, or pulmonary hypertension). The combination of gold-standard anatomic characterization of cardiac structure, major vessel, and extracardiac findings with tissue characterization offers enhanced ability to exclude other pathologic conditions that may mimic ARVC.[87]

Cardiovascular Magnetic Resonance for Risk Stratification of Patients with Arrhythmogenic Cardiomyopathy

Although the process of risk stratification for ICD implantation is complex, CMR may be of benefit in determining ICD suitability. The severity of the RV and LV disease seems to be associated with major arrhythmic risk. One study identified LVSD as a major predictor of subsequent arrhythmic death in patients with ARVC.[88] Although LVSD can be detected on a range of imaging modalities, it is widely recognized that CMR is more sensitive in identifying mild impairment. A study of 69 patients with ARVC-associated mutations and no prior sustained ventricular arrhythmia found that the coexistence of electrical abnormalities with abnormalities on CMR offered incremental value in detecting patients with incident sustained major arrhythmic events.[89]

Cardiovascular Magnetic Resonance in the Clinical Management of Arrhythmogenic Cardiomyopathy

Beyond aiding decisions regarding ICD implantation, the scope for using CMR to guide therapy for patients with ARVC is relatively narrow. One application is in characterizing scar substrate to optimize ventricular tachycardia ablation procedures, although further data are required to determine whether this improves safety and procedural success.[90] As CMR access for patients with devices continues to improve, there is potential for further development of CMR-guided therapy in the future.

CARDIOVASCULAR MAGNETIC RESONANCE IN OTHER FORMS OF HERITABLE CARDIOMYOPATHY
Restrictive Cardiomyopathy

Restrictive cardiomyopathy (RCM) encompasses a diverse group of myocardial diseases that may result from inherited or acquired predisposition or as part of systemic disease. Morphologically RCM is typically characterized by a nondilated left ventricle with diastolic dysfunction.[91] The variation within this group is such that complete coverage is beyond the scope of this review. With specific focus on inherited RCM, CMR plays an important role in excluding cardiac amyloidosis, sarcoidosis, Anderson-Fabry disease, and cardiac iron loading through LGE and parametric mapping techniques (as described previously), as all of these conditions can present with an RCM phenotype.[92]

Left Ventricular Noncompaction

Excessive trabeculation of the left ventricle occurs as an independent entity and as part of a spectrum of pathologic and physiologic conditions. There may be a genetic predisposition. LV noncompaction (LVNC) has historically been defined by prominent LV trabeculation, thin compacted myocardium, and deep myocardial recesses.[81] The role of CMR is principally in the identification and evaluation of trabeculation. Four CMR-based diagnostic criteria for LVNC exist. The Petersen method evaluates the ratio of noncompacted to compacted myocardium in diastole[93]; the Stacey method evaluates the same ratio in systole[94]; the Jacquier method uses the mass ratio between total and trabeculae mass[95]; and the Captur method uses a quantitative measure of trabecular complexity.[96] It is important to note that the existing CMR-based diagnostic criteria may over-diagnose LVNC and such strategies should be adopted in the context of other supporting features such as myocardial dysfunction, family history, ECG abnormalities, or LGE..[97] The existing literature does seem to support an association between LGE and adverse cardiovascular outcomes in LVNC, although larger studies are required for better understanding of whether this association affects clinical management.[98] The extent of trabeculation, however, does not seem to be associated with adverse outcomes.[99]

SUMMARY

The inherited cardiomyopathies are a heterogeneous group of conditions with a significant global burden of disease. Early identification, accurate risk stratification, and close monitoring of disease progression are of paramount importance in improving disease outcomes. As primary diseases of the heart muscle, the ability to intricately characterize the myocardial substrate is essential. CMR is the only imaging modality that combines gold-standard volumetric analysis with myocardial tissue characterization, and thus offers the most comprehensive investigative tool for patients with cardiomyopathy. As CMR services expand, it is anticipated that access to this modality will improve. Future research should focus on the growing applications of CMR to guide therapies and the rapidly expanding interface between advanced cardiac imaging and artificial intelligence.

DISCLOSURE

The authors have nothing to disclose.

REFERENCES

1. Elliott P, Andersson B, Arbustini E, et al. Classification of the cardiomyopathies: a position statement from the European Society Of Cardiology Working Group on Myocardial and Pericardial Diseases. Eur Heart J 2008;29(2):270–6.
2. Japp AG, Gulati A, Cook SA, et al. The diagnosis and evaluation of dilated cardiomyopathy. J Am Coll Cardiol 2016;67(25):2996–3010.
3. Maceira AM, Prasad SK, Khan M, et al. Normalized left ventricular systolic and diastolic function by steady state free precession cardiovascular magnetic resonance. J Cardiovasc Magn Reson 2006;8(3):417–26.
4. Bellenger NG, Burgess MI, Ray SG, et al. Comparison of left ventricular ejection fraction and volumes in heart failure by echocardiography, radionuclide ventriculography and cardiovascular magnetic resonance. Are they interchangeable? Eur Heart J 2000;21(16):1387–96.
5. Mahrholdt H, Wagner A, Judd RM, et al. Delayed enhancement cardiovascular magnetic resonance assessment of non-ischaemic cardiomyopathies. Eur Heart J 2005;26(15):1461–74.
6. Gulati A, Jabbour A, Ismail TF, et al. Association of fibrosis with mortality and sudden cardiac death in patients with nonischemic dilated cardiomyopathy. J Am Med Assoc 2013;309(9):896–908.
7. Moravsky G, Ofek E, Rakowski H, et al. Myocardial fibrosis in hypertrophic cardiomyopathy: Accurate reflection of histopathological findings by CMR. JACC Cardiovasc Imaging 2013;6(5):587–96.
8. Iles LM, Ellims AH, Llewellyn H, et al. Histological validation of cardiac magnetic resonance analysis of regional and diffuse interstitial myocardial fibrosis. Eur Heart J Cardiovasc Imaging 2015;16(1):14–22.
9. McCrohon JA, Moon JCC, Prasad SK, et al. Differentiation of heart failure related to dilated cardiomyopathy and coronary artery disease using gadolinium-enhanced cardiovascular magnetic resonance. Circulation 2003;108(1):54–9.
10. Ho CY, Abbasi SA, Neilan TG, et al. T1 measurements identify extracellular volume expansion in hypertrophic cardiomyopathy sarcomere mutation carriers with and without left ventricular hypertrophy. Circ Cardiovasc Imaging 2013;6(3):415–22.
11. Salerno M, Kramer CM. Advances in parametric mapping with CMR imaging. JACC Cardiovasc Imaging 2013;6(7):806–22.
12. Flett AS, Hayward MP, Ashworth MT, et al. Equilibrium contrast cardiovascular magnetic resonance for the measurement of diffuse myocardial fibrosis: preliminary validation in humans. Circulation 2010;122(2):138–44.

13. Bull S, White SK, Piechnik SK, et al. Human non-contrast T1 values and correlation with histology in diffuse fibrosis. Heart 2013;99(13):932–7.

14. Miller CA, Naish JH, Bishop P, et al. Comprehensive validation of cardiovascular magnetic resonance techniques for the assessment of myocardial extracellular volume. Circ Cardiovasc Imaging 2013; 6(3):373–83.

15. Sibley CT, Noureldin RA, Gai N, et al. T1 mapping in cardiomyopathy at cardiac MR: Comparison with endomyocardial biopsy. Radiology 2012;265(3): 724–32.

16. Buckberg G, Hoffman JIE, Mahajan A, et al. Cardiac mechanics revisited: the relationship of cardiac architecture to ventricular function. Circulation 2008; 118(24):2571–87.

17. Claus P, Omar AMS, Pedrizzetti G, et al. Tissue tracking technology for assessing cardiac mechanics: principles, normal values, and clinical applications. JACC Cardiovasc Imaging 2015;8(12): 1444–60.

18. Brown J, Jenkins C, Marwick TH. Use of myocardial strain to assess global left ventricular function: A comparison with cardiac magnetic resonance and 3-dimensional echocardiography. Am Heart J 2009;157(1):102.e1-5.

19. Pinto YM, Elliott PM, Arbustini E, et al. Proposal for a revised definition of dilated cardiomyopathy, hypokinetic non-dilated cardiomyopathy, and its implications for clinical practice: A position statement of the ESC working group on myocardial and pericardial diseases. Eur Heart J 2016; 37(23):1850–8.

20. Ware JS, Li J, Mazaika E, et al. Shared genetic predisposition in peripartum and dilated cardiomyopathies. N Engl J Med 2016;374(3):233–41.

21. Ware JS, Amor-Salamanca A, Tayal U, et al. Genetic etiology for alcohol-induced cardiac toxicity. J Am Coll Cardiol 2018;71(20):2293–302.

22. Petretta M, Pirozzi F, Sasso L, et al. Review and metaanalysis of the frequency of familial dilated cardiomyopathy. Am J Cardiol 2011;108(8):1171–6.

23. Tayal U, Prasad S, Cook SA. Genetics and genomics of dilated cardiomyopathy and systolic heart failure. Genome Med 2017;9(1):20.

24. Felker GM, Thompson RE, Hare JM, et al. Underlying causes and long-term survival in patients with initially unexplained cardiomyopathy. N Engl J Med 2000;342(15):1077–84.

25. Køber L, Thune JJ, Nielsen JC, et al. Defibrillator implantation in patients with nonischemic systolic heart failure. N Engl J Med 2016;375(13):1221–30.

26. Assomull RG, Shakespeare C, Kalra PR, et al. Role of cardiovascular magnetic resonance as a gatekeeper to invasive coronary angiography in patients presenting with heart failure of unknown etiology. Circulation 2011;124(12):1351–60.

27. Friedrich MG, Sechtem U, Schulz-Menger J, et al. Cardiovascular magnetic resonance in myocarditis: a JACC white paper. J Am Coll Cardiol 2009; 53(17):1475–87.

28. Birnie DH, Sauer WH, Bogun F, et al. HRS expert consensus statement on the diagnosis and management of arrhythmias associated with cardiac sarcoidosis. Heart Rhythm 2014;11(7):1304–23.

29. Kandolin R, Lehtonen J, Airaksinen J, et al. Cardiac sarcoidosis: epidemiology, characteristics, and outcome over 25 years in a nationwide study. Circulation 2015;131(7):624–32.

30. Kouranos V, Tzelepis GE, Rapti A, et al. Complementary role of CMR to conventional screening in the diagnosis and prognosis of cardiac sarcoidosis. JACC Cardiovasc Imaging 2017;10(12):1437–47.

31. Gujja P, Rosing DR, Tripodi DJ, et al. Iron overload cardiomyopathy: better understanding of an increasing disorder. J Am Coll Cardiol 2010;56(13): 1001–12.

32. Anderson LJ, Westwood MA, Holden S, et al. Myocardial iron clearance during reversal of siderotic cardiomyopathy with intravenous desferrioxamine: a prospective study using T2* cardiovascular magnetic resonance. Br J Haematol 2004;127(3):348–55.

33. Kirk P, Roughton M, Porter JB, et al. Cardiac T2* magnetic resonance for prediction of cardiac complications in thalassemia major. Circulation 2009; 120(20):1961–8.

34. Pennell DJ, Udelson JE, Arai AE, et al. Cardiovascular function and treatment in β-thalassemia major: a consensus statement from the American Heart Association. Circulation 2013;128(3): 281–308.

35. Augusto JB, Eiros R, Nakou E, et al. Dilated cardiomyopathy and arrhythmogenic left ventricular cardiomyopathy: a comprehensive genotype-imaging phenotype study. Eur Heart J Cardiovasc Imaging 2020;21(3):326–36.

36. Tayal U, Newsome S, Buchan R, et al. Phenotype and clinical outcomes of titin cardiomyopathy. J Am Coll Cardiol 2017;70(18):2264–74.

37. Hasselberg NE, Haland TF, Saberniak J, et al. Lamin A/C cardiomyopathy: young onset, high penetrance, and frequent need for heart transplantation. Eur Heart J 2018;39(10):853–60.

38. Holmström M, Kivistö S, Heliö T, et al. Late gadolinium enhanced cardiovascular magnetic resonance of lamin A/C gene mutation related dilated cardiomyopathy. J Cardiovasc Magn Reson 2011; 13(1):30.

39. Raman SV, Sparks EA, Baker PM, et al. Mid-myocardial fibrosis by cardiac magnetic resonance in patients with lamin A/C cardiomyopathy: possible substrate for diastolic dysfunction. J Cardiovasc Magn Reson 2007;9(6):907–13.

40. Assomull RG, Prasad SK, Lyne J, et al. Cardiovascular magnetic resonance, fibrosis, and prognosis in dilated cardiomyopathy. J Am Coll Cardiol 2006; 48(10):1977–85.

41. Neilan TG, Coelho-Filho OR, Danik SB, et al. CMR quantification of myocardial scar provides additive prognostic information in nonischemic cardiomyopathy. JACC Cardiovasc Imaging 2013;6(9):944–54.

42. Masci PG, Doulaptsis C, Bertella E, et al. Incremental prognostic value of myocardial fibrosis in patients with non-ischemic cardiomyopathy without congestive heart failure. Circ Heart Fail 2014;7(3):448–56.

43. Leyva F, Taylor RJ, Foley PWX, et al. Left ventricular midwall fibrosis as a predictor of mortality and morbidity after cardiac resynchronization therapy in patients with nonischemic cardiomyopathy. J Am Coll Cardiol 2012;60(17):1659–67.

44. Alba AC, Gaztañaga J, Foroutan F, et al. Prognostic value of late gadolinium enhancement for the prediction of cardiovascular outcomes in dilated cardiomyopathy: an international, multi-institutional study of the MINICOR group. Circ Cardiovasc Imaging 2020;13(4):e010105.

45. Halliday BP, Baksi AJ, Gulati A, et al. Outcome in dilated cardiomyopathy related to the extent, location, and pattern of late gadolinium enhancement. JACC Cardiovasc Imaging 2018. https://doi.org/10.1016/j.jcmg.2018.07.015.

46. Halliday BP, Gulati A, Ali A, et al. Association between midwall late gadolinium enhancement and sudden cardiac death in patients with dilated cardiomyopathy and mild and moderate left ventricular systolic dysfunction. Circulation 2017;135(22): 2106–15.

47. Puntmann VO, Carr-White G, Jabbour A, et al. T1-mapping and outcome in nonischemic cardiomyopathy all-cause mortality and heart failure. JACC Cardiovasc Imaging 2016;9(1):40–50.

48. Chen Z, Sohal M, Voigt T, et al. Myocardial tissue characterization by cardiac magnetic resonance imaging using T1 mapping predicts ventricular arrhythmia in ischemic and non-ischemic cardiomyopathy patients with implantable cardioverter-defibrillators. Heart Rhythm 2015;12(4):792–801.

49. Romano S, Judd RM, Kim RJ, et al. Feature-tracking global longitudinal strain predicts death in a multicenter population of patients with ischemic and non-ischemic dilated cardiomyopathy incremental to ejection fraction and late gadolinium enhancement. JACC Cardiovasc Imaging 2018. https://doi.org/10.1016/j.jcmg.2017.10.024.

50. Ponikowski P, Voors AA, Anker SD, et al. 2016 ESC Guidelines for the diagnosis and treatment of acute and chronic heart failure. Eur Heart J 2016;37(27): 2129–2200m.

51. Leyva F, Foley PWX, Chalil S, et al. Cardiac resynchronization therapy guided by late gadolinium-enhancement cardiovascular magnetic resonance. J Cardiovasc Magn Reson 2011;13(1):1–9.

52. Leong DP, Chakrabarty A, Shipp N, et al. Effects of myocardial fibrosis and ventricular dyssynchrony on response to therapy in new-presentation idiopathic dilated cardiomyopathy: insights from cardiovascular magnetic resonance and echocardiography. Eur Heart J 2012;33(5):640–8.

53. Kubanek M, Sramko M, Maluskova J, et al. Novel predictors of left ventricular reverse remodeling in individuals with recent-onset dilated cardiomyopathy. J Am Coll Cardiol 2013;61(1):54–63.

54. Masci PG, Schuurman R, Andrea B, et al. Myocardial fibrosis as a key determinant of left ventricular remodeling in idiopathic dilated cardiomyopathy: A contrast-enhanced cardiovascular magnetic study. Circ Cardiovasc Imaging 2013;6(5):790–9.

55. Zamorano JL, Anastasakis A, Borger MA, et al. 2014 ESC guidelines on diagnosis and management of hypertrophic cardiomyopathy: The task force for the diagnosis and management of hypertrophic cardiomyopathy of the European Society of Cardiology (ESC). Eur Heart J 2014;35(39):2733–79.

56. Seferović PM, Polovina M, Bauersachs J, et al. Heart failure in cardiomyopathies: a position paper from the Heart Failure Association of the European Society of Cardiology. Eur J Heart Fail 2019;21(5): 553–76.

57. Maron BJ, Gardin JM, Flack JM, et al. Prevalence of hypertrophic cardiomyopathy in a general population of young adults. Circulation 1995;92(4): 785–9.

58. Semsarian C, Ingles J, Maron MS, et al. New perspectives on the prevalence of hypertrophic cardiomyopathy. J Am Coll Cardiol 2015;65(12):1249–54.

59. Maron BJ, Ommen SR, Semsarian C, et al. Hypertrophic cardiomyopathy: present and future, with translation into contemporary cardiovascular medicine. J Am Coll Cardiol 2014;64(1):83–99.

60. Maron BJ, Rowin EJ, Casey SA, et al. Hypertrophic cardiomyopathy in adulthood associated with low cardiovascular mortality with contemporary management strategies. J Am Coll Cardiol 2015;65(18): 1915–28.

61. Maron MS, Rowin EJ, Maron BJ. How to image hypertrophic cardiomyopathy. Circ Cardiovasc Imaging 2017;10(7):1–15.

62. Valente AM, Lakdawala NK, Powell AJ, et al. Comparison of echocardiographic and cardiac magnetic resonance imaging in hypertrophic cardiomyopathy sarcomere mutation carriers without left ventricular hypertrophy. Circ Cardiovasc Genet 2013;6(3): 230–7.

63. Rickers C, Wilke NM, Jerosch-Herold M, et al. Utility of cardiac magnetic resonance imaging in the diagnosis of hypertrophic cardiomyopathy. Circulation 2005;112(6):855–61.

64. Myerson SG, Bellenger NG, Pennell DJ. Assessment of left ventricular mass by cardiovascular magnetic resonance. Hypertension 2002;39(3):750–5.

65. Moon JCC, Fisher NG, McKenna WJ, et al. Detection of apical hypertrophic cardiomyopathy by cardiovascular magnetic resonance in patients with non-diagnostic echocardiography. Heart 2004;90(6): 645–9.

66. Maron MS, Finley JJ, Bos JM, et al. Prevalence, clinical significance, and natural history of left ventricular apical aneurysms in hypertrophic cardiomyopathy. Circulation 2008;118(15):1541–9.

67. Cardim N, Galderisi M, Edvardsen T, et al. Role of multimodality cardiac imaging in the management of patients with hypertrophic cardiomyopathy: An expert consensus of the European Association of Cardiovascular Imaging endorsed by the Saudi Heart Association. Eur Heart J Cardiovasc Imaging 2015;16(3):280.

68. Rudolph A, Abdel-Aty H, Bohl S, et al. Noninvasive detection of fibrosis applying contrast-enhanced cardiac magnetic resonance in different forms of left ventricular hypertrophy. relation to remodeling. J Am Coll Cardiol 2009; 53(3):284–91.

69. Dass S, Suttie JJ, Piechnik SK, et al. Myocardial tissue characterization using magnetic resonance non-contrast T1 mapping in hypertrophic and dilated cardiomyopathy. Circ Cardiovasc Imaging 2012; 5(6):726–33.

70. Puntmann VO, Voigt T, Chen Z, et al. Native T1 mapping in differentiation of normal myocardium from diffuse disease in hypertrophic and dilated cardiomyopathy. JACC Cardiovasc Imaging 2013;6(4): 475–84.

71. Sado DM, White SK, Piechnik SK, et al. Identification and assessment of anderson-fabry disease by cardiovascular magnetic resonance noncontrast myocardial T1 mapping. Circ Cardiovasc Imaging 2013;6(3):392–8.

72. Moon JCC, Sachdev B, Elkington AG, et al. Gadolinium enhanced cardiovascular magnetic resonance in Anderson-Fabry disease: evidence for a disease specific abnormality of the myocardial interstitium. Eur Heart J 2003;24(23):2151–5.

73. Pöyhönen P, Hiippala A, Ollila L, et al. Cardiovascular magnetic resonance findings in patients with PRKAG2 gene mutations. J Cardiovasc Magn Reson 2015;17(1). https://doi.org/10.1186/s12968-015-0192-3.

74. Syed IS, Glockner JF, Feng DL, et al. Role of cardiac magnetic resonance imaging in the detection of cardiac amyloidosis. JACC Cardiovasc Imaging 2010; 3(2):155–64.

75. Weng Z, Yao J, Chan RH, et al. Prognostic value of LGE-CMR in HCM: a meta-analysis. JACC Cardiovasc Imaging 2016;9(12):1392–402.

76. Chan RH, Maron BJ, Olivotto I, et al. Prognostic value of quantitative contrast-enhanced cardiovascular magnetic resonance for the evaluation of sudden death risk in patients with hypertrophic cardiomyopathy. Circulation 2014;130(6):484–95.

77. Raman B, Ariga R, Spartera M, et al. Progression of myocardial fibrosis in hypertrophic cardiomyopathy: mechanisms and clinical implications. Eur Heart J Cardiovasc Imaging 2019;20(2):157–67.

78. Kramer CM, Appelbaum E, Desai MY, et al. Hypertrophic Cardiomyopathy Registry: the rationale and design of an international, observational study of hypertrophic cardiomyopathy. Am Heart J 2015; 170(2):223–30.

79. Valeti US, Nishimura RA, Holmes DR, et al. Comparison of surgical septal myectomy and alcohol septal ablation with cardiac magnetic resonance imaging in patients with hypertrophic obstructive cardiomyopathy. J Am Coll Cardiol 2007;49(3):350–7.

80. Lu M, Du H, Gao Z, et al. Predictors of outcome after alcohol septal ablation for hypertrophic obstructive cardiomyopathy: an echocardiography and cardiovascular magnetic resonance imaging study. Circ Cardiovasc Interv 2016;9(3):1–12.

81. Towbin JA, McKenna WJ, Abrams DJ, et al. 2019 HRS expert consensus statement on evaluation, risk stratification, and management of arrhythmogenic cardiomyopathy. Heart Rhythm 2019;16(11): e301–72.

82. Marcus FI, McKenna WJ, Sherrill D, et al. Diagnosis of arrhythmogenic right ventricular cardiomyopathy/dysplasia: proposed modification of the task force criteria. Circulation 2010;121(13):1533–41.

83. Borgquist R, Haugaa KH, Gilljam T, et al. The diagnostic performance of imaging methods in ARVC using the 2010 Task Force criteria. Eur Heart J Cardiovasc Imaging 2014;15(11):1219–25.

84. Dalal D, Tandri H, Judge DP, et al. Morphologic variants of familial arrhythmogenic right ventricular dysplasia/cardiomyopathy. a genetics-magnetic resonance imaging correlation study. J Am Coll Cardiol 2009;53(15):1289–99.

85. Rastegar N, Burt JR, Corona-Villalobos CP, et al. Cardiac MR findings and potential diagnostic pitfalls in patients evaluated for arrhythmogenic right ventricular cardiomyopathy. Radiographics 2014;34(6): 1553–71.

86. Hunold P, Wieneke H, Bruder O, et al. Late enhancement: A new feature in MRI of arrhythmogenic right ventricular cardiomyopathy? J Cardiovasc Magn Reson 2005;7(4):649–55.

87. Amadu AM, Baritussio A, Dastidar AG, et al. Arrhythmogenic right ventricular cardiomyopathy (ARVC) mimics: the knot unravelled by cardiovascular MRI. Clin Radiol 2019;74(3):228–34.

88. Brun F, Groeneweg JA, Gear K, et al. Risk stratification in arrhythmic right ventricular cardiomyopathy

without implantable cardioverter-defibrillators. JACC Clin Electrophysiol 2016;2(5):558–64.

89. Te Riele ASJM, Bhonsale A, James CA, et al. Incremental value of cardiac magnetic resonance imaging in arrhythmic risk stratification of arrhythmogenic right ventricular dysplasia/cardiomyopathy- associated desmosomal mutation carriers. J Am Coll Cardiol 2013;62(19):1761–9.

90. Yamashita S, Sacher F, Mahida S, et al. Image integration to guide catheter ablation in scar-related ventricular tachycardia. J Cardiovasc Electrophysiol 2016;27(6):699–708.

91. Muchtar E, Blauwet LA, Gertz MA. Restrictive cardiomyopathy: genetics, pathogenesis, clinical manifestations, diagnosis, and therapy. Circ Res 2017; 121(7):819–37.

92. Habib G, Bucciarelli-Ducci C, Caforio ALP, et al. Multimodality imaging in restrictive cardiomyopathies: An EACVI expert consensus document in collaboration with the "Working Group on myocardial and pericardial diseases" of the European Society of Cardiology endorsed by The Indian Academy of Echocardiography. Eur Heart J Cardiovasc Imaging 2017;18(10):1090–1.

93. Petersen SE, Selvanayagam JB, Wiesmann F, et al. Left ventricular non-compaction: Insights from cardiovascular magnetic resonance imaging. J Am Coll Cardiol 2005;46(1):101–5.

94. Stacey RB, Andersen MM, St. Clair M, et al. Comparison of systolic and diastolic criteria for isolated LV noncompaction in CMR. JACC Cardiovasc Imaging 2013;6(9):931–40.

95. Jacquier A, Thuny F, Jop B, et al. Measurement of trabeculated left ventricular mass using cardiac magnetic resonance imaging in the diagnosis of left ventricular non-compaction. Eur Heart J 2010; 31(9):1098–104.

96. Captur G, Muthurangu V, Cook C, et al. Quantification of left ventricular trabeculae using fractal analysis. J Cardiovasc Magn Reson 2013;15(1):1.

97. Ross SB, Jones K, Blanch B, et al. A systematic review and meta-analysis of the prevalence of left ventricular non-compaction in adults. Eur Heart J 2020; 41(14):1428–1436b.

98. Grigoratos C, Barison A, Ivanov A, et al. Meta-analysis of the prognostic role of late gadolinium enhancement and global systolic impairment in left ventricular noncompaction. JACC Cardiovasc Imaging 2019;12(11P1):2141–51.

99. Aung N, Doimo S, Ricci F, et al. Prognostic significance of left ventricular noncompaction: Systematic review and meta-analysis of observational studies. Circ Cardiovasc Imaging 2020;1–14. https://doi.org/10.1161/CIRCIMAGING.119.009712.

Role of Cardiovascular Magnetic Resonance in Ischemic Cardiomyopathy

Aneesh S. Dhore-Patil, MD[a], Ashish Aneja, MD, FSCMR[b],*

KEYWORDS

- Cardiac magnetic resonance • Ischemic cardiomyopathy • Stress CMR • Microvascular obstruction
- Viability

KEY POINTS

- Cardiac magnetic resonance (CMR) is integral to comprehensive cardiac structural and functional assessment.
- Stress CMR is a reliable and highly accurate method for the noninvasive assessment of coronary artery disease.
- Late gadolinium enhancement CMR has revolutionized the assessment of myocardial infarction (MI) using CMR.
- Microvascular obstruction and intramyocardial hemorrhage may hold the key for improved risk stratification in MI.
- Viability assessment using CMR is critical in the determining the utility of revascularization in ischemic cardiomyopathy patients.

INTRODUCTION

Ischemic heart disease is the most common cause of cardiovascular morbidity and mortality. Although echocardiography is the backbone of cardiovascular imaging, cardiac magnetic resonance (CMR) is integral to comprehensive cardiac structural and functional assessment. At the various stages of ischemic heart disease, CMR can accurately quantify infarct acuity, size, and complications; guide therapy; and prognosticate recovery. Many cardiologists consider CMR a noninvasive biopsy, using a combination of legacy and emerging techniques, validated by invasive biopsy data.

ROLE OF CARDIAC MAGNETIC RESONANCE FOR THE DIAGNOSIS OF ISCHEMIC HEART DISEASE

Stress CMR is highly sensitive and specific to evaluate for coronary artery disease (CAD). The primary technique consists of stress testing (with various stressor agents) and assessment of myocardial viability by delayed gadolinium enhancement or late gadolinium enhancement (LGE) imaging.

Stress Cardiac Magnetic Resonance

Stress CMR has been used since 1987[1] to diagnose myocardial ischemia,[2] quantify myocardial contractile reserve,[3] and identify patients at risk

[a] Tulane University Heart and Vascular Center, Tulane University, 1415 Tulane Avenue, New Orleans, LA 70112, USA; [b] Department of Cardiovascular Diseases, Case Western Reserve University, MetroHealth Medical Center, 2500 MetroHealth Drive, Cleveland, OH 44109, USA
* Corresponding author.
E-mail address: aaneja@metrohealth.org

Heart Failure Clin 17 (2021) 41–56
https://doi.org/10.1016/j.hfc.2020.08.005
1551-7136/21/© 2020 Elsevier Inc. All rights reserved.

for adverse cardiovascular outcomes.[4] Stress CMR relies on the principle of detecting wall motion abnormalities (WMAs) provoked by a primary stress agent (dobutamine) and the single-photon emission computed tomography (SPECT) principle of detecting perfusion defects with administration of a vasodilator (adenosine/regadenoson or dipyridamole). Dobutamine stress CMR (DS-CMR) has higher sensitivity and specificity compared with dobutamine stress echocardiography (DS-E) because of independence from acoustic windows and availability of viability data.[5] Vasodilator CMR imaging is associated with higher sensitivity but lower specificity.[6] Exercise CMR stress testing (with a bicycle ergometer or treadmill) has limited availability in clinical practice because of complex logistics resulting from the powerful magnetic field. Techniques, such as tissue tagging and feature tracking, may improve the sensitivity and specificity but not employed widely in clinical practice.[7–10]

Dobutamine stress cardiac magnetic resonance

DS-CMR compared with DS-E has a higher sensitivity (86% vs 74%, respectively), specificity (86% vs 70%, respectively), and accuracy (86% vs 73%, respectively).[7] As discussed previously, this is the result of superior spatial resolution and endocardial border delineation. Stress echocardiography also is less reliable in patients with baseline WMAs from prior myocardial infarction(s) (MI[s]). In a study of 160 patients, Wahl and colleagues[11] showed that DS-CMR had a sensitivity of 89% and specificity of 84% at detecting greater than 50% coronary artery luminal narrowing. In the same study, the sensitivities of showing luminal narrowing of 1 or 2 or 3 epicardial arteries were 87%, 91%, and 100%, respectively. Furthermore, universal adoption of balanced steady-state free precession as the standard protocol for rest and stress cine imaging has reduced scan times and increased sensitivity (89%) when compared with previous protocols.[12]

Safety of dobutamine stress cardiac magnetic resonance Patient discomfort and a legitimate concern for adverse events associated with dobutamine and atropine have stymied widespread use of DS-CMR. Because ST segment changes are uninterpretable in the magnetic field, reliance is placed on real-time cine imaging. This is acceptable because WMAs with stress generally precede ST segment changes. Patient comfort issues notwithstanding, in a 1000-patient DS-CMR study, Wahl and colleagues[11] showed a safety profile comparable to DS-E. In this study, 54% patients needed atropine, 64% had minor events,

6% had major events, and only 1 patient had sustained ventricular tachycardia requiring defibrillation. There were no deaths or MIs.

Vasodilator perfusion cardiac magnetic resonance

Vasodilator perfusion CMR can be performed using either adenosine, dipyridamole, or regadenoson as the stressor agent (**Fig. 1**). After injection of the vasodilator, gadolinium (Gd) is used as the first-pass perfusion (FFP) agent. Areas of prior infarction and ischemia have a slower rate of contrast uptake due to absent or decreased myocardial blood flow. Vasodilator imaging has 2 unique advantages over inotropes, such as dobutamine: first, perfusion defects tend to develop before WMAs, and, second, the protocol is significantly shorter, leading to improved accuracy of image capture (3–6 minutes for infusion and 1 minute for imaging). Vasodilator CMR has been validated by numerous studies.[13–16] It has a higher sensitivity (93% vs 82%, respectively) and lower specificity (66% vs 96%, respectively) compared head to head with DS-CMR.[6] The lower specificity of perfusion testing may result from a hypointense artifact (Gibbs ringing artifact), which appears along the myocardial blood-pool interface imitating a subendocardial perfusion defect. Using a 3T magnet can lower contrast dose and the false-positive rate. Image quality, however, with 3T is adversely affected by a nonhomogeneous magnetic field. A quantitative approach to perfusion imaging also improves accuracy.[17–21]

The CE-MARC and MR-INFORM trials

Accurate risk stratification and determining appropriateness of revascularization in patients with cardiac chest pain remain in evolution. Traditionally, coronary angiography has fulfilled this role and emerged as the gold standard by adopting fractional flow reserve (FFR) measurements. Imaging modalities, such as SPECT perfusion and computed tomography (CT) angiography without and with noninvasively derived FFR, are being used to make revascularization decisions but have significant limitations. The CE-MARC[17] was a landmark trial that compared a combination of adenosine stress CMR, cine CMR, LGE, and magnetic resonance angiography to SPECT using coronary angiography as the gold standard. In the 752 patients, CMR had a statistically significant higher sensitivity (86.5% vs 66.5%, respectively) and negative predictive value (90.5% vs 79.1%, respectively) compared with SPECT. Specificity (83.4% vs 82.6%, respectively) and positive predictive value (77.2% vs 71.4%, respectively), although not significant, were higher in the CMR

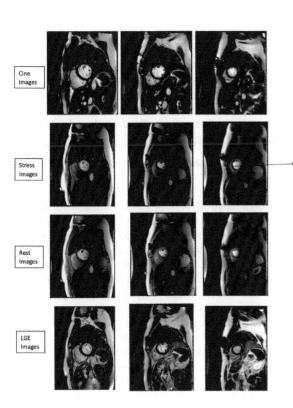

Fig. 1. Vasodilator perfusion CMR showing from top to bottom cines, stress perfusion, rest perfusion, and LGE imaging with ischemia in the left anterior descending territory.

group versus the SPECT group. This trial helped establish the utility of CMR in a large clinical setting. In a subsequent cost-effectiveness analysis, the combination of stress testing and CMR was more cost effective than exercise testing with SPECT.[22,23] Emerging clinical trial data with vasodilator CMR are showing a high concordance with FFR. This was evaluated in the MR-INFORM trial, which compared adenosine CMR to invasive FFR. Index revascularization occurred in 35.7% of the CMR group and 45% of the FFR group, a highly statistically significant difference ($P = .005$). The primary outcome of death, nonfatal MI or target vessel revascularization, and number of patients free of angina at 12 months were similar in both groups.

The CE-MARC2,[24] in follow-up to CE-MARC, investigated the utility of stress CMR for coronary angiography utilization. The 1202 patients recruited were randomized to standard of care, CMR stress, and stress myocardial perfusion imaging (MPI) arms (240:481:481). The results demonstrated that unnecessary angiography was performed in 28.8% of the standard-of-care arm versus 7.5% in CMR and 7.1% in the MPI arms, respectively. The occurrence of major adverse cardiovascular events (MACEs) at 12 months was similar in the 3 arms (1.7% vs 2.5% vs

2.5%, respectively). The investigators concluded stress CMR led to a lower probability of unnecessary testing than standard of care and was equally as effective as MPI. There are no large head-to-head trials comparing quantitative stress CMR with other modalities, but preliminary data are encouraging.[25]

ROLE OF CARDIAC MAGNETIC RESONANCE IN MYOCARDIAL INFARCTION

CMR is an underutilized imaging modality in the evaluation of acute MI (AMI). Delayed gadolinium enhancement or LGE is the gold standard for detecting scar ischemic and nonischemic scar resulting from prior injury and provides valuable prognostic information. The relatively novel parametric mapping techniques, such as T1, T2, T2*, and extracellular volume fraction estimation, can supplement diagnostic and prognostic data obtained from LGE imaging. The presence of microvascular obstruction (MVO) after a MI is detected most accurately and reliably by LGE CMR and intramyocardial hemorrhage (IMH) with T2* imaging. Finally, CMR is the gold standard technique to diagnose and quantify complications of AMI, such as left ventricular (LV) thrombus, LV dysfunction, aneurysm, pseudoaneurysm, ventricular septal defect formation, and valvular complications.

Cardiac Magnetic Resonance for the Detection of Acute Coronary Syndromes and Acute Myocardial Infarction

Cine CMR is a powerful tool to assess regional WMAs with great accuracy because of excellent spatial and temporal resolution. Even in the urgent setting of ACS, cine CMR within 6 hours of presentation can detect a non–ST elevation MI (NSTEMI) with 89% and ischemic heart disease with 98% sensitivity.[26] When combined with LGE, the sensitivity for AMI detection is increased to 100%.

Late Gd imaging is the gold standard for detecting myocardial scar. It has been validated by multiple animal studies by comparing to histopathology,[27] through clinical trials comparing the size of infarction with biomarker elevation,[28–30] extent of transmural infarction and recovery of ventricular function,[28,29,31–33] and finally for viability imaging in patients undergoing revascularization.[34] It is important to understand the mechanism of Gd uptake and hyperenhancement in AMI. After intravenous administration, Gd-based agents rapidly enter the interstitium in-between cardiac myocytes but not across an intact cell membrane. This leads to significant T1 shortening in areas of contrast uptake, leading to increased signal. In noninfarcted myocardium, which consists of myocardial cells with intact cell membranes, Gd-based agents are excluded from the intracellular space. Hence, these intracellular spaces have a longer T1 and appear dark. Using Look-Locker or scout sequences, which rely on inversion recovery methods,[35] the correct inversion time can be determined to null the normal myocardium, which appears dark on LGE images. In cases of damaged tissue or infarcted myocardium, the loss of cell membrane integrity leads to intracellular infiltration of the Gd agents leading to a high-signal or hyperenhancement in both extracellular and intracellular spaces in the setting of a properly nulled myocardium. Intense LGE in the area of infarction also is seen in chronic infarcts.[36–38] Tissue in chronic infarcts is composed mainly of fibroblasts and collagen fibrils with large intracellular spaces. This allows for easy diffusion of Gd agents in comparison to normal myocardium, which is tightly packed. A sufficient time delay should be used when LGE images are acquired, such that the blood pool signal intensity is lower than the brighter subendocardial infarcted myocardium, allowing for reliable differentiation between these layers. Late Gd imaging also is more sensitive for AMI compared with SPECT. In AMI, CMR can detect small infarcts, such as those with lower troponin elevations or infarcts in the circumflex territory, significantly better than SPECT,[39–42] making CMR especially valuable for the evaluation of MI with normal coronary arteries. In addition, the significantly better spatial resolution markedly improves the ability to detect subendocardial infarcts.[40]

T1 and T2 imaging for acute myocardial infarction

Using T1 and T2 imaging it is possible to create quantitative pixel-wise maps of the myocardium with embedded information.[43] The application of these maps in AMI has made it possible to differentiate infarcted, salvaged, and remote myocardium. T1 mapping refers to pixel-wise measurement of absolute T1 relaxation times on a quantitative map.[44] Myocardial edema, which is an early consequence of myocardial necrosis, can be seen on T1 maps as prolonged relaxation times.[45] T1 mapping can detect myocardial edema as it develops within minutes of coronary occlusion and resolves weeks or months after the MI. This has been studied with native T1 showing a high sensitivity (96%) and specificity (91%) at detecting AMI.[44,46] This can be used in both ST elevation MI (STEMI) and NSTEMI, in patients with smaller infarcts.[46]

T2-weighted imaging is highly sensitive in detecting myocardial edema/inflammation.[47] Using rapid pulse sequences, T2-weighted spin-echo images can be used to differentiate between edematous and normal myocardium[48] (**Fig. 2**). T2 maps also can be used to characterize area at risk. Originally done using dark-blood imaging,[49] bright blood methods have improved its diagnostic reliability[50,51] and can detect IMH[52] as well.

T1 and T2 mapping techniques are improving rapidly. Both have had advancements in motion correction methods that eliminate the need for breath holds.[53,54] They have been validated for area at risk imaging against reference standards of microspheres,[55] fluorescent dyes, and CT perfusion images[56,57] and are expected to become routine parts of clinical CMR imaging.

Microvascular Obstruction After Myocardial Infarction

Restoration of blood flow after prolonged occlusion may result in MVO and its related no-reflow phenomenon, important in determining the morbidity and ventricular function recovery after an AMI. Regions of no-reflow or MVO can be imaged by angiography, SPECT, PET, and echocardiography (with ultrasound-enhancing agents) but are best evaluated by CMR (**Fig. 3**). It has

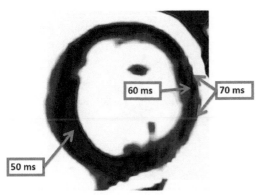

Fig. 2. T2 maps demonstrating lower relaxation times in areas of myocardial edema/infarction (60–70 ms) compared with the normal of approximately 50 ms in the septum.

been posited that initial ischemic injury leads to endothelial damage at the capillary level leading to extravasation of red blood cells (RBCs) into the extravascular space surrounding the myocardium. Free radical injury from iron in the RBCs leads to myocardial damage and capillary plugging with necrotic endothelium and RBC stasis leads to no reperfusion to the core of the infarct despite restoration of epicardial blood flow.[58] Actually, the damage is compounded by revascularization, which leads to reperfusion injury from oxygen free radicals. These regions of MVO or

no reflow can be imaged by CMR using FFP and LGE imaging. FFP imaging (FPP-CMR)[59–61] involves dynamic imaging of multiple imaging planes after an intravenous contrast bolus. On FPP-CMR, areas of MVO are hypoenhanced, which persists for greater than 2 minutes compared with increased signal intensity in normal and infarcted myocardium. With LGE-CMR,[62,63] although infarcted myocardium appears hyperenhanced, regions of MVO are hypoenhanced within the hyperenhanced regions. Early Gd enhancement imaging, obtained within 2 minutes to 5 minutes of Gd injection at a high inversion time (approximately 500 ms), identifies a larger area of MVO than LGE. Thus, early MVO (EMVO) imaging is sensitive and late MVO (LMVO) specific for no-reflow. Upon comparison, FPP-CMR appears more sensitive[62] for the detection of MVO and correlates better with histopathologic analysis.[64] LGE-CMR tends to underestimate the extent of MVO and may miss smaller regions due to slower penetration of contrast.[42] The presence of MVO has been shown on multiple occasions to portend poor cardiovascular outcomes. Initial studies revealed that EMVO predicts transmurality of infarcts and ventricular remodeling and is an independent prognostic marker for the occurrence of MACEs.[59] Initial studies indicated that EMVO played a greater role in predicting worse outcomes following STEMI[59] but a meta-analysis suggested that both early and LMVO predict poor

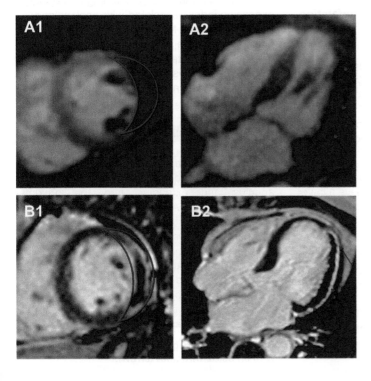

Fig. 3. Cine and LGE images showing MVO in the circumflex territory. (A1) cine short axis view; (A2) cine horizontal axis view; (B1) LGE short axis view; and (B2) LGE horizontal axis view. *Crescents* and *arrows* pointing towards areas of MVO.

outcomes.[65] LMVO appears to indicate a greater risk with an increased odds ratio (4.3 vs 2.6, respectively) compared with EMVO.[65] This may be due to higher specificity for no-reflow zones or the identification of IMH, which represents more significant injury.

Intramyocardial hemorrhage

A longer duration of ischemia leads to more extensive endothelial necrosis, which can lead to IMH. IMH is observed in areas of no reflow and requires T2*-weighted imaging (**Fig. 4**) because contrast-enhanced CMR cannot differentiate between MVO and IMH.[66–68] Evidence suggests that IMH's association with MACE results from a larger infarct size, smaller salvage index, larger ventricular volumes, and lower LVEF.[65] Eitel and colleagues[69] in a study of 346 patients (122 with IMH) explored the relationship of IMH and LMVO with MACE in STEMI patients with reperfusion within 12 hours. On multivariate analysis, IMH was determined to be an independent predictor of MACE 6 months post-AMI (HR 2.04) whereas LMVO was not.[70] Another recent study evaluated IMH and its relationship with MACE in 264 patients and found similar results on multivariate analysis (HR 2.7), with IMH better than MVO for predicting MACE.[70] Studies also have demonstrated iron deposits in the regions of IMH, which could explain their pathogenesis and point toward a potential target for therapy.[71,72] Further studies are needed to explore IMH and its role in AMI.

Complications of Acute Myocardial Infarction

Formation of an LV thrombus is a relatively common and morbid complication. CMR is the gold standard for imaging LV thrombi (**Fig. 5**). LGE-CMR has significantly higher sensitivity then transthoracic echocardiography (TTE) and transesophageal echocardiography (TEE) (88% vs 23% [TTE] and 40% [TEE]) and equal specificity (96% all) in patients with ischemic cardiomyopathy.[73–75] Contrast-aided echocardiography improves the sensitivity and accuracy of TTE (61% vs 33%, respectively, and 92% vs 82%, respectively) but still misses a substantial number of thrombi.[76] Given the lower cost and convenience, TTE is preferred, but CMR is highly reliable for confirmation.

The mechanical complications of AMI have become less frequent but remain associated with high morbidity and mortality.[77] The most frequent mechanical complications include ventricular aneurysm (**Fig. 6**), pseudoaneurysm (**Fig. 7**), free wall rupture, infarct-related ventricular septal defects, and papillary muscle rupture with associated mitral regurgitation.

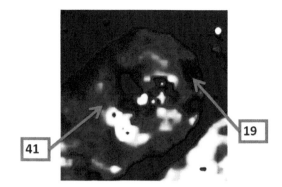

Fig. 4. T2* map indicating low signal intensity in areas of iron deposition from IMH.

Role of Cardiac Magnetic Resonance in Evaluating Therapies for Ischemic Cardiomyopathy

The focus of management for MI always has been reduction in hard clinical endpoints, such as cardiac death and development of heart failure.[78] Before large-scale interventions can be undertaken, however, smaller proof of concept studies with surrogate endpoints are performed to gauge treatment efficacy. Because CMR allows detection of small areas of myocardial injury reproducibly and accurately, it can significantly reduce the investigational sample size.[79–81] These advantages have helped CMR shape therapies. In 1995, Schulman and colleagues[82] were able to show reduced infarct segment length and infarct expansion index associated with enalaprilat therapy 1 month post-MI utilizing CMR. Johnson and colleagues[83] were able to use CMR to assess the effect of angiotensin-converting enzyme inhibitor therapy on post-MI LV mass in patients with LVEF greater than 40%. The ramipril arm (43

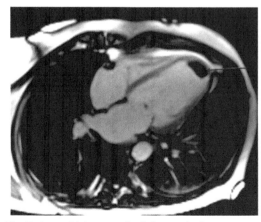

Fig. 5. Long T1 image of a left ventricular aneurysm with an apical thrombus (*arrow*).

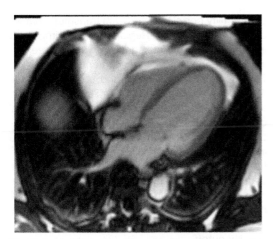

Fig. 6. Long T1 image of an apical aneurysm.

patients) was associated with a decrease in LV mass with no change in the control group (35 patients). β-Blocker therapy also has been studied using CMR. The METOCARD-CINC trial (270 patients)[84] was able to a show a smaller infarct size and improved LVEF in the active treatment arm compared with placebo. In MERIT-HF[85] (41 patients), metoprolol succinate was able to show a significant decrease in LV volumes and an increase in LVEF in patients with chronic heart failure with no change in the placebo group. In the CHRISTMAS trial,[86] a double-blind trial with 34 participants utilizing CMR, carvedilol therapy led to significant reduction in ventricular volumes and improved function in chronic systolic heart failure patients.

VIABILITY

Myocardial viability is defined as the presence alive cardiomyocytes in an area of myocardial

ischemia or underperfusion.[87] These cardiomyocytes show severe dysfunction at baseline but have the potential to recover myocardial function.[88,89]

Using Cardiac Magnetic Resonance to Assess Myocardial Viability

When using CMR for viability testing, a systematic approach is needed. This begins with characterizing cardiac shape, size, wall thickness, estimation of chamber volumes, and myocardial mass.

Transmural scar identification by cine cardiac magnetic resonance

Cine CMR is well established for assessing LV contractility. Severe wall thinning, often seen with long-standing transmural infarcts is suggestive of nonviability. On the contrary, the presence of normal wall thickness in diastole with known infarction may suggest the presence of viable myocardium. Because ventricular remodeling could take up to 4 months, however, preserved wall thickness at end diastole cannot be used as a marker of viability in infarcts less than 4 months old. This was studied by Baer and colleagues,[90] when they compared CMR findings to PET and SPECT in identical myocardial regions. An end-diastolic wall thickness of 5.5 mm was used to define transmural scar because it corresponded well with histopathologic studies of transmural scars.[91] They found that areas with mean wall thickness less than 5.5 mm had significantly reduced uptake of fluorodeoxyglucose (FDG). In 83% of the patients, the diagnosis of viability based on FDG-PET and CMR was identical. Another study tested patients who underwent CMR 3 months after revascularization versus controls.[92] In 43 patients, 9.6% segments with wall thickness of less than 5.5 mm improved with

Fig. 7. Late Gd enhancement images with an inferior pseudoaneurysm with a thrombus.

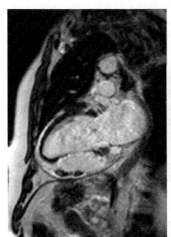
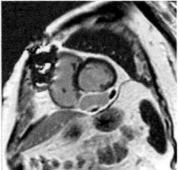

revascularization (90% negative predictive value). In segments with wall thickness exceeding 5.5 mm, 62.4% segments with preserved wall thickness (>5.5 mm) improved (62% positive predictive value). Ejection fraction (EF) increased significantly in patients with dobutamine-induced systolic wall thickening greater than 2 mm versus those graded as having predominantly scar (14% ± 9% vs 3% ± 10%, respectively; P<.0003). Measurement of myocardial thickness is important but may be insufficient in predicting viability. In a large observational study, Shah and colleagues[93] observed that even regions less than 5.5 mm in thickness and no scar and LGE could recover contractile function after revascularization. The number of such segments in this study, however, was relatively small.

Dobutamine stress cardiac magnetic resonance

Functional cine dobutamine magnetic resonance is an option for viability assessment. DS-CMR works on the basic principle of myocardial responsiveness to sympathomimetic agents. For this purpose, improvement in myocardial contractility in previously infarcted or hypokinetic hibernating myocardial segments with low-dose dobutamine infusion suggests potential for functional recovery with revascularization.[94] This technique is not clinically popular, however, because LGE imaging is highly accurate without the need for initiating an infusion and cardiac monitoring.

Late gadolinium enhancement imaging

LGE imaging is the current gold standard for detecting myocardial scar as well as MVO and no reflow. The distinct advantage of LGE CMR lies in its ability to distinguish between transmural and nontransmural scar, which generally is not possible with SPECT, PET, or echocardiography. Observing the extent of the scar and its location also helps differentiate ischemic cardiomyopathy from nonischemic cardiomyopathy.[38]

Prediction of myocardial response to revascularization remains the ultimate goal of viability testing, which was been studied with LGE CMR. An initial study by Kim and colleagues[34] demonstrated an inverse relationship between transmural extent of infarction and functional recovery after revascularization. A study by Selvanayagam and colleagues[30] further strengthened the relationship between transmural extent of infarction and predicting response to revascularization. In their 52-patient study involving patients undergoing multivessel coronary artery bypass graft (CABG), they performed preoperative (day 6) and postoperative CMR (6 months) for comparison. In the segments with hyperenhancement on LGE, recovery of contractility correlated well with transmural nature of the infarct (P<.001). Regional function improved in the vast majority of segments with no preexisting hyperenhancement. In segments with 51% to 75% scar, 25% recovered and only a miniscule 4% recovered with greater than 76% scar. Importantly, the degree of preoperative segmental dysfunction did not influence the relationship between the transmural extent of scar and the improvement in function. Pegg and colleagues[95] then performed a secondary analysis on these same patients and found that the 21/33 patients who had an EF improvement greater than 3% had greater than or equal to 10/16 viable or normal segments as defined by less than 50% transmural viability cutoff.

Patients with severely reduced EF are the most challenging because surgical risk is formidable. Gerber and colleagues[96] investigated this in a study that extended the findings of Kim and colleagues[34] (EF 43% ± 13%) and Selvanayagam and colleagues[30] (EF 62% ± 12%) to patients with lower EFs (EF 24% ± 7%). This study was nonrandomized, and all patients underwent LGE CMR. Of the 144 patients included, 86 underwent complete revascularization (92% CABG) and 58 received medical therapy. At 3 years of follow-up, the medical therapy group with viable segments had a significantly higher mortality compared with those with nonviable segments (survival 48% vs 77%, respectively; P 0.02). Conversely, in the revascularization group, viable segments were not associated with a statistically significant improvement in survival. When patients with viable segments in the revascularized group were compared with the medical therapy group, medical therapy alone was associated with hazard ratio of 4.56 for death. Thus, the investigators concluded that the presence of dysfunctional viable myocardium (detected by LGE CMR) without revascularization was an independent predictor of mortality in ischemic cardiomyopathy. These findings strengthened findings from a prior metanalysis,[97] which suggests that patients with viability testing prior to revascularization could result in a significant improvement in mortality compared with medical therapy alone. Patients without viability had intermediate mortality regardless of revascularization.

Cardiac magnetic resonance compared with other imaging modalities for viability testing

Despite the evidence, viability testing–guided revascularization is controversial. Modalities currently used namely SPECT, LV angiography, PET, echocardiography, and finally CMR have highly variable predictive values (**Table 1**). A

Table 1
Various modalities for viability testing

Testing Modality	Assessment of Viability	Sensitivity (%)	Specificity (%)	Positive Predictive Value (%)	Negative Predictive Value (%)	Advantages	Disadvantages
CMR	Contractile reserve	84	63	72	78	• Best spatial resolution • No radiation exposure • Best scar quantification	• Avoid in eGFR <30 mL/kg/min[a] • Avoid in cardiac devices[b] • Not widely available • Body habitus
SPECT thallium	Sarcolemmal integrity	87	54	67	79	• Cost • Widely available	• Highest radiation exposure • Low spatial resolution
SPECT technetium	Mitochondrial membrane integrity	83	65	74	76	• Cost • Widely available	• Radiation exposure • Low spatial resolution
PET	Cellular glucose uptake capacity	93	63	74	87	• Highest sensitivity	• Radiation exposure • Better than SPECT but inferior to CMR for spatial resolution
Dobutamine echocardiography	Contractile reserve	80	78	75	83	• Cost • Widely available • No radiation exposure	• Limited by acoustic windows • High interobserver variability

[a] Relative contraindication.
[b] Acceptable in magnetic resonance conditional devices.

systematic comparison of these modalities requires clarification of the contextual definitions of sensitivity and specificity. Sensitivity is the ability of an imaging modality to accurately identify viable/healthy myocardium whereas specificity is the ability to characterize myocardial scar. Prior studies have validated the use of CMR for viability testing by comparing it with SPECT thallium[98] and with FDG-PET.[99] In summary, CMR is superior with significantly higher spatial resolution and accurate resolution of transmural and subendocardial scar.

Surgical treatment for ischemic heart failure trial

Prediction of LV recovery after revascularization requires a careful risk benefit analysis balancing procedure risk and potential surgical benefit versus excellent medical therapy. The Surgical Treatment for Ischemic Heart Failure[100] was a unique trial geared toward testing the role of revascularization (CABG) in the management of ischemic cardiomyopathy. A substudy of the original trial explored the relationship of viability testing with revascularization. Of the 1212 patients enrolled, 601 patients underwent viability testing. Of these, 298 patients received CABG plus medical therapy and 303 received medical therapy. During the median follow-up of 5.1 years, patients with viable myocardium experienced a 37% mortality whereas those with nonviable myocardium, 41%. On univariate analysis, patients with viable myocardium had a HR of 0.64 ($P = .003$) for death but this association no longer was significant after adjustment. The trial was a landmark in assessing medical therapy versus CABG plus medical therapy but was for the following reasons. First, patients selected to undergo viability testing were not chosen randomly. Moreover, viability status was not assigned randomly between treatment groups, leading to significant differences in the baseline characteristics of patients. Second, SPECT and dobutamine echocardiogram were used to assess viability. Although SPECT and dobutamine stress echocardiogram are similar in performance, they are insensitive techniques. Third, on reanalysis, more than 20% of the patients had an EF greater than 35%—a higher EF may reduce the benefit of revascularization. Finally, even in the patients undergoing revascularization, the completeness of revascularization was uncertain. Retrospectively speaking, it not clear whether PET or CMR use would have altered STICH trial results. In addition, advancements in medical therapy may have blunted viability-based revascularization benefit. This is evident from the lower mortality in the medical therapy arms of

the STICH trial compared with a prior metanalysis.[97] Hence, the results of the trial should be interpreted cautiously and the decision to revascularize contingent on variables, such as EF, complexity of coronary anatomy, age, comorbidities, and viability status.[101]

FUTURE DIRECTIONS—NONCONTRAST CARDIAC MAGNETIC RESONANCE TECHNOLOGIES
Blood Oxygen Level–Dependent Imaging

Blood oxygen level–dependent (BOLD) CMR relies on the paramagnetic properties of deoxyhemoglobin as an endogenous contrast agent. Increasing deoxyhemoglobin content of tissue leads to signal reduction on T2* or T2 images. Hence, BOLD CMR can be used to determine myocardial oxygenation.[102,103] Successful demonstrations of the efficacy of BOLD in animal studies led to extensive studies in the ischemic heart disease.[104–107] Manka and colleagues,[108] in a 46-patient study, were able to demonstrate the feasibility of BOLD CMR with 3T in patients who underwent a clinically indicated coronary angiography after BOLD CMR. In the 23 patients who had significant CAD, BOLD CMR at rest revealed significantly lower T2* signal for ischemic segments compared with normal and nonischemic segments. After adenosine stress, T2* signal increased significantly in normal segments. Another study by Arnold and colleagues[109] compared BOLD imaging to coronary angiography in a prospective study involving 60 patients with and without known CAD and found that BOLD imaging had an accuracy of 84%, a sensitivity of 92% and a specificity of 72% for detecting myocardial ischemia. The two-dimensional cardiac phase–resolved BOLD CMR (CP-BOLD CMR) was a 9-patient feasibility study.[110] When compared with thallium SPECT, CP-BOLD CMR performed well at detecting significant differences between stress and rest images in healthy, mildly involved, and severely involved coronary segments ($P<.05$). More recently, it was studied in 37 patients with CAD with FFR measurement.[111] This study showed that in patients with FFR less than 0.8, the sensitivity and specificity for detecting a perfusion defect were 86% and 92%, respectively. Improved visualization can be achieved by strategies to overcome flow/motion artifacts, but these still need to be studied in a clinical setting.[112,113]

BOLD imaging has the potential of being able to quantify myocardial oxygenation without the need for contrast use. Quantifying myocardial oxygenation would help risk-stratify all patients with CAD specifically those with balanced ischemia secondary to multivessel CAD. Improvements in technique and adoption of recent advances of CMR could help establish BOLD CMR as a safe alternative in the early detection and monitoring of ischemic heart disease.

Spectroscopy

Magnetic resonance spectroscopy can be used as well to detect viability. Adenosine triphosphate (ATP) is critical to cardiomyocyte function. After severe ischemic injury, ATP, myocardial creatine, and phosphocreatine are depleted rapidly. [114] ^{31}P magnetic resonance can be used to measure the amount of phosphocreatine and ATP in cardiomyocytes. [114] In viable myocardium, the absolute concentration of ATP is relatively normal compared with reduced concentrations in nonviable/scar myocardium. Although attractive, spectroscopy is not used clinically, given a high dependence on operator skill and inadequate spatial and temporal resolution. With improvement in techniques and technology, this imaging modality has promise to enter clinical practice due to high diagnostic accuracy. [115]

T1 rho Imaging

Magnetic resonance imaging using spin locking radiofrequency pulses (T1 rho) has become of interest in the visualization of ischemic heart disease. The spin-locking sequences radiofrequency pulse increases the sensitivity for low-frequency interactions between macromolecules (amines, amides, and hydroxyl groups) and water, which helps obtain important molecular information from diseased myocardium without the use of contrast. Like T1 and T2-weighted imaging, T1 rho also relies on signal enhancement due to myocardial edema in AMI. Infarcted myocardium has a stronger signal intensity than normal myocardium, which correlates well with LGE. [116] In preclinical studies with a swine model, T1 rho was comparable to LGE for chronic myocardial scar. [117]

Overall, T1 rho is promising noncontrast modality for characterization of the myocardium. Advancements in technique, such as correction of field heterogeneity and incorporation of parallel imaging, will improve the modality and allow for wider application after appropriate clinical validation.

SUMMARY AND FUTURE DIRECTIONS

CMR imaging provides a highly accurate, robust, and noninvasive modality for the evaluation of ischemic heart disease. It improves on other noninvasive modalities, such as echocardiography, SPECT, and PET, in the detection, assessment, and long-term prognostication of ischemic heart disease. The superior accuracy of CMR has proved to be pivotal in research and its incorporation in clinical trials allows for smaller patient samples without the sacrifice of power needed to demonstrate clinical effect. With emerging data linking phenomenon, such as MVO and IMH, to clinical outcomes, LGE CMR may improve risk stratification of patients with AMI. Finally, timing of revascularization remains the holy grail of ischemic heart disease and viability assessment using CMR may be the missing link needed to help reduce morbidity and mortality associated with the disease. Furthermore, emerging advances in parametric mapping, BOLD, and spectroscopy may change the CMR landscape by effectively eliminating Gd-based contrast use.

DISCLOSURE

Dr. Aneja serves on Advisory Board of MyoKardia, Inc. Dr. Dhore-Patil has nothing to disclose.

REFERENCES

1. Sechtem U, Sommerhoff BA, Markiewicz W, et al. Regional left ventricular wall thickening by magnetic resonance imaging: evaluation in normal persons and patients with global and regional dysfunction. Am J Cardiol 1987;59(1):145–51, 2949575.
2. Pattynama PM, de Roos A. MR evaluation of myocardial ischemia and infarction. Top Magn Reson Imaging 1995;7(4):218–31, 8534493.
3. Dendale PA, Franken PR, Waldman GJ, et al. Low-dosage dobutamine magnetic resonance imaging as an alternative to echocardiography in the detection of viable myocardium after acute infarction. Am Heart J 1995;130(1):134–40, 7611103.
4. Jahnke C, Nagel E, Gebker R, et al. Prognostic value of cardiac magnetic resonance stress tests: adenosine stress perfusion and dobutamine stress wall motion imaging. Circulation 2007;115(13):1769–76, 17353441.
5. Nagel E, Lehmkuhl HB, Bocksch W, et al. Noninvasive diagnosis of ischemia-induced wall motion abnormalities with the use of high-dose dobutamine stress MRI: comparison with dobutamine stress echocardiography. Circulation 1999;99:763–70.
6. Pingitore A, Lombardi M, Scattini B, et al. Head to head comparison between perfusion and function during accelerated high-dose dipyridamole magnetic resonance stress for the detection of coronary artery disease. Am J Cardiol 2008;101(1):8–14, 18157957.

7. Ibrahim E. Myocardial tagging by Cardiovascular Magnetic Resonance: evolution of techniques–pulse sequences, analysis algorithms, and applications. J Cardiovasc Magn Reson 2011;13(1):36.

8. Rosen BD, Saad MF, Arnett DK, et al. Hypertension and smoking are associated with reduced regional left ventricular function in asymptomatic: individuals the Multi-Ethnic Study of Atherosclerosis. J Am Coll Cardiol 2006;47(6):1150–8.

9. Osman NF, Kerwin WS, McVeigh ER, et al. Cardiac motion tracking using CINE harmonic phase (HARP) magnetic resonance imaging. Magn Reson Med 1999;42(6):1048–60.

10. Korosoglou G, Lehrke S, Wochele A, et al. Strain-encoded CMR for the detection of inducible ischemia during intermediate stress. JACC Cardiovasc Imaging 2010;3(4):361–71, 20394897.

11. Wahl A, Paetsch I, Roethemeyer S, et al. High-dose dobutamine-atropine stress cardiovascular MR imaging after coronary revascularization in patients with wall motion abnormalities at rest. Radiology 2004;233(1):210–6, 15304662.

12. Paetsch I, Jahnke C, Wahl A, et al. Comparison of dobutamine stress magnetic resonance, adenosine stress magnetic resonance, and adenosine stress magnetic resonance perfusion. Circulation 2004;110(7):835–42, 15289384.

13. Pennell DJ, Underwood SR, Ell PJ, et al. Dipyridamole magnetic resonance imaging: a comparison with thallium-201 emission tomography. Br Heart J 1990;64(6):362–9, 2271342.

14. Hamon M, Fau G, Hamon M. Meta-analysis of the diagnostic performance of stress perfusion cardiovascular magnetic resonance for detection of coronary artery disease. J Cardiovasc Magn Reson 2010;12(1).

15. Heitner J, Kim R, Judd R. Prognostic Value of Vasodilator Stress Cardiac Magnetic Resonance Imaging. JAMA Cardiol 2019;4(3):256.

16. Wu H, Kwong R. Cardiac magnetic resonance imaging in patients with coronary disease. 2020.

17. Greenwood J, Maredia N, Younger J, et al. Cardiovascular magnetic resonance and single-photon emission computed tomography for diagnosis of coronary heart disease (CE-MARC): a prospective trial. Lancet 2012;379:453–60, 22196944.

18. Giang T, Nanz D, Coulden R, et al. Detection of coronary artery disease by magnetic resonance myocardial perfusion imaging with various contrast medium doses: first European multicenter experience. Eur Heart J 2004;25:1657–65, 15351166.

19. Wolff S, Schwitter J, Coulden R, et al. Myocardial first-pass perfusion magnetic resonance imaging: a multicenter dose-ranging study. Circulation 2004;110:732–7, 15289374.

20. Schwitter J, Wacker CM, van Rossum AC, et al. MR-IMPACT: magnetic resonance imaging for myocardial perfusion assessment in coronary artery disease trial: comparison of perfusion CMR with single photon emission computed tomography for the detection of coronary artery disease in a multicenter, multivendor, randomized trial. Eur Heart J 2008;29:480–9, 18208849.

21. Schwitter J, Wacker CM, Wilke N, et al. Superior diagnostic performance of perfusion-CMR versus SPECT to detect coronary artery disease: the secondary endpoints of the multicenter multivendor MR-IMPACT II. J Cardiovasc Magn Reson 2012;14:61–71, 22938651.

22. Walker S, Greenwood J, Sculpher M. Cost-effectiveness of cardiovascular magnetic resonance in the diagnosis of coronary heart disease: an economic evaluation using data from the CE-MARC study. Heart 2013;99(12):873–81.

23. Nagel E, Greenwood J, McCann G, et al. Magnetic Resonance Perfusion or Fractional Flow Reserve in Coronary Disease. N Engl J Med 2019;380(25):2418–28.

24. Greenwood J, Ripley D, Everett C, et al. Effect of Care Guided by Cardiovascular Magnetic Resonance, Myocardial Perfusion Scintigraphy, or NICE Guidelines on Subsequent Unnecessary Angiography Rates. JAMA 2016;316(10):1051.

25. Sammut EC, Villa ADM, Di Giovine G, et al. Prognostic Value of Quantitative Stress Perfusion Cardiac Magnetic Resonance. JACC Cardiovasc Imaging 2018;11(5):686–94.

26. Kwong RY, Schussheim AE, Rekhraj S, et al. Detecting acute coronary syndrome in the emergency department with cardiac magnetic resonance imaging. Circulation 2003;107:531–7, 12566362.

27. Kim RJ, Fieno DS, Parrish TB, et al. Relationship of MRI delayed contrast enhancement to irreversible injury, infarct age, and contractile function. Circulation 1999;100:1992–2002, 10556226.

28. Choi KM, Kim RJ, Gubernikoff G, et al. Transmural extent of acute myocardial infarction predicts long-term improvement in contractile function. Circulation 2001;104:1101–7, 11535563.

29. Ingkanisorn WP, Rhoads KL, Aletras AH, et al. Gadolinium delayed enhancement cardiovascular magnetic resonance correlates with clinical measures of myocardial infarction. J Am Coll Cardiol 2004;43:2253–9, 15193689.

30. Selvanayagam JB, Kardos A, Francis JM, et al. Value of delayed-enhancement cardiovascular magnetic resonance imaging in predicting myocardial viability after surgical revascularization. Circulation 2004;110:1535–41, 15353496.

31. Baks T, van Geuns RJ, Biagini E, et al. Recovery of left ventricular function after primary angioplasty for acute myocardial infarction. Eur Heart J 2005;26:1070–7, 15716283.

32. Beek AM, Kuhl HP, Bondarenko O, et al. Delayed contrast-enhanced magnetic resonance imaging

for the prediction of regional functional improvement after acute myocardial infarction. J Am Coll Cardiol 2003;42:895–901, 12957439.

33. Gerber BL, Garot J, Bluemke DA, et al. Accuracy of contrast-enhanced magnetic resonance imaging in predicting improvement of regional myocardial function in patients after acute myocardial infarction. Circulation 2002;106:1083–9, 12196333.

34. Kim RJ, Wu E, Rafael A, et al. The use of contrast-enhanced magnetic resonance imaging to identify reversible myocardial dysfunction. N Engl J Med 2000;343:1445–53, 11078769.

35. Simonetti OP, Kim RJ, Fieno DS, et al. An improved MR imaging technique for the visualization of myocardial infarction. Radiology 2001;218:215–23, 11152805.

36. Grover S, Srinivasan G, Selvanayagam JB. Evaluation of myocardial viability with cardiac magnetic resonance imaging. Prog Cardiovasc Dis 2011;54:204–14, 22014488.

37. Ramani K, Judd RM, Holly TA, et al. Contrast magnetic resonance imaging in the assessment of myocardial viability in patients with stable coronary artery disease and left ventricular dysfunction. Circulation 1998;98:26872694, 9851954.

38. Wu E, Judd RM, Vargas JD, et al. Visualisation of presence, location, and transmural extent of healed Q-wave and non-Q-wave myocardial infarction. Lancet 2001;357:21–8, 11197356.

39. Wagner A, Mahrholdt H, Holly TA, et al. Contrast-enhanced MRI and routine single photon emission computed tomography (SPECT) perfusion imaging for detection of subendocardial myocardial infarcts: an imaging study. Lancet 2003;361:374–9, 12573373.

40. Ibrahim T, Bulow HP, Hackl T, et al. Diagnostic value of contrast-enhanced magnetic resonance imaging and single-photon emission computed tomography for detection of myocardial necrosis early after acute myocardial infarction. J Am Coll Cardiol 2007;49:208–16, 17222732.

41. Ibrahim T, Nekolla SG, Hornke M, et al. Quantitative measurement of infarct size by contrast-enhanced magnetic resonance imaging early after acute myocardial infarction: comparison with single-photon emission tomography using Tc99m-sestamibi. J Am Coll Cardiol 2005;45:544–52, 15708702.

42. Lund GK, Stork A, Saeed M, et al. Acute myocardial infarction: evaluation with first-pass enhancement and delayed enhancement MR imaging compared with 201Tl SPECT imaging. Radiology 2004;232:49–57, 15166320.

43. Messroghli DR, Moon JC, Ferreira VM, et al. Clinical recommendations for cardiovascular magnetic resonance mapping of T1, T2, T2* and extracellular volume: a consensus statement by the Society for Cardiovascular Magnetic Resonance (SCMR) endorsed by the European Association for Cardiovascular Imaging (EACVI). J Cardiovasc Magn Reson 2017;19:75, 28992817.

44. Haaf P, Garg P, Messroghli DR, et al. Cardiac T1 Mapping and Extracellular Volume (ECV) in clinical practice: a comprehensive review. J Cardiovasc Magn Reson 2016;18:89.

45. Walls MC, Verhaert D, Min JK, et al. Myocardial edema imaging in acute coronary syndromes. J Magn Reson Imaging 2011;34:1243–50, 22102557.

46. Dall'Armellina E, Choudhury R, Karamitsos T, et al. Cardiovascular magnetic resonance by non contrast T1-mapping allows assessment of severity of injury in acute myocardial infarction. J Cardiovasc Magn Reson 2012;14(1):15.

47. Abdel-Aty H, Zagrosek A, Schulz-Menger J, et al. Delayed enhancement and T2-weighted cardiovascular magnetic resonance imaging differentiate acute from chronic myocardial infarction. Circulation 2004;109:2411–6, 15123531.

48. Abdel-Aty H, Boye P, Zagrosek A, et al. Diagnostic performance of cardiovascular magnetic resonance in patients with suspected acute myocarditis: comparison of different approaches. J Am Coll Cardiol 2005;45:1815–22, 15936612.

49. Carlsson M, Ubachs JF, E Hedstrom, et al. Myocardium at risk after acute infarction in humans on cardiac magnetic resonance: quantitative assessment during follow-up and validation with single-photon emission computed tomography. JACC Cardiovasc Imaging 2009;2:569–76, 19442942.

50. Kellman P, Aletras AH, Mancini C, et al. T2-prepared SSFP improves diagnostic confidence in edema imaging in acute myocardial infarction compared to turbo spin echo. Magn Reson Med 2007;57:891–7, 17457880.

51. Aletras AH, Kellman P, Derbyshire JA, et al. ACUT2E TSE-SSFP: a hybrid method for T2-weighted imaging of edema in the heart. Magn Reson Med 2008;59:229–35, 18228588.

52. Payne AR, Berry C, Kellman P, et al. Bright-blood T(2)-weighted MRI has high diagnostic accuracy for myocardial hemorrhage in myocardial infarction: a preclinical validation study in swine. Circ Cardiovasc Imaging 2011;4:738–45, 21930836.

53. Messroghli DR, Radjenovic A, Kozerke S, et al. Modified Look-Locker inversion recovery (MOLLI) for high-resolution T1 mapping of the heart. Magn Reson Med 2004;52:141–6, 15236377.

54. Giri S, Shah S, Xue H, et al. Myocardial T(2) mapping with respiratory navigator and automatic nonrigid motion correction. Magn Reson Med 2012;68:1570–8, 22851292.

55. Ugander M, Bagi PS, Oki AJ, et al. Myocardial edema as detected by pre-contrast T1 and T2

CMR delineates area at risk associated with acute myocardial infarction. JACC Cardiovasc Imaging 2012;5:596–603, 22698528.

56. Bulluck H, White SK, Frohlich GM, et al. Quantifying the area at risk in reperfused ST-segment-elevation myocardial infarction patients using hybrid cardiac positron emission tomography-magnetic resonance imaging. Circ Cardiovasc Imaging 2016;9: e003900, 26926269.

57. Dall'Armellina E, Karia N, Lindsay AC, et al. Dynamic changes of edema and late gadolinium enhancement after acute myocardial infarction and their relationship to functional recovery and salvage index. Circ Cardiovasc Imaging 2011;4: 228–36, 21447711.

58. Reffelmann T, Kloner RA. The no-reflow phenomenon: a basic mechanism of myocardial ischemia and reperfusion. Basic Res Cardiol 2006;101(5): 359–72, 16915531.

59. Wu KC, Zerhouni EA, Judd RM, et al. Prognostic significance of microvascular obstruction by magnetic resonance imaging in patients with acute myocardial infarction. Circulation 1998;97:765–72.

60. Lima JA, udd RM, Bazille A, et al. Regional heterogeneity of human myocardial infarcts demonstrated by contrast-enhanced MRI: Potential mechanisms. Circulation 1995;92:1117–25.

61. Orn S, Manhenke C, Greve OJ, et al. Microvascular obstruction is a major determinant of infarct healing and subsequent left ventricular remodelling following primary percutaneous coronary intervention. Eur Heart J 2009;30:1978–85.

62. Nijveldt R, Hofman MB, Hirsch A, et al. Assessment of microvascular obstruction and prediction of short-term remodeling after acute myocardial infarction: cardiac MR imaging study. Radiology 2009;250:363–70.

63. Yan AT, Gibson CM, Larose E, et al. Characterization of microvascular dysfunction after acute myocardial infarction by cardiovascular magnetic resonance first-pass perfusion and late gadolinium enhancement imaging. J Cardiovasc Magn Reson 2006;8:831–7.

64. Wu KC, Kim RJ, Bluemke DA, et al. Quantification and time course of microvascular obstruction by contrast-enhanced echocardiography and magnetic resonance imaging following acute myocardial infarction and reperfusion. J Am Coll Cardiol 1998;32:1756–64.

65. Hamirani YS, Wong A, Kramer CM, et al. Effect of microvascular obstruction and intramyocardial hemorrhage by CMR on LV remodeling and outcomes after myocardial infarction: a systematic review and meta-analysis. JACC Cardiovasc Imaging 2014;7(9):940–52, 25212800.

66. Kumar A, Green JD, Sykes JM, et al. Detection and Quantification of Myocardial Reperfusion Hemorrhage Using T2*-Weighted CMR. JACC Cardiovasc Imaging 2011;4(12):1274–83, 22172784.

67. Kali A, Tang RLQ, Kumar A, et al. Detection of acute reperfusion myocardial hemorrhage with cardiac MR imaging: T2 versus T2. Radiology 2013; 269(2):387–95, 23847253.

68. Kandler D, Lucke C, Grothoff M, et al. The relation between hypointense core, microvascular obstruction and intramyocardial haemorrhage in acute reperfused myocardial infarction assessed by cardiac magnetic resonance imaging. Eur Radiol 2014;24(12):3277–88, 25097126.

69. Eitel I, Kubusch K, Strohm O, et al. Prognostic value and determinants of a hypointense infarct core in T2-weighted cardiac magnetic resonance in acute reperfused ST-elevation-myocardial infarction. Circ Cardiovasc Imaging 2011;4(4):354–62, 21518773.

70. Reinstadler S, Reindl M, Eitel I, et al. Intramyocardial haemorrhage and prognosis after ST-elevation myocardial infarction. Eur Heart J Cardiovasc Imaging 2018;20(2):138–46.

71. Bulluck H, White SK, Rosmini S, et al. Chronic iron deposit and left ventricular remodeling in reperfused STEMI patients. J Cardiovasc Magn Reson 2016;18(Suppl 1):P230.

72. Bulluck H, Rosmini S, Abdel-Gadir A, et al. Residual Myocardial Iron Following Intramyocardial Hemorrhage During the Convalescent Phase of Reperfused ST-Segment-Elevation Myocardial Infarction and Adverse Left Ventricular Remodeling. Circ Cardiovasc Imaging 2016;9(10):e004940.

73. AU Srichai MB, Junor C, Smedira NG, et al. Clinical, imaging, and pathological characteristics of left ventricular thrombus: a comparison of contrast-enhanced magnetic resonance imaging, transthoracic echocardiography, and transesophageal echocardiography with surgical or pathological validation. Am Heart J 2006;152(1):75.

74. Mollet N, Dymarkowski S, Rademakers F, et al. Visualization of Ventricular Thrombi With Contrast-Enhanced Magnetic Resonance Imaging in Patients With Ischemic Heart Disease. Circulation 2002;106(23):2873–6.

75. Barkhausen J, Hunold P, Erbel R, et al. Detection and Characterization of Intracardiac Thrombi on MR Imaging. Am J Roentgenol 2002;179(6): 1539–44.

76. Weinsaft JW, Kim RJ, Ross M, et al. Contrast-enhanced anatomic imaging as compared to contrast-enhanced tissue characterization for detection of left ventricular thrombus. JACC Cardiovasc Imaging 2009;2(8):969–79.

77. Puerto E, Viana-Tejedor A, Martín-Asenjo R, et al. Temporal Trends in Mechanical Complications of Acute Myocardial Infarction in the Elderly. J Am Coll Cardiol 2018;72(9):959–66.

78. Baritussio A, Scatteia A, Bucciarelli-Ducci C. Role of cardiovascular magnetic resonance in acute and chronic ischemic heart disease. Int J Cardiovasc Imaging 2018;34(1):67–80.

79. Nicolosi GL, Latini R, Marino P, et al. The prognostic value of predischarge quantitative two-dimensional echocardiographic measurements and the effects of early lisinopril treatment on left ventricular structure and function after acute myocardial infarction in the GISSI-3 Trial. Gruppo Italia. Eur Heart J 1996;17(11):1646–56, 8922912.

80. Bellenger NG, Davies LC, Francis JM, et al. Reduction in sample size for studies of remodeling in heart failure by the use of cardiovascular magnetic resonance. J Cardiovasc Magn Reson 2000;2(4):271–8, 11545126.

81. Engblom H, Heiberg E, Erlinge D, et al. Sample size in clinical cardioprotection trials using myocardial salvage index, infarct size, or biochemical markers as endpoint. J Am Heart Assoc 2016;5(3):e002708, 26961520.

82. Schulman SP, Weiss JL, Becker LC, et al. Effect of early enalapril therapy on left ventricular function and structure in acute myocardial infarction. Am J Cardiol 1995;76(11):764–70, 7572651.

83. Johnson DB, Foster RE, Barilla F, et al. Angiotensin-converting enzyme inhibitor therapy affects left ventricular mass in patients with ejection fraction >40% after acute myocardial infarction. J Am Coll Cardiol 1997;29(1):49–54, 8996294.

84. Ibanez B, Macaya C, Sánchez-Brunete V, et al. Effect of early metoprolol on infarct size in st-segment-elevation myocardial infarction patients undergoing primary percutaneous coronary intervention: the Effect of Metoprolol in Cardioprotection During an Acute Myocardial Infarction (METO-CARD-CNIC) trial. Circulation 2013;128(14):1495–503, 24002794.

85. Groenning BA, Nilsson JC, Sondergaard L, et al. Antiremodeling effects on the left ventricle during beta-blockade with metoprolol in the treatment of chronic heart failure. J Am Coll Cardiol 2000;36(7):2072–80, 11127443.

86. Pennell D, Burgess M, Atkinson P, et al. The Carvedilol Hibernation Reversible Ischaemia Trial, Marker of Success (CHRISTMAS) study. Int J Cardiol 2000;72(3):265–74.

87. Chareonthaitawee P, Gersh BJ, Araoz PA, et al. Revascularization in severe left ventricular dysfunction: the role of viability testing. J Am Coll Cardiol 2005;46:567–74.

88. Braunwald E, Kloner RA. The stunned myocardium: prolonged, postischemic ventricular dysfunction. Circulation 1982;66:1146–9, 6754130.

89. Heusch G, Schulz R. Hibernating myocardium: a review. J Mol Cell Cardiol 1996;28:2359–72, 9004153.

90. Baer FM, Smolarz K, Jungehulsing M, et al. Chronic myocardial infarction: assessment of morphology, function, and perfusion by gradient echo magnetic resonance imaging and 99mTc-methoxyisobutyl-isonitrile SPECT. Am Heart J 1992;123:636–45, 1539515.

91. Pirolo JS, Hutchins GM, Moore GW. Infarct expansion: pathologic analysis of 204 patients with a single myocardial infarct. J Am Coll Cardiol 1986;7:349–54, 2935567.

92. Baer FM, Theissen P, Schneider CA, et al. Dobutamine magnetic resonance imaging predicts contractile recovery of chronically dysfunctional myocardium after successful revascularization. J Am Coll Cardiol 1998;31:1040–8, 9562005.

93. Shah DJ, Kim HW, James O, et al. Prevalence of regional myocardial thinning and relationship with myocardial scarring in patients with coronary artery disease. JAMA 2013;309:909–18, 23462787.

94. Cigarroa CG, deFilippi CR, Brickner ME, et al. Dobutamine stress echocardiography identifies hibernating myocardium and predicts recovery of left ventricular function after coronary revascularization. Circulation 1993;88:430–6, 8339406.

95. Pegg TJ, Selvanayagam JB, Jennifer J, et al. Prediction of global left ventricular functional recovery in patients with heart failure undergoing surgical revascularisation, based on late gadolinium enhancement cardiovascular magnetic resonance. J Cardiovasc Magn Reson 2010;12:56, 20929540.

96. Gerber BL, Rousseau MF, Ahn SA, et al. Prognostic value of myocardial viability by delayed-enhanced magnetic resonance in patients with coronary artery disease and low ejection fraction: impact of revascularization therapy. J Am Coll Cardiol 2012;59:825–35, 22361403.

97. Allman KC, Shaw LJ, Hachamovitch R, et al. Myocardial viability testing and impact of revascularization on prognosis in patients with coronary artery disease and left ventricular dysfunction: a meta-analysis. J Am Coll Cardiol 2002;39:1151–8, 11923039.

98. Ansari M, Araoz PA, Gerard SK, et al. Comparison of late enhancement cardiovascular magnetic resonance and thallium SPECT in patients with coronary disease and left ventricular dysfunction. J Cardiovasc Magn Reson 2004;6:549–56, 15137339.

99. Klein C, Nekolla SG, Bengel FM, et al. Assessment of myocardial viability with contrast-enhanced magnetic resonance imaging: comparison with positron emission tomography. Circulation 2002;105:162–7, 11790695.

100. Velazquez E, Lee K, Bonow R, et al. Coronary-Artery Bypass Surgery in Patients with Left Ventricular Dysfunction. N Engl J Med 2011;364(17):1607–16.

101. Bonow RO, Holly TA. Myocardial viability testing: still viable after stich? J Nucl Cardiol 2011;18: 991–4, 21913051.

102. Wacker C, Bock M, Hartlep A, et al. Changes in myocardial oxygenation and perfusion under pharmacological stress with dipyridamole: Assessment usingT*2 andT1 measurements. Magn Reson Med 1999;41(4):686–95.

103. Bauer W, Wacker C, Hartlep A, et al. The relationship between the BOLD-induced T2 and T2*: A theoretical approach for the vasculature of myocardium. Magn Reson Med 1999;42(6):1004–10.

104. Atalay MK, Reeder SB, Zerhouni EA, et al. Blood oxygenation dependence of T1 and T2 in the isolated, perfused rabbit heart at 4.7T. Magn Reson Med 1995;34:623–7, 8524032.

105. Wright KB, Klocke FJ, Deshpande VS, et al. Assessment of regional differences in myocardial blood flow using t2-weighted 3D BOLD imaging. Magn Reson Med 2001;46:573–8, 11550251.

106. Foltz WD, Huang H, Fort S, et al. Vasodilator response assessment in porcine myocardium with magnetic resonance relaxometry. Circulation 2002;106:2714–9, 12438298.

107. Shea SM, Fieno DS, Schirf BE, et al. T2-prepared steady-state free precession blood oxygen level-dependent MR imaging of myocardial perfusion in a dog stenosis model. Radiology 2005;236: 503–9, 16040907.

108. Manka R, Paetsch I, Schnackenburg B, et al. BOLD cardiovascular magnetic resonance at 3.0 tesla in myocardial ischemia. J Cardiovasc Magn Reson 2010;12(1):54.

109. Arnold J, Karamitsos T, Rimoldi O, et al. Myocardial Oxygenation in Coronary Artery Disease. J Am Coll Cardiol 2012;59(22):1954–64.

110. Dharmakumar R, Green J, Flewitt J, et al. Imaging for probing the myocardial perfusion reserves of patients with coronary artery disease: a feasibility study. Los Angeles (CA): Society for Cardiovascular Magnetic Resonance; 2008.

111. Luu JM, Friedrich MG, Harker J, et al. Relationship of vasodilator-induced changes in myocardial oxygenation with the severity of coronary artery stenosis: a study using oxygenation-sensitive cardiovascular magnetic resonance. Eur Heart J Cardiovasc Imaging 2014;15:1358–67.

112. Zhou X, Tsaftaris SA, Liu Y, et al. Artifact-reduced two-dimensional cine steady state free precession for myocardial blood-oxygen-level-dependent imaging. J Magn Reson Imaging 2010;31:863–71, 20373430.

113. Oksuz I, Mukhopadhyay A, Dharmakumar R. Unsupervised myocardial segmentation for cardiac BOLD. IEEE Trans Med Imaging 2017;36: 2228–38, 28708550.

114. Yabe T, Mitsunami K, Inubushi T, et al. Quantitative measurements of cardiac phosphorus metabolites in coronary artery disease by 31P magnetic resonance spectroscopy. Circulation 1995;92:15–23, 7788910.

115. Kim H, Lee D, Pohost G. 31P cardiovascular magnetic resonance spectroscopy: a unique approach to the assessment of the myocardium. Future Cardiol 2009;5(6):523–7.

116. Muthupillai R, Flamm S, Wilson J, et al. Acute Myocardial Infarction: Tissue Characterization with T1ρ-weighted MR Imaging—Initial Experience. Radiology 2004;232(2):606–10.

117. Witschey WR, Pilla JJ, Ferrari G, et al. Rotating frame spin lattice relaxation in a swine model of chronic, left ventricular myocardial infarction. Magn Reson Med 2010;64(5):1453–60.

Cardiovascular Magnetic Resonance in Right Heart and Pulmonary Circulation Disorders

Carla Contaldi, MD, PhD[a],*, Francesco Capuano, PhD[b], Luigia Romano, MD[c],
Brigida Ranieri, PhD[d], Francesco Ferrara, MD, PhD[a], Gaetano Mirto[e],
Salvatore Rega[f,1], Rosangela Cocchia, MD[g], Anna Agnese Stanziola, MD[h],
Ellen Ostenfield, MD, PhD[i,2], Santo Dellegrottaglie, MD, PhD[j],
Eduardo Bossone, MD, PhD, FCCP, FESC[g], Robert O. Bonow, MD, FAHA, FESC[k]

KEYWORDS

- Cardiac magnetic resonance • Right heart and pulmonary circulation disorders • Diagnosis
- Prognosis • Therapeutic management

KEY POINTS

- Cardiac magnetic resonance (CMR) allows accurate multiplanar assessment of right ventricle (RV) volume, global and regional systolic function, tissue characterization, and evaluation of right heart and pulmonary artery blood flows.
- The aim of this paper is to review the role of CMR in RV pressure-overload and volume-overload disorders and RV cardiomyopathies.
- The clinical utility of CMR in diagnosis, prognosis, and therapeutic management of the right heart and pulmonary circulation disorders is discussed.

INTRODUCTION

Cardiac magnetic resonance (CMR) provides a noninvasive morphologic and functional assessment, tissue characterization, and blood flow evaluation of the right heart and pulmonary circulation.[1]

Right heart and pulmonary circulation disorders are generally caused by right ventricle (RV) pressure overload, volume overload, and cardiomyopathy and they are associated with distinct clinical courses and therapeutic approaches, although they often may coexist.[2]

[a] Department of Cardiology, University Hospital of Salerno, Via Enrico de Marinis, Cava de' Tirreni, Salerno 84013, Italy; [b] Department of Industrial Engineering, Federico II University of Naples, Via Claudio 21, Naples 80125, Italy; [c] General and Emergency Radiology Division, A Cardarelli Hospital, Via Cardarelli 9, Naples I-80131, Italy; [d] IRCCS SDN, Via Gianturco 113, Naples I-80142, Italy; [e] Clinical Engineering Division, A Cardarelli Hospital, Via Cardarelli 9, Naples I-80131, Italy; [f] Medical School, Federico II University of Naples, Via Pansini 5, Naples I-80131, Italy; [g] Cardiology Division, A Cardarelli Hospital, Via Cardarelli 9, Naples I-80131, Italy; [h] Department of Respiratory Diseases, Monaldi Hospital, University "Federico II", Via Leonardo Bianchi, Naples 80131, Italy; [i] Department of Medical Imaging and Physiology, Cardiac Imaging, Skåne University Hospital, Entrégatan 7, Lund 222 42, Sweden; [j] Division of Cardiology, Clinica Villa dei Fiori, C.so Italia 157, 80011, Acerra, Naples, Italy; [k] Department of Medicine-Cardiology, Northwestern University Feinberg School of Medicine, 676 North St. Clair Street, Arkes Suite 2330, Chicago, IL 60611, USA
[1] Present address: Via Ima 3, 83023 Lauro (AV), Italy.
[2] Present address: Sö lvegatan 19-BMC F12, Lund, Sweden.
* Corresponding author.
E-mail address: contaldi.carla@gmail.com

Heart Failure Clin 17 (2021) 57–75
https://doi.org/10.1016/j.hfc.2020.08.006
1551-7136/21/© 2020 Elsevier Inc. All rights reserved.

This paper reviews CMR application in imaging of the right heart and pulmonary circulation and discusses its current and future application for the management of patients with right heart and pulmonary circulation disorders.

THE NORMAL RIGHT HEART AND PULMONARY CIRCULATION

The RV appears crescent shaped in cross-section, so it cannot be characterized using geometric assumptions. In normal conditions, the interventricular septum is concave toward the left ventricle (LV) throughout the cardiac cycle (**Fig. 1**).[2,3] The RV can be described in terms of the inlet region, the trabeculated apical myocardium and the infundibulum or RV outflow tract (RVOT).[2,3] The RV free wall is thinner than the LV wall.[2,3] The superficial RV wall layer is composed of myocardial fibers arranged more circumferentially than in the LV and it is responsible for inward contraction. The subendocardial RV layer is composed of preferentially arranged longitudinal myocardial fibers that causes systolic contraction of the base toward the apex. Shortening of the RV is greater longitudinally (75% of RV contraction) than radially, and twisting and rotational movements do not contribute significantly to contraction.[2,3] The RV and LV are closely interrelated through the septum, epicardial circumferential myocytes, and the pericardial space, which are the anatomic basis for biventricular functional interdependence. RV is more compliant of accommodating increased preload, but has heightened sensitivity to afterload change (it is unable to cope with brisk increments in pulmonary artery [PA] pressures).[2,3]

THE ROLE OF CARDIAC MAGNETIC RESONANCE

Strengths and weakness of imaging modalities in the evaluation of structure and function of right heart and pulmonary circulation unit are illustrated in **Table 1**.[1,4-6]

CMR is the gold standard modality for noninvasive RV imaging. It allows multiplanar imaging of the RV, gives accurate quantitative assessment of several parameters (ventricular volumes, myocardial mass, ejection fraction [EF], stroke volume [SV], and cardiac output [CO]), and qualitative assessment of RV regional function with a low intraobserver and interobserver variability and good interstudy reproducibility.[5,6] CMR allows also tissue characterization and evaluation of vascular abnormalities.[1,5,6] Limitations of CMR may include low availability, high cost, breath hold requirement, claustrophobia, safety in patients with ferromagnetic implants, and use of gadolinium in patients with severe chronic renal failure.[1]

CARDIAC MAGNETIC RESONANCE IMAGING PROTOCOL

Routine CMR scans include cine, phase contrast (PC), and postcontrast sequences. For cine imaging, balanced steady-state free precession (b-SSFP) is the sequence of choice for assessment of LV and RV size and function due to its excellent contrast-to-noise ratio between cardiac structures and high reproducibility and reliability. Stacks of cardiac short-axis and transaxial images are acquired for a complete volumetric coverage of the RV.[7] Also, PC imaging of PA, including main (MPA), right (RPA), and left (LPA), can be obtained to assess PA hemodynamic variables and dimensions. Using this technique, pulmonary flow (QP) and systemic flow (QS) ratio and valve regurgitation severity can be quantified. Then, contrast-enhanced magnetic resonance angiography (ce-MRA) allows accurate visualization of central, lobar, and segmental pulmonary vessels. In patients for whom gadolinium is contraindicated, 3D whole-heart MRA (or 3D-SSFP) can be used instead. Finally, late gadolinium enhancement (LGE) imaging, obtained 10 to 15 min after administration of intravenous gadolinium contrast agent,

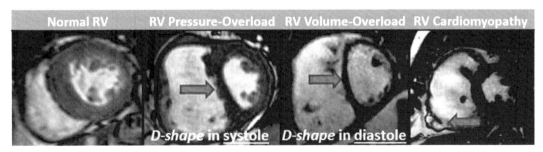

Fig. 1. Normal RV (normal RV dimension and septum concave toward LV), RV pressure-overload (RV hypertrophy and D shape of LV in "systole"), RV volume-overload (RV dilatation and D shape of LV in "diastole"), RV arrhythmogenic cardiomyopathy (RV dilatation and aneurysms). LV, left ventricle; RV, right ventricle.

Table 1
Relative strengths and weaknesses of different multimodality imaging techniques in the evaluation of structure and function of right heart and pulmonary circulation

	Echo	CMR	CT	Nuclear Imaging
Availability	++++	++	+++	++
Portability	++++	–	–	–
Cost	Low	High	Medium	Medium
Speed of acquisition	++++	++	++++	+
Radiation risk	–	–	+++[a]	++++
Suitability for sick or claustrophobic patients	++++	+	++	+/–
Contrast agents	+/–	+	++++	–
Temporal resolution	++++	+++	++	–[b]
Spatial resolution	++	+++	++++	+
Right heart structure	+++	++++	++	–
Right ventricular function	+++	++++	++	++
Tissue characterization	+	++++	++	+
Myocardial viability	+	++++	+	+++
First-pass perfusion	++	++++	+	++++
Coronary artery imaging	+	++	+++	–
Assessment of pressure gradients	++++	++	–	–
Clinical application	• Allows to assess right heart structure, function, and pressures at rest and during exercise • 2D echo can be used as a screening tool • 3D echo is more accurate and reproducible in evaluating RV size and systolic function	• Is the gold standard in evaluating right heart structure and function • Allows tissue characterization and evaluation of vascular abnormalities • Ruling out underlying CAD	• Allows quantitative 3D RV assessment and fatty infiltration when CMR is unavailable or unsuitable • Ruling out underlying CAD and lung disease (interstitial, COPD, CTEPH, cancer)	• Allows assessment of myocardial ischemia and viability in underlying suspected CAD

(continued on next page)

Table 1
(continued)

	Echo	CMR	CT	Nuclear Imaging
Limitations	• Highly operator dependent • Inadequate imaging window • Limited evaluation of right ventricle and pulmonary circulation	• Safety in patients with ferromagnetic implants • Use of gadolinium in patients with severe chronic renal failure • Breath holding • No portability • Higher cost • Claustrophobia	• Radiation exposure • Use of iodinated contrast • No portability • Higher cost • Claustrophobia	• Radiation exposure • No portability • Low spatial resolution • Long scanning time • Significantly higher cost

+ denotes a positive remark and − denotes a negative remark. The number of signs indicates the estimated potential value.

Abbreviations: CAD, coronary artery disease; CMR, cardiovascular magnetic resonance; COPD, chronic obstructive pulmonary disease; CT, computed tomography; CTEPH, chronic thromboembolic pulmonary hypertension; RV, right ventricle.

[a] Radiation risk is significantly higher when the cine ventricular function and fist pass perfusion are performed.

[b] Temporal resolution for nuclear techniques is variable and depends on the radiotracer and counts.

Modified from Zhou X, Ferrara F, Contaldi C, et al. Right ventricular size and function in chronic heart failure: not to be forgotten. Heart Fail Clin 2019;15:210; with permission.

permits visualization and quantification of myocardial reparative fibrosis (scar).[5,6] When indicated, other optional CMR techniques can be used (**Table 2**).

PRESSURE-OVERLOAD DISORDERS

RV pressure overload leads to RV hypertrophy, predominantly end-systolic and early-diastolic flattening of the interventricular septum and "D shape" of the LV in systole (see **Fig. 1**). In the setting of chronic pressure overload, the RV initially responds with preserved volumes and function and compensatory "concentric" hypertrophy, successively, with "eccentric" hypertrophy, progressive RV dilatation, dyssynchrony, fibrosis, and reduced CO, leading to deterioration of exercise capacity and ultimately clinical decompensation. The RV becomes less dependent on longitudinal shortening.[2] The most common chronic RV pressure-overload disorders are described in the following paragraphs.

Table 2
Cardiac magnetic resonance protocol for right heart and pulmonary circulation

Technique	Information
CINE (b-SSFP)	• RV and LV dimension, mass, regional and global function • Atrial dimension • Interventricular septal changes • MPA, LPA, RPA dimension • Pulmonary valve direct planimetry
Phase contrast	• QP and QS • Cardiac output and PA flow profile • Pulmonary valve direct regurgitant volume • PA stiffness and pulsatility
LGE	• Ventricular myocardial reparative fibrosis • Ventricular myocardial microvascular obstruction
ce-MRA	• Vascular anatomy • Pulmonary perfusion
3D whole-heart MRA or 3D SSFP	• Vascular anatomy
Black blood images with and without fat suppression (when indicated)	• Fat infiltration
T2w STIR (when indicated)	• Myocardial edema • Myocardial hemorrhage
T1-Mapping (optional)	• Diffuse myocardial fibrosis
T2-Mapping (optional)	• Myocardial edema
Tagging technique/feature tracking (optional)	• Strain and strain rate analysis • Interventricular asynchrony
4D Flow (optional)	• RV and PA 3D flow patterns • PA vortex • PA wall shear stress and energy loss • RV kinetic energy work density

Abbreviations: b-SSFP, balanced steady-state free precession; ce-MRA, contrast-enhanced magnetic resonance angiography; LPA, left pulmonary artery; LV, left ventricle; MPA, main pulmonary artery; PA, pulmonary artery; QP, pulmonary flow; QS, systemic flow; RPA, right pulmonary artery; RV, right ventricle.

Pulmonary Hypertension

Pulmonary hypertension (PH) is a pathophysiological condition defined as an increase in mean PA pressure (mPAP) $\geq$25 mm Hg at rest by right heart catheterization (RHC). It is hemodynamically categorized into 2 groups: precapillary and postcapillary. In particular, pulmonary arterial hypertension (PAH) is defined as a group of precapillary PH and pulmonary vascular resistance (PVR) >3 Wood units in absence of the other causes of precapillary PH.[8] The PH diagnostic algorithm with the specific role of noninvasive imaging is illustrated in **Fig. 2**.

ROLE OF CARDIAC MAGNETIC RESONANCE IN PULMONARY HYPERTENSION
Diagnosis and Cause

The most accurate tools by cine-CMR, for the identification of PH are the ventricular mass index, which expresses the degree of chronic RV pressure overload,[9] the increased area and thickness of basal segment of the septomarginal band,[10] and the interventricular septum curvature ratio, which is an accurate and reproducible index of RV systolic pressure.[11] Cine-CMR also allows visualization of the degree of flattening of the interventricular septum and a "D-shaped" LV in the presence of severe PH (see **Fig. 1**).[2]

Using 2D-PC, peak PA systolic pressure can be derived using the modified Bernoulli equation and reduced pulmonary average velocities, blood flow, and distensibility can be evaluated in patients with PH.[12] Average velocity in the MPA has a high degree of reliability in detecting PH and it has also a strong inverse correlation with PAP and PVR.[13] Relative area change (RAC) can be used as a marker of MPA stiffness. RAC increases early in PH and may detect exercise-induced PH before overt pressure increases occur at rest.[14]

LGE-CMR shows areas of LGE induced by chronic ventricular overload frequently in the RV insertion points of the interventricular septum corresponding to higher fiber stress zones (**Fig. 3**, **Table 3**).[15,16] However, no single CMR parameter can exclude PH.

In identifying the cause of PH due to left heart disease, CMR can quantify LV volumes and EF accurately, identify valvular heart disease, and differentiate between ischemic and nonischemic cardiomyopathy by the pattern of LGE.[1] If coronary artery disease is suspected, stress perfusion CMR can evaluate LV and RV function, perfusion, and myocardial scar. In chronic thromboembolic PH, ce-MRA may allow accurate visualization of the lobar and segmental pulmonary vessels, and 3D whole-heart MRA may measure regional changes in segmental or subsegmental lung perfusion.[1,5,6] In patients with PAH secondary to congenital heart disease, CMR provides complete evaluation of cardiac and extracardiac structures and may be useful in diagnosis, treatment planning and follow-up[5,6] (see **Fig. 2**).

Risk Stratification, Prognosis, and Monitor Treatment Efficacy

Cine-CMR is useful in clinical management. An increased RV end-diastolic volume (EDV) indexed to body surface area (RV EDVI) is the most reliable marker for RV failure and a valuable predictor of poor survival. The correlation of RV dilatation to mortality is stronger than RV hypertrophy[17]; however, ventricular mass index has been suggested to be a predictor of decreased survival.[18] RV EF is the strongest predictor of mortality[19,20] and severity of right atrial (RA) volume dilation is associated with disease progression and prognosis.[21,22] PC-CMR measurements reflecting stiffness of the proximal pulmonary vasculature[23] are independent predictors of outcome. LGE at the RV insertion point seems to be associated with more advanced PH, especially if the LGE is including the septum (**Table 4**).[16,24]

For the monitoring of drug therapy in patients with PH, RV mass and RV EF by cine-CMR might be used.[19,25] In patients with PH, the addition of sildenafil to bosentan therapy reduces RV mass and this effect is associated with improvements of symptoms and NT-proBNP[25]; after 1 year of therapy, reduced RV EF is associated with poor outcome, even in patients with PAH with PVR improvement[19] (**Table 5**).

NOVEL CARDIAC MAGNETIC RESONANCE TECHNIQUES IN PULMONARY HYPERTENSION
T1-Mapping

T1-mapping has been developed to quantify diffuse myocardial fibrosis directly measuring the T1 relaxation times. Native T1 reflects both the intracellular and extracellular compartments.[26] The extracellular contrast volume (ECV) (calculated taking into account myocardial and blood T1 values precontrast and postcontrast) provides a direct measure of the of myocardium occupied by extracellular space.[26]

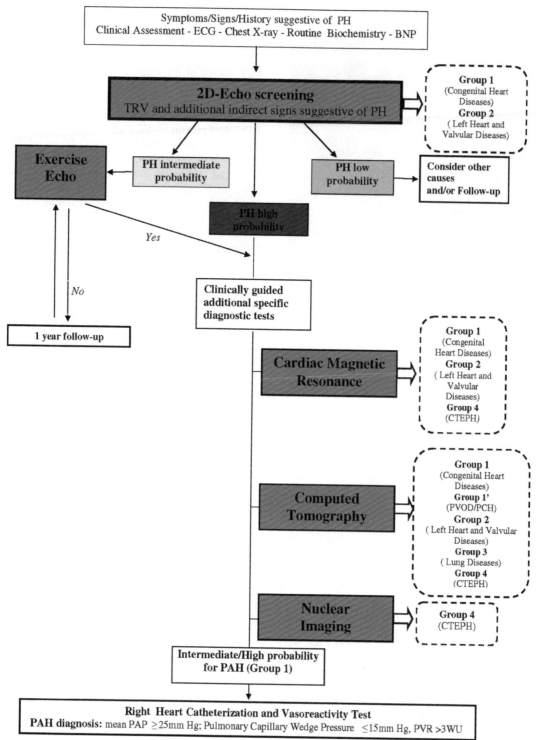

Fig. 2. Flowchart of PH diagnostic algorithm with the specific role of noninvasive imaging. CTEPH, chronic thromboembolic pulmonary hypertension; PAH, pulmonary arterial hypertension; PAP, pulmonary artery pressure; PCH, pulmonary capillary hemangiomatosis; PH, pulmonary hypertension; PVOD, pulmonary veno-occlusive disease; PVR, pulmonary vascular resistance; TRV, transtricuspid valve regurgitation velocity; WU, Wood units.

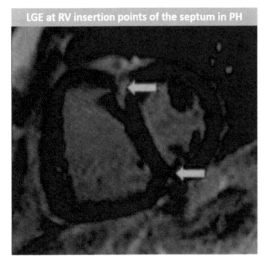

LGE at RV insertion points of the septum in PH

Fig. 3. An example of LGE (*blue arrows*) at RV insertion point spreading into the septum in a patient with PH. LGE, late gadolinium enhancement; PH, pulmonary hypertension; RV, right ventricle.

In patients with precapillary PH, native T1 values of RV insertion points are significantly increased and are related to PH severity.[27] In patients with PH, RV ECV is increased. Both native T1 and ECV values at RV insertion points are increased and show significant correlations with pulmonary hemodynamics, RV arterial coupling, and RV performance. ECV is increased before overt RV systolic dysfunction.[28] ECV is useful in detecting myocardial involvement in early stages of PH, can guide management, and serve as a therapeutic target. However, caution should be emphasized in interpreting T1 values in the thin and highly trabeculated RV free wall, as partial volume effects and inclusion of fat or blood (erroneously, however easily done) in the region of interest are major caveats to the measurements.

Strain Analysis

Fast strain encoded (SENC) is a through-plane CMR-tagging technique that allows direct

Table 3
The main cardiac magnetic resonance diagnostic parameters in pulmonary hypertension

Diagnostic CMR Variable	Cutoff Value	Detection of PH Sensitivity (%)	Specificity (%)	Reference
Cine-CMR				
VMI (RV mass/LV mass)	≥0.4	81	88	Swift et al,[9] 2012
LV septal to free wall curvature ratio	≤0.67	87	100	Dellegrottaglie et al,[11] 2007
RV EDVI	≥75 mL/m²	67	50	Swift et al,[9] 2012
RV mass index	≥20 g/m²	83	84	Swift et al,[9] 2012
RV EF	≤35%	67	71	Swift et al,[9] 2012
RV RAC	≤30%	61	81	Swift et al,[9] 2012
TAPSE	≤2 cm	76	64	Swift et al,[9] 2012
PC-CMR				
PA RAC (max MPA CSA–min MPA CSA/min MPA CSA)	≥15%	84	74	Swift et al,[14] 2012
PA average velocity	<11.7 cm/s	93	82	Sanz et al,[13] 2007
Retrograde flow	≥0.3 L/min/m²	83	71	Swift et al,[9] 2012
LGE-CMR				
RV insertion site LGE	Present	83	94	Swift et al,[9] 2012
4D-Flow-CMR				
MPA vortical blood flow (t_{vortex})[a]	≥14.3%	97	96	Reiter et al,[33] 2015

Abbreviations: CSA, cross-sectional area; EDVI, end-diastolic volume index; EF, ejection fraction; LV, left ventricle; MPA, main pulmonary artery; RAC, relative area change; RV, right ventricle; VMI, ventricular mass index.
[a] t_{vortex}:the percentage of cardiac phases with vortex present.
Modified from Swift AJ, Rajaram S, Condliffe R, et al. Diagnostic accuracy of cardiovascular magnetic resonance imaging of right ventricular morphology and function in the assessment of suspected pulmonary hypertension results from the ASPIRE registry. J Cardiovasc Magn Reson. 2012;14(1):40.

Table 4
The main cardiac magnetic resonance prognostic parameters in pulmonary hypertension

Prognostic CMR Variable	Cutoff Value	Comment	Reference
Cine-CMR			
RV EDVI	$\geq$84 mL/m^2	Predictor of RV failure and mortality	Van Wolferen et al,[17] 2007
RV EF	$\leq$35%	Predictor of poor outcome and mortality	van de Veerdonk et al,[19] 2011
Ventricular mass index (RV end-diastolic mass/LV end-diastolic mass)	$\geq$0.7	Predictor of decreased 2-y survival	Hagger et al,[18] 2009
RA volume	Increased	Associated with disease progression and prognosis	Sato et al,[21] 2013
PC-CMR			
Pulmonary artery relative area change	$\leq$16%	Predictor of poor outcome and mortality	Gan et al,[23] 2007
SVI	$\leq$25 mL/m^2	Predictor of RV failure and mortality	Van Wolferen et al,[17] 2007
LGE-CMR			
RV insertion site LGE	Present	Predictor of poor prognosis	Freed et al,[16] 2012
Feature tracking CMR			
RV GLS and GLSR	Reduced	Associated with poor outcome	Menezes de Siqueira et al,[30] 2016
RV GCSR	> -0.8 s^{-1}	Predictor of events	Menezes de Siqueira et al,[30] 2016
LV GLS	> -14.2%	Predictor of poor outcome and mortality in precapillary PH	Padervinskienė et al,[31] 2019

Abbreviations: EDVI, end-diastolic volume index; EF, ejection fraction; GCSR, global circumferential strain rate; GLS, global longitudinal strain; GLSR, global longitudinal strain rate; LV, left ventricle; RV, right ventricle; SVI, stroke volume index.

measurement of regional function by using a free-breathing single-heartbeat real-time acquisition. It allows direct measurement of longitudinal strain by using short-axis images. Fast SENC identifies significantly reduced RV longitudinal contractility at basal-mid anterior septal insertions and mid anterior RV wall in patients with PAH with normal global RV function.[29]

Feature tracking (FT) is a novel method that allows quantification of myocardial deformation from cine-CMR images. Patients with PH show significant reductions in global longitudinal strain (GLS), global circumferential strain (GCS), global longitudinal strain rate (GLSR), and global circumferential strain rate (GCSR). GLS, GLSR, and GCSR are independently associated with outcome.[30] LV GLS also shows correlation with RV dysfunction and is associated with poor clinical outcome and mortality.[31] Therefore, in PH, quantification of RV and LV strain by FT-CMR is feasible, correlates with disease severity, and is independently associated with poor outcome (see **Table 4**).

Blood Flow Imaging

4D Flow CMR is an evolving imaging technique that provides in-vivo assessment of 3-directional blood flow within 3D vascular structures throughout the cardiac cycle. RV volume, function, and mass can be quantified with interobserver agreement comparable with cine-CMR SSFP sequences.[32] Whole-heart 4D flow CMR enables detection and visualization of both normal and abnormal right heart flow patterns. In patients with PH, vortex of blood flow in the MPA from 4D flow CMR is present and the vortex duration has been related with mPAP (**Fig. 4**, see **Table 3**).[33] Vorticity is decreased in the RPA of patients with PH and it correlates with an increase in PVR.[34] 4D flow CMR can also estimate wall shear stress (WSS), a measure of viscous hemodynamic forces

Table 5
Role of cardiac magnetic resonance in right heart and pulmonary circulation disorders

Pulmonary Hypertension	Pulmonary Valve Stenosis	Tricuspid Valve Regurgitation	Pulmonary Valve Regurgitation	Systemic-to-Pulmonary Shunt	RV Infarction	Arrhythmogenic Cardiomyopathy	Other Nonischemic Cardiomyopathies (*Hypertrophy, Dilated, Noncompaction, Tako-Tsubo, Amyloidosis, Sarcoidosis, Myocarditis*)
Diagnosis	Accurate assessment of valve stenosis severity: prefer *planimetry*	Accurate assessment of valve regurgitation severity: prefer *indirect method*	Accurate assessment of valve regurgitation severity: prefer *direct method*	Size, location, and number of communications between pulmonary and systemic circulations: *intra- and extracardiac*	Evaluation of RV ischemic injury: • RV anatomic and functional assessment • Tissue characterization	Early diagnosis	Early RV/LV involvement
Cause	Hemodynamic consequences	Hemodynamic consequences	Hemodynamic consequences	Hemodynamic consequences	RV infarction complications	Disease classification	Prognosis
Prognosis	Identify sub- or supravalvular stenosis	Prognosis	Prognosis	Accurate QP/QS ratio quantification	Prognosis	Prognosis	Detection of eventual associated systemic alterations, ie, enlarged lymph nodes
Monitor treatment efficacy	Secondary PA dilatation		Timing of reintervention: in previous surgery for congenital heart diseases	Atrial septal defect rims		Follow-up in *definite, borderline, or possible arrhythmogenic cardiomyopathy*	

Guidance to pulmonic valvuloplasty-valve replacement	Indication to pulmonary valve replacement		Family screening
Indication to percutaneous valve treatment			Differential diagnosis

Abbreviations: LV, left ventricle; PA, pulmonary artery; RV, right ventricle; QP, pulmonary flow; QS, systolic flow.

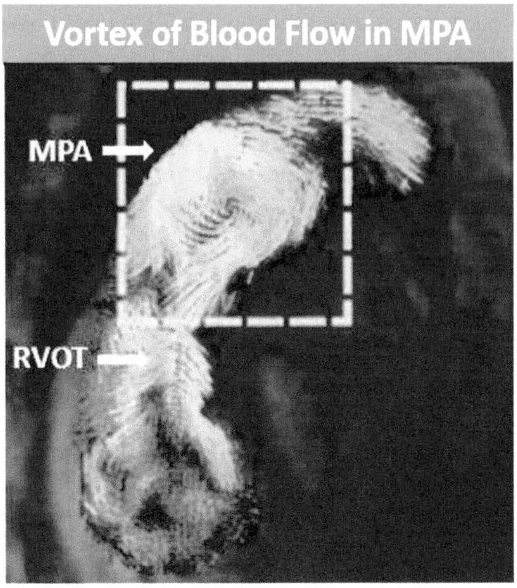

Fig. 4. An example of a vortex of blood flow in the MPA in a patient with PH by 4D flow CMR. CMR, cardiac magnetic resonance; MPA, main pulmonary artery; PH, pulmonary hypertension.

acting on the vessel walls (risk factor of endothelial degeneration) and energy loss (EL), the energy dissipation caused by abnormal 3D blood flow (associated with high cardiac workload) in aortic disease.[35] EL is a possible predictor of heart failure.[36] In patients with PH, 4D flow CMR at the MPA, RPA, and LPA shows significantly lower WSS, independent of the 4D flow CMR acquisition strategy.[37] In addition, PA WSS is reduced in both children and adults with PAH associated with the degree of vessel dilation and stiffness. EL, instead, is increased in PAH without difference between adults and pediatric patients.[38] In patients with PAH, increase in RV kinetic energy work density and in PA percent EL seem to be promising markers for RV dysfunction.[39]

Computational fluid dynamics (CFD) modeling, is another novel technology that generates equations of fluid dynamics in a computer using patient-specific vascular or heart chambers geometries and physiologic flow or pressure conditions. The geometries are reconstructed from segmentation of CMR or computed tomography (CT) images (**Fig. 5**). This technique has high temporal and spatial resolution and can also be used to reproduce the virtual flow that would be realized in hypothetical postsurgical conditions, therefore adding predictive capabilities to modern flow imaging.[40] A CFD combined with CMR study has demonstrated for the first time that WSS is altered in PAH, showing reduced WSS in

the proximal PAs, as reported successively by 4D flow CMR.[41] The prognostic value of these novel technologies for blood flow imaging remain to be proven; however, in the future they could offer a noninvasive alternative to RHC and could help in early detection of PH.

FUTURE PERSPECTIVES OF CARDIAC MAGNETIC RESONANCE IN PULMONARY HYPERTENSION

Exercise Cardiac Magnetic Resonance

CMR during exercise permits highly reproducible and accurate measurements of RV volumes and function, and CO is comparable with that obtained by the direct Fick method.[42] Assessment of RV function with CMR during exercise stratifies patients with PAH currently perceived as having a low risk of mortality into different degrees of RV inotropic reserve. Reduced RV SV during exercise CMR is a plausible marker of increased risk of decompensation, possibly warranting targeted therapy intensification to restore RV functional reserve.[43]

CMR during exercise is currently performed in very few centers because of difficulties in running adequate exercise sessions in the magnetic resonance environment.

Cardiac Magnetic Resonance-Guided Right Heart Catheterization

CMR-guided RHC (CMR-RHC) can combine the benefits of CMR and invasive cardiac catheterization.

CMR-RHC, using passive catheters, is an attractive modality for comprehensive hemodynamic characterization of cardiovascular conditions, such as PAH. After baseline CMR for cardiac function, transfemoral catheters are navigated into the superior vena cava (SVC), and thereafter from the right atrium into the RV and one or both pulmonary arteries. Patients with suspected PAH can be screened using first-pass contrast lung perfusion. Procedure time increases with worsening PAH.[44,45] CMR-RHC applications are still in the primordial phase of clinical application, with few advanced centers equipped with hybrid-invasive CMR facilities. However, in the future CMR-RHC might be incorporated into routine clinical practice for the investigation of PAH.

Pulmonary valve stenosis

Pulmonary valve stenosis (PS) is another cause of RV pressure overload and it is usually an isolated congenital abnormality but may be associated with other conditions (tetralogy of Fallot,

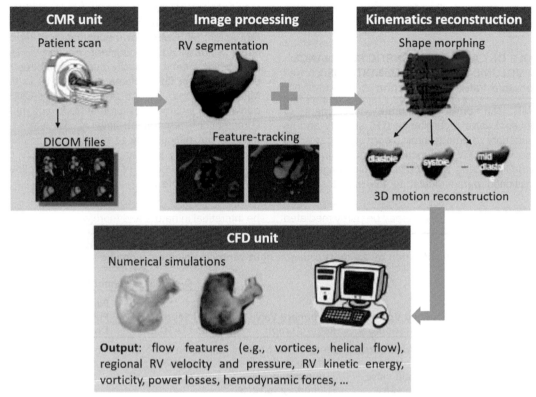

Fig. 5. A workflow from clinical imaging to numerical simulation of RV flow using CFD. (1) Acquisition of cine-CMR SSFP images; (2) FT-CMR to automatically extract the time evolution of the RV endocardium and a fine 3D triangulated surface mesh of the geometry of the RV obtained through a segmentation process; (3) reconstruction of 3D RV motion using an image registration technique; (4) numerical simulations performed using CFD to solve the flow equations inside the previously computed moving geometry. CFD, computational fluid dynamics; CMR, cardiac magnetic resonance; FT-CMR, feature tracking cardiac magnetic resonance; RV, right ventricle; SSFP, steady-state free precession.

congenital rubella, and Noonan syndrome). PS may be secondary to carcinoid syndrome, rheumatic heart disease, thrombus, or cardiac surgery. PS is also associated with secondary dilation of MPA and LPA (less so the RPA) and with abnormalities of the structure of PA wall.[46,47]

ROLE OF CARDIAC MAGNETIC RESONANCE IN PULMONARY VALVE STENOSIS

Imaging the pulmonary valve requires an RVOT view and potentially a second view perpendicular to this plane.[46–48] Cine-CMR shows doming of the leaflets, a high-velocity jet across the pulmonary valve and subvalvular or supravalvular stenosis. Short-axis cine imaging through the valve tips in systole provides direct planimetry of the valve orifice for accurate determination of anatomic orifice area. Multiple parallel thin slices may be helpful to locate the optimal slice. Cine-CMR can also quantify the hemodynamic

consequences of PS.[46,48] PC-CMR quantifies the peak velocity and the peak gradient is calculated using the modified Bernoulli equation.[48] CMR can also provide a functional/effective orifice area (similar to the continuity equation by echocardiography), but direct planimetry is usually more reliable.[47] CMR can be useful to select patients eligible for percutaneous valve replacement. Valvuloplasty and valve replacement may be performed under CMR guidance (see **Table 5**).[47]

VOLUME-OVERLOAD DISORDERS

RV volume overload leads to RV dilatation and hypertrophy with increased free wall mass but preserved thickness and predominantly diastolic leftward septal shift with "D shape" of LV in diastole (see **Fig. 1**). In the setting of chronic volume overload, RV contractility remains preserved for long time periods, although contractile reserve may be compromised.[2,3] The most common RV volume-overload disorders[2,3,48–51] are listed in **Table 6**.

ROLE OF CARDIAC MAGNETIC RESONANCE IN VOLUME-OVERLOAD CONDITIONS
Tricuspid Valve Regurgitation

CMR can provide accurate assessment of tricuspid valve regurgitation (TR) severity and its secondary hemodynamic consequences and also identify RV dysfunction. Standard long-axis cine-CMR views with additional thin image slices positioned perpendicular to the leaflet sections may help to visualize the detailed anatomy/function. PC-CMR in-plane is helpful to identify the regurgitant jet. CMR allows quantitation of *regurgitant volume* and *regurgitant fraction*.[48] The *regurgitant volume* is usually calculated indirectly, subtracting the flow volume by PC-CMR in the MPA from the SV obtained by cine-CMR-derived RV volume measurements. Direct measurement of regurgitant flow at the valve is feasible but difficult due to mobile valve leaflets and high-velocity jets. An increased RV EDV by cine-CMR can predict RV dysfunction at follow-up[48–50] (see **Table 5**).

Table 6
Definition and classification of the most common right ventricle volume-overload disorders

	Tricuspid Valve Regurgitation	Pulmonary Valve Regurgitation	Systemic-to-Pulmonary Shunt	
			Atrial Septal Defect (ASD)	Partial Anomalous Pulmonary Vein Drainage (PAPVC)
Definition	Blood flows back through the tricuspid valve *Tricuspid valve complex:* large tricuspid annulus, 3 leaflets (anterior, posterior, and septal), 3 independent papillary muscles, and chordae tendineae	Blood flows back through the pulmonary valve *Pulmonary valve:* 3 semilunar leaflets (anterior, left, and right)	Defect in the interatrial septum	Anomalous connection of 1 or more pulmonary veins to the systemic venous system
Classification	Primary anatomic valvular problems: • Iatrogenic • Endocarditis • Rheumatic valve disease • Carcinoid • Congenital heart disease (ie, Ebstein anomaly) Functional (more common): • Annular dilatation due to RA and/or RV dilatation and papillary muscle displacement	Native valve (rare) Primary anatomic problems: • Endocarditis • Carcinoid Secondary to: • Surgical valvotomy/valvectomy or balloon pulmonary valvuloplasty for pulmonary stenosis (eg, tetralogy of Fallot) Functional: • PA dilatation • Severe PAH	Ostium secundum (80%) *Ostium primum (15%):* ± atrioventricular valve defects Sinus venous (5%): • Near the SVC • ± PAPVC (ie, upper right PV in SVC or RA) Coronary sinus (<1%)	The first most common type: • Right upper and middle PV into SVC • Often + superior sinus venosus ASD The second most common type: • Left upper PV into the left innominate vein via a vertical vein Scimitar syndrome: • All right-sided PVs into RA, IVC or hepatic veins

Abbreviations: IVC, inferior vena cava; PA, pulmonary artery; PAH, pulmonary arterial hypertension; PV, pulmonary vein; RA, right atrium; RV, right ventricle; SVC, superior vena cava.

Pulmonary Valve Regurgitation

CMR is the most accurate method for quantifying pulmonary valve regurgitation (PR) and its secondary hemodynamic consequences, and it plays a crucial role in the timing of reintervention in patients with previous surgery for congenital heart diseases (ie, tetralogy of Fallot). Cine-CMR can show a dark jet of dephasing during diastole extending into the RVOT. PC-CMR quantifies PR using a through-plane positioned just above the valve and the measurement of regurgitant volume is usually direct (**Fig. 6**). The regurgitant volume or regurgitant fraction and RV EDV have been shown to be highly predictive of the development of symptoms and the need for surgery[46,48,51] (see **Table 5**).

Systemic-to-Pulmonary Shunt

Cine-CMR can provide intracardiac and extracardiac anatomy, size, location, and number of communications between pulmonary and systemic circulations, ventricular volumes and function, and PA dimensions. In atrial septal defect (ASD), cine-CMR can show low-intensity flow jets between the atria. SSFP images in multiple axial and short-axis planes perpendicular to ASD provide an assessment of the defect location and size throughout the cardiac cycle. PC-CMR is the noninvasive gold standard for quantifying QP and QS, independent of the location of the shunt.[48,51] In a PC-cine acquisition with a very low velocity-encoding limit, the flow via the ASD can lead to aliasing and clear demarcation of the defect, allowing measurement of the ASD rims for evaluation of eligibility to percutaneous closure. Ce-MRA details extracardiac shunts[48,51] (see **Table 5**).

RIGHT VENTRICLE CARDIOMYOPATHIES
Right Ventricle Infarction

The RV can be involved frequently in inferior acute myocardial infarction (AMI) (up to 50%) and less often in anterior AMI. Isolated RV AMI is rare (<3%). The RV is more resistant to prolonged ischemia than the LV thanks to its more favorable oxygen demand/supply profile; however, lack of RV recovery is associated with persistent hemodynamic compromise and high mortality.[2]

Role of cardiac magnetic resonance in RV infarction

In RV infarction, CMR is clinically useful because it allows detailed anatomic and functional assessment of RV and provides tissue characterization. Axial and short-axis cine-CMR can assess accurately eventual increased RV volume, reduced EF, and regional function alterations. In acute RV infarction, T_2 STIR sequences can show RV edema and eventual hemorrhage. LGE-CMR can show, in the RV and frequently in the territory of right coronary artery, subendocardial or transmural LGE, microvascular obstruction (in the acute setting) (**Fig. 7**), and RV thrombi. LGE of the RV is feasible, but challenging as the RV wall is thin and may require a different time inversion than that used to assess LV LGE. RV LGE has strong prognostic relevance[52] (see **Table 5**).

Arrhythmogenic Cardiomyopathy

Arrhythmogenic cardiomyopathy (ARVC) is a genetically determined cardiomyopathy, characterized by the replacement of the ventricular myocardium by fibro-fatty tissue, from the epicardium toward the endocardium. The RV can be primarily affected with RV dilatation and altered regional and/or global function (see **Fig. 1**); however, the LV can also be involved, although LV dimensions or function can be normal. Isolated or predominant LV involvement can also be present, usually limited to the subepicardium or midmural layers of the posterolateral wall. ARVC can be a cause of sudden cardiac death due to ventricular fibrillation in young adults, so early diagnosis can be very important.[53,54]

Role of cardiac magnetic resonance in arrhythmogenic cardiomyopathy

CMR is the imaging modality of choice for early diagnosis of ARVC, as it allows RV multiplanar imaging and tissue characterization. Axial and short-axis cine-CMR are useful for assessment of RV wall motion abnormalities (regional RV akinesia or dyskinesia or dyssynchronous RV contraction) in addition to increased RV volumes and reduced RV EF, which are the CMR diagnostic criteria included in the last 2010 Task Force Criteria (see **Fig. 1**).[53] Axial and short-axis LGE images are useful for assessment of RV and LV LGE. LV LGE (present in up to 25% of patients with ARVC), instead, has diagnostic value. LGE has mostly a subepicardial/midwall distribution involving especially the posterolateral wall and may be the only sign of LV involvement (**Fig. 8**). On the basis of LGE, the classification of ARVC has been revised to include the *traditional RV form*, morpho-functional RV abnormalities with or without RV LGE; *LV-dominant form*, LV LGE; *biventricular form*, RV involvement with LV LGE, without LV decreased systolic function; and finally the *end-stage form*, biventricular involvement characterized by both morpho-functional abnormalities with biventricular heart failure and tissue characterization abnormalities of both ventricles.[53–55] Currently, no imaging

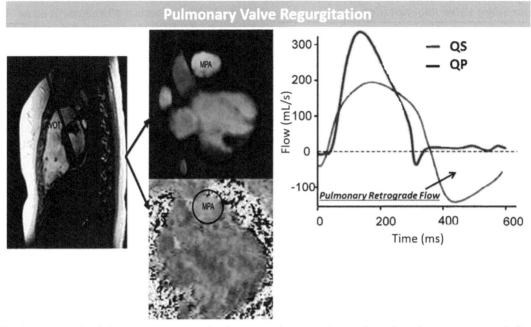

Fig. 6. An example of direct measurement of pulmonary valve regurgitant volume by pulmonary retrograde flow using PC-CMR. PC-CMR, phase contrast cardiac magnetic resonance; QP, pulmonary flow; QS, systemic flow.

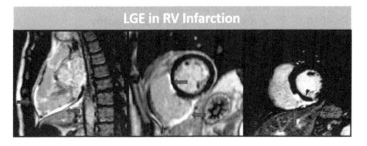

Fig. 7. RV myocardial infarct (*blue arrows*) with involvement of LV inferior wall and microvascular obstruction (*black arrowhead*) demonstrated by LGE-CMR. LGE-CMR, late gadolinium enhancement-cardiac magnetic resonance; LV, left ventricle; RV, right ventricle.

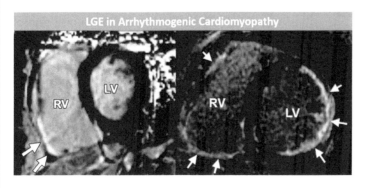

Fig. 8. Examples of LGE in arrhythmogenic cardiomyopathy involving RV and LV (*white arrows*). LGE, late gadolinium enhancement; LV, left ventricle; RV, right ventricle.

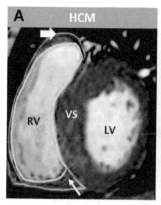
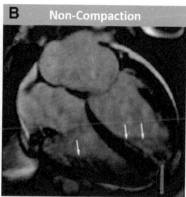

Fig. 9. Short axis showing increased wall thickness in the superior segment and inferior segment (*white arrows*) of the RV wall in hypertrophic cardiomyopathy (*A*) and horizontal long axis showing marked trabeculations in both the LV and RV and an LV thrombus (*blue arrow*) in noncompaction cardiomyopathy (*B*). HCM, hypertrophic cardiomyopathy; LV, left ventricle; RV, right ventricle; VS, ventricular septum.

modality alone (including CMR) can diagnose ARVC.[53] However, CMR evidence of LV involvement is a strong independent predictor of cardiac events in patients with a definite, borderline or possible ARVC diagnosis[54,55] (see **Table 5**).

Other Nonischemic Cardiomyopathies

The RV may also be affected in other nonischemic cardiomyopathies, in which CMR allows early detection of RV involvement[1,2] (**Fig. 9**, see **Table 5**).

SUMMARY

CMR allows accurate and reproducible multiplanar anatomic and functional assessment of the RV, tissue characterization, and blood flow evaluation of the right heart and pulmonary circulation. It also adds precision to evaluation valvular heart disease and shunt severity.

CMR has shown increasing clinical utility in diagnosis, risk stratification, prognosis, and therapeutic management in disorders of the right heart and pulmonary circulation.

CLINICS CARE POINTS

- CMR is the gold standard modality for noninvasive RV imaging.
- CMR is useful in diagnosis, risk stratification, prognosis and therapeutic management in disorders of the right heart and pulmonary circulation.
- Limitations of CMR may include low availability, high cost, claustrophobia, safety in patients with ferromagnetic implants and use of gadolinium in patients with severe chronic renal failure.

DISCLOSURE

Funding: This research did not receive any specific grant from funding agencies in the public, commercial, ornot-for-profit sectors.

REFERENCES

1. Zhou X, Ferrara F, Contaldi C, et al. Right ventricular size and function in chronic heart failure: not to be forgotten. Heart Fail Clin 2019;15:205–17.
2. Sanz J, Sánchez-Quintana D, Bossone E, et al. Anatomy, function, and dysfunction of the right ventricle: JACC State-of-the-Art Review. J Am Coll Cardiol 2019;73:1463–82.
3. Konstam MA, Kiernan MS, Bernstein D, et al. Evaluation and management of right-sided heart failure: a scientific statement from the American Heart Association. Circulation 2018;137:e578–622.
4. Lang RM, Badano LP, Mor-Avi V, et al. Recommendations for cardiac chamber quantification by echocardiography in adults: an update from the American Society of Echocardiography and the European Association of Cardiovascular Imaging. J Am Soc Echocardiogr 2015;28:1–39.e14.
5. Bossone E, Dellegrottaglie S, Patel S, et al. Multimodality imaging in pulmonary hypertension. Can J Cardiol 2015;31:440–59.
6. Dellegrottaglie S, Ostenfeld E, Sanz J, et al. Imaging the right heart-pulmonary circulation unit: the role of MRI and computed tomography. Heart Fail Clin 2018;14:377–91.
7. Thiele H, Nagel E, Paetsch I, et al. Functional cardiac MR imaging with steady-state free precession (SSFP) significantly improves endocardial border delineation without contrast agents. J Magn Reson Imaging 2001;14:362–7.
8. Galiè N, Humbert M, Vachiery JL, et al, ESC Scientific Document Group. 2015 ESC/ERS Guidelines for the diagnosis and treatment of pulmonary hypertension: The Joint Task Force for the Diagnosis and Treatment

of Pulmonary Hypertension of the European Society of Cardiology (ESC) and the European Respiratory Society (ERS): Endorsed by: Association for European Paediatric and Congenital Cardiology (AEPC), International Society for Heart and Lung Transplantation (ISHLT). Eur Heart J 2016;37:67–119.

9. Swift AJ, Rajaram S, Condliffe R, et al. Diagnostic accuracy of cardiovascular magnetic resonance imaging of right ventricular morphology and function in the assessment of suspected pulmonary hypertension results from the ASPIRE registry. J Cardiovasc Magn Reson 2012;14:40.

10. Karakus G, Zencirci E, Degirmencioglu A, et al. Easily measurable, noninvasive, and novel finding for pulmonary hypertension: hypertrophy of the basal segment of septomarginal trabeculation of right ventricle. Echocardiography 2017;34: 290–5.

11. Dellegrottaglie S, Sanz J, Poon M, et al. Pulmonary hypertension: accuracy of detection with left ventricular septal-to-free wall curvature ratio measured at cardiac MR. Radiology 2007;243:63–9.

12. Reiter G, Reiter U, Kovacs G, et al. Magnetic resonance-derived 3-dimensional blood flow patterns in the main pulmonary artery as a marker of pulmonary hypertension and a measure of elevated mean pulmonary arterial pressure. Circ Cardiovasc Imaging 2008;1:23–30.

13. Sanz J, Kuschnir P, Rius T, et al. Pulmonary arterial hypertension: noninvasive detection with phase-contrast MR imaging. Radiology 2007;243:70–9.

14. Swift AJ, Rajaram S, Condliffe R, et al. Pulmonary artery relative area change detects mild elevations in pulmonary vascular resistance and predicts adverse outcome in pulmonary hypertension. Invest Radiol 2012;47:571–7.

15. Bradlow WM, Assomull R, Kilner PJ, et al. Understanding late gadolinium enhancement in pulmonary hypertension. Circ Cardiovasc Imaging 2010;3: 501–3.

16. Freed BH, Gomberg-Maitland M, Chandra S, et al. Late gadolinium enhancement cardiovascular magnetic resonance predicts clinical worsening in patients with pulmonary hypertension. J Cardiovasc Magn Reson 2012;1:14.

17. Van Wolferen SA, Marcus JT, Boonstra A, et al. Prognostic value of right ventricular mass, volume, and function in idiopathic pulmonary arterial hypertension. Eur Heart J 2007;28:1250–7.

18. Hagger D, Condliffe R, Woodhouse N, et al. Ventricular mass index correlates with pulmonary artery pressure and predicts survival in suspected systemic sclerosis-associated pulmonary arterial hypertension. Rheumatology 2009;48:1137–42.

19. van de Veerdonk MC, Kind T, Marcus J, et al. Progressive right ventricular dysfunction in patients with pulmonary arterial hypertension responding to therapy. J Am Coll Cardiol 2011;58:2511–9.

20. Baggen VJ, Leiner T, Post MC, et al. Cardiac magnetic resonance findings predicting mortality in patients with pulmonary arterial hypertension: a systematic review and meta-analysis. Eur Radiol 2016;26:3771–80.

21. Sato T, Tsujinog I, Oyama-Manabe N, et al. Right atrial volume and phasic function in pulmonary hypertension. Int J Cardiol 2013;168:420–6.

22. Bredfelt A, Rådegran G, Hesselstrand R, et al. Increased right atrial volume measured with cardiac magnetic resonance is associated with worse clinical outcome in patients with pre-capillary pulmonary hypertension. ESC Heart Fail 2018;5:864–75.

23. Gan CT, Lankhaar JW, Westerhof N, et al. Noninvasively assessed pulmonary artery stiffness predicts mortality in pulmonary arterial hypertension. Chest 2007;132:1906–12.

24. Swift AJ, Rajaram S, Capener D, et al. LGE patterns in pulmonary hypertension do not impact overall mortality. JACC Cardiovasc Imaging 2014;7: 1209–17.

25. van Wolferen SA, Boonstra A, Marcus JT, et al. Right ventricular reverse remodeling after sildenafil in pulmonary arterial hypertension. Heart 2006;92: 1860–1.

26. Moon JC, Messroghli DR, Kellman P, et al. Society for Cardiovascular Magnetic Resonance Imaging; Cardiovascular Magnetic Resonance Working Group of the European Society of Cardiology. Myocardial T1 mapping and extracellular volume quantification: a Society for Cardiovascular Magnetic Resonance (SCMR) and CMR Working Group of the European Society of Cardiology consensus statement. J Cardiovasc Magn Reson 2013;15:92.

27. Spruijt OA, Vissers L, Bogaard HJ, et al. Increased native T1-values at the interventricular insertion regions in precapillary pulmonary hypertension. Int J Cardiovasc Imaging 2016;32:451–9.

28. García-Álvarez A, García-Lunar I, Pereda D, et al. Association of myocardial T1-mapping CMR with hemodynamics and RV performance in pulmonary hypertension. JACC Cardiovasc Imaging 2015;8: 76–82.

29. Shehata ML, Harouni AA, Skrok J, et al. Regional and global biventricular function in pulmonary arterial hypertension: a cardiac MR imaging study. Radiology 2013;266:114–22.

30. Menezes de Siqueira ME, Pozo E, Fernandes VR, et al. Characterization and clinical significance of right ventricular mechanics in pulmonary hypertension evaluated with cardiovascular magnetic resonance feature tracking. J Cardiovasc Magn Reson 2016;18:39.

31. Padervinskienė L, Krivickiene A, Hoppenot D, et al. Prognostic value of left ventricular function and mechanics in pulmonary hypertension: a pilot cardiovascular magnetic resonance feature tracking study. Medicina (Kaunas) 2019;55:E73.

32. Hanneman K, Kino A, Chenget JY, et al. Assessment of the precision and reproducibility of ventricular volume, function, and mass measurements with ferumoxytol-enhanced 4D Flow MRI. J Magn Reson Imaging 2016;44:383–9.

33. Reiter G, Reiter U, Kovacs G, et al. Blood flow vortices along the main pulmonary artery measured with MR imaging for diagnosis of pulmonary hypertension. Radiology 2015;275:71–9.

34. Kheyfets VO, Schafer M, Podgorski CA, et al. 4D magnetic resonance flow imaging for estimating pulmonary vascular resistance in pulmonary hypertension. J Magn Reson Imaging 2016;44:914–22.

35. Garcia J, Barker AJ, Markl M. The role of imaging of flow patterns by 4D Flow MRI in aortic stenosis. JACC Cardiovasc Imaging 2019;12:252–66.

36. van Ooij P, Allen BD, Contaldi C, et al. 4D flow MRI and T1-mapping: assessment of altered cardiac hemodynamics and extracellular volume fraction in hypertrophic cardiomyopathy. J Magn Reson Imaging 2016;43:107–14.

37. Barker AJ, Roldan-Alzate A, Entezari P, et al. Four-dimensional flow assessment of pulmonary artery flow and wall shear stress in adult pulmonary arterial hypertension: results from two institutions. Magn Reson Med 2015;73:1904–13.

38. Truong U, Fonseca B, Dunning J, et al. Wall shear stress measured by phase contrast cardiovascular magnetic resonance in children and adolescents with pulmonary arterial hypertension. J Cardiovasc Magn Reson 2013;15:81.

39. Han QJ, Witschey WRT, Fang-Yen CM, et al. Altered right ventricular kinetic energy work density and viscous energy dissipation in patients with pulmonary arterial hypertension: a pilot study using 4D flow MRI. PLoS One 2015;10:e0138365.

40. Itatani K, Miyazaki S, Furusawa T, et al. New imaging tools in cardiovascular medicine: computational fluid dynamics and 4D flow MRI. Gen Thorac Cardiovasc Surg 2017;65:611–21.

41. Tang BT, Pickard SS, Chan FP, et al. Wall shear stress is decreased computational fluid dynamics study. Pulm Circ 2012;2:470–6.

42. La Gerche A, Claessen G, Van de Bruaene A, et al. Cardiac MRI: a new gold standard for ventricular volume quantification during high-intensity exercise. Circ Cardiovasc Imaging 2013;6:329–38.

43. Göransson C, Vejlstrup N, Carlsen J. Exercise cardiovascular magnetic resonance imaging allows differentiation of low-risk pulmonary arterial hypertension. J Heart Lung Transplant 2019;38:627–35.

44. Knight DS, Kotecha T, Martinez-Naharro A, et al. Cardiovascular magnetic resonance-guided right heart catheterization in a conventional CMR environment—predictors of procedure success and duration in pulmonary artery hypertension. J Cardiovasc Magn Reson 2019;21:57.

45. Ratnayaka K, Faranesh AZ, Hansen MS, et al. Real-time MRI-guided right heart catheterization in adults using passive catheters. Eur Heart J 2013;34:380–9.

46. Rajiah P, Nazarian J, Vogelius E, et al. CT and MRI of pulmonary valvular abnormalities. Clin Radiol 2014;69:630–8.

47. Garcia MJ. Evaluation of valvular heart disease by cardiac magnetic resonance and computed tomography. In: Otto CM, Bonow RO, editors. Valvular heart disease: a companion to Braunwald's heart disease. 4th edition. Philadelphia: Elsevier; 2014. p. 109–12.

48. Cavalcante JL, von Knobelsdor F, Myerson S. Valve Disease. In: Lombardi M, Plain S, Petersen S, et al, editors. The EACVI textbook of cardiovascular magnetic resonance. 1st edition. Oxford: Oxford University Press; 2018. p. 444–54.

49. Khalique OK, Cavalcante JL, Shah D, et al. Multimodality imaging of the tricuspid valve and right heart anatomy. JACC Cardiovasc Imaging 2019;12:516–31.

50. Martin-Garcia AC, Dimopoulos K, Boutsikou M, et al. Tricuspid regurgitation severity after atrial septal defect closure or pulmonic valve replacement. Heart 2020;106:455–61.

51. Di Salvo G, Miller O, Babu Narayan S, et al. 2016–2018 EACVI Scientific Documents Committee. Imaging the adult with congenital heart disease: a multimodality imaging approach-position paper from the EACVI. Eur Heart J Cardiovasc Imaging 2018;19:1077–98.

52. Masci PG, Francone M, Desmet W, et al. Right ventricular ischemic injury in patients with acute ST-segment elevation myocardial infarction: characterization with cardiovascular magnetic resonance. Circulation 2010;122:1405–12.

53. Marcus FI, McKenna WJ, Sherrill D, et al. Diagnosis of arrhythmogenic right ventricular cardiomyopathy/dysplasia: proposed modification of the Task Force Criteria. Eur Heart J 2010;31:806–14.

54. Basso C, Bauce B, Corrado D, et al. Pathophysiology of arrhythmogenic cardiomyopathy. Nat Rev Cardiol 2011;9:223–33.

55. Haugaa KH, Basso C, Badano LP, et al. EACVI Scientific Documents Committee, EACVI Board members and external reviewers; EACVI Scientific Documents Committee, EACVI Board members and external reviewers. Comprehensive multimodality imaging approach in arrhythmogenic cardiomyopathy—an expert consensus document of the European Association of Cardiovascular Imaging. Eur Heart J Cardiovasc Imaging 2017;18:237–53.

Cardiovascular Magnetic Resonance of Myocardial Fibrosis, Edema, and Infiltrates in Heart Failure

Kate Liang, MBBCh[a,b], Anna Baritussio, MD, PhD[c],
Alberto Palazzuoli, MD, PhD[d], Matthew Williams, MBChB, BSc[a,b],
Estefania De Garate, MD[a,b], Iwan Harries, MBBCh, BSc[a,b],
Chiara Bucciarelli-Ducci, MD, PhD[a,b,e],*

KEYWORDS

- Cardiac MRI • Tissue characterisation • Mapping • Gadolinium enhancement • Myocardial edema
- Myocardial fibrosis

KEY POINTS

- Cardiac magnetic resonance (CMR) is a unique imaging modality for noninvasive tissue characterization.
- Distribution patterns of myocardial edema and fibrosis guide the differential diagnosis and aid the identification of the underlying condition.
- Novel CMR techniques of parametric mapping increasingly are recognized and utilized as part of the diagnostic capability for tissue characterization.

INTRODUCTION

Cardiac magnetic resonance (CMR) is a novel and unique imaging tool providing noninvasive tissue characterization. In particular, it can assess the presence and extent of myocardial fibrosis, edema, and infiltrates of various etiologies. The ability to assess etiology based on various imaging sequences demonstrates the noninvasive diagnostic capability of cardiac magnetic resonance imaging (MRI), which is particularly relevant in heart failure patients.

Different types of sequences are employed to image these different aspects of myocardial composition. Typically, the CMR test begins with anatomic and functional cine imaging using a steady-state free precession sequence, providing information on the size of the cardiac chambers as well as the regional and global function of the left and right ventricles and valve assessment. T2-weighted imaging is added to assess the presence and extent of myocardial edema or inflammation, typically using a short tau inversion recovery sequence (STIR). Tissue characterization for myocardial fibrosis is achieved with a T1-weighted sequence after the administration of a gadolinium-chelate contrast agent (GBCA). This technique can image infarct fibrosis, replacement fibrosis, and infiltration.

[a] Department of Cardiology, Bristol Heart Institute, University Hospitals Bristol and Weston NHS Foundation Trust, Bristol, UK; [b] Bristol Medical School, Translational Health Sciences, University of Bristol, Bristol, UK; [c] Department of Cardiac, Thoracic, Vascular Sciences and Public Health, University Hospital Padua, Padua, Italy; [d] Cardiovascular Diseases Unit, Department of Internal Medicine, Le Scotte Hospital, University of Siena, Siena 53100, Italy; [e] Bristol National Institute of Health Research (NIHR) Centre University of Bristol and University Hospitals Bristol NHS Foundation Trust, Bristol, UK
* Corresponding author. Department of Cardiology, Bristol Heart Institute, University Hospitals Bristol and Weston NHS Foundation Trust, Bristol, UK.
E-mail address: C.bucciarelli-ducci@bristol.ac.uk

The newer CMR relaxometry techniques, such as T1 mapping, T2 mapping, and extracellular volume (ECV), add a semiquantitative dimension to the assessment of myocardial fibrosis and edema. Uniquely, ECV allows the determination of interstitial myocardial fibrosis. These sequences are available for both 1.5T and 3.0T scanners.

These sequences are described and the imaging patterns relevant for clinical practice focused on. The advantages and disadvantages of each technique are appraised briefly and related each to common etiologies of heart failure with their associated patterns of myocardial edema, fibrosis, and infiltrates.

IMAGING MYOCARDIAL EDEMA

Edema can be imaged using T2-weighted imaging sequences. T2-weighted (T2-STIR) is the sequence used most commonly to image myocardial edema and inflammation. It is a breath-held black-blood segmented turbo spin-echo technique using triple inversion-recovery preparation module to suppress signal from flowing blood and fat.[1] On CMR, it is used to identify myocyte swelling and interstitial edema. The T2 sequences need to be acquired before the administration of GBCA, which not only shortens the T1 properties of the myocardium but also alters its T2 properties.

It is important, therefore, to adequately protocol each clinical request to include T2 imaging (when indicated) prior to contrast administration, if relevant to the clinical question.

It is an important technique to help differentiate between acute and chronic infarction, to identify the area at risk (AAR),[2,3] and to determine the acute phase of nonischemic processes, such as acute versus chronic myocarditis and acute versus chronic sarcoidosis.[1]

There are alternative sequences to image myocardial edema and inflammation. Acquisition for cardiac unified T2 edema imaging is a hybrid turbo spin-echo SSFP pulse sequence that does not require a black-blood preparation or a T2 preparation.[4] This combination of sequences into 1 imaging sequence leads to better differentiation of edema whilst delineating blood-pool and myocardium in acute infarctions.

The newer T2 mapping increasingly is recognized and utilized in clinical practice and guidelines.[5,6] It is a balanced SSFP breath-held technique allowing direct quantification of myocardial inflammation and edema, overcoming the limitations of T2-STIR and other sequences, such as blood pooling and loss of signal due to cardiac movement during acquisition. Images are formed in a pixel-related color map with a color scale indicating the different T2 values.

Early gadolinium enhancement (EGE) is a breath-held gradient-echo sequence usually acquired 1 minute to 3 minutes after administration of GBCA.[7] EGE demonstrates hyperemia, which is a marker of acute inflammation. EGE images, however, also are useful to identify states of markedly reduced or absent perfusion, such as microvascular obstruction in the context of acute myocardial infarction, or the presence of intracavity thrombus, both entities appearing as hypoenhanced areas.[8]

A comparative study of 4 available methods to imaging myocardial edema has concluded that T2 mapping is the most reproducible method.[9]

Validation of Cardiac Magnetic Resonance in Myocardial Edema Imaging

The ability of CMR to detect myocardial edema has been validated against histology. Kim and colleagues[10] demonstrated that in vivo measurement of infarct size by ^{23}Na-MRI correlated with triphenyl tetrazolium chloride staining, with increases in Na$^+$ levels secondary to myocardial ischemia and to edema-related extracellular space expansion. More recently, T2-weighted sequences and contrast-enhanced cine-SSFP sequences for the measurement of the AAR and final infarct size showed comparable results to histologic analysis with Evan blue dye and triphenyl tetrazolium chloride staining, respectively.[11] It also has been shown that the AAR measured by fluorescent microspheres at the time of coronary occlusion in an animal model correlated with the size of increased signal intensity on T2-weighted imaging.[12] Finally, in a human study on acute myocardial infarction, myocardium at risk as measured on T2-weighted images correlated with that measured on single-photon emission computed tomography performed early after reperfusion.[13]

IMAGING MYOCARDIAL FIBROSIS AND INFILTRATES

Myocardial fibrosis and infiltrates are defined most commonly with T1-weighted imaging post-GBCA administration. Imaging of fibrosis is important because it often conveys relevant information in disease prognostication.[14]

Late gadolinium enhancement (LGE) imaging is performed 5 minutes to 15 minutes after administration of GBCAs. It is a major part of tissue characterization on CMR. Gadolinium-chelate contrast is an extracellular agent that accumulates in abnormal myocardium where extracellular space has increased due to pathology. The accumulation of GBCAs shortens T1-values leading to higher signal on T1-weighted images. Because washout of the contrast agent from abnormal myocardium is delayed, these areas re-enhance and appear bright. The patterns of LGE, alongside edema imaging, can differentiate between ischemic and nonischemic pathology. Ischemic etiologies typically show subendocardial to transmural enhancement, reflecting the wavefront of the ischemic damage. Midmyocardial or subepicardial patterns are hallmarks of nonischemic pathologies of different etiologies.[15]

Fibrosis imaging in both ischemic and nonischemic pathology is advanced further by the inclusion of CMR relaxometry techniques, namely T1-mapping[16,17] and ECV. There are various sequences available to perform T1 mapping and ECV, with the majority utilizing single shot balanced SSFP imaging. The most common method for T1-mapping is the modified Look-Locker inversion recovery (MOLLI) sequence.[18] Other available sequences include saturation recovery single-shot acquisition[19] and a shortened sequence (ShMOLLI),[20] which allows quicker acquisition of data without a detrimental impact on image quality. ECV is calculated as the ratio of native (precontract) T1-mapping and postcontrast T1 mapping, which is a validated surrogate marker for interstitial fibrosis[21] Blood hematocrit needs to be included in the ECV formula in order to correct for the red blood cell density in the blood pool, but recent research suggested novel methods of synthetic hematocrit allowing ECV calculations without the need for serum blood haematocrit.[22,23]

Diffuse infiltrative processes also will prolong T1 values and, therefore, the specificity of T1 mapping in these scenarios is reduced.[7]

T2* imaging is a multiecho gradient-echo sequence used at 1.5T and best performed with dark-blood sequences.[24,25] It is used most commonly for assessment of iron loading and is performed with a single breath-hold.[26,27] Simultaneous evaluation of the liver and myocardium can be done allowing assessment of both hepatic and myocardial iron loading. This should be performed only on 1.5T scanning with a 3-tier grading system.[28] Reference to prior scans should be made in order to assess serial measurements.

Validation of Cardiac Magnetic Resonance in Imaging Myocardial Fibrosis

CMR fibrosis imaging techniques have been widely validated with recognition of its importance in disease prognostication.[29] Histologic correlation of ischemic scar and LGE on CMR has been demonstrated in both animal and human studies and compares favorably against SPECT.[13,30–32] CMR has demonstrated both histologic correlation and clinical validity in both ischemic and nonischemic pathologies[33,34] with the use of CMR fibrosis imaging being explored in valvular heart disease.[35] The advent of T1-mapping techniques provides additional diagnostic quantification of myocardial fibrosis in nonischemic pathologies with increasing recognition of its relevance and validity in clinical practice.[36–38]

CLINICAL PATTERNS OF DISEASE

The unique capability of tissue characterization by CMR can aid differential diagnosis of etiologies of heart failure. These can be separated into ischemic and nonischemic with specific patterns recognized in each. The combination of both T2-weighted and T1-weighted imaging helps identifying diagnosis as well as the chronicity of disease.

Edema is a hallmark of an acute myocardial insult, with fibrosis more reflective of a chronic process. Edema usually resolves within 3 months, both in ischemic and nonischemic etiologies.[39] The presence of fibrosis in different heart failure etiologies often is correlated with poorer prognosis.

Features of both edema and fibrosis imaging are summarized in **Fig. 1**. Cardiovascular diseases and patterns of recognition of myocardial edema and fibrosis are summarized briefly but addressed specifically in the other contributions to this issue.

Ischemic Conditions

As discussed in the Aneesh S. Dhore-Patil and Ashish Aneja's article, "Role of Cardiovascular Magnetic Resonance in Ischemic Cardiomyopathy," section of this issue, ischemic patterns of LGE follow the ischemic wavefront, with subendocardial or transmural enhancement, in cases of full-thickness myocardial infarction.[15] The subendocardial predominance is unique to ischemic damage and generally not seen in nonischemic etiologies of heart failure, with the exception of amyloidosis and endomyocardial fibrosis.

Nonischemic Conditions

Myocarditis
Imaging in acute myocarditis demonstrates edema with increased myocardial signal on T2-weighted imaging, which is the most used method. Generally, edema changes in acute myocarditis follow a noncoronary distribution with a subepicardial/midwall predominance. It often is seen in the lateral wall[40] but may be seen in up to 70% of

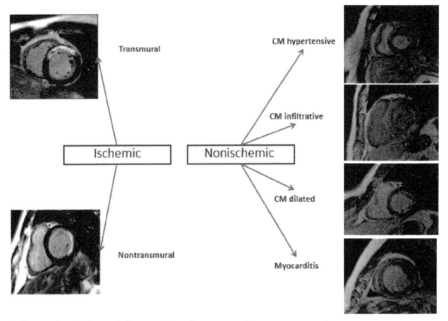

Fig. 1. Clinical scenarios of heart failure and cardiac magnetic resonance patterns.

patients as a diffuse pattern, particularly on T2-mapping. New diagnostic criteria for acute myocarditis require 1 T1-weighted and 1 T2-weighted criterion to be met, either by standard weighted sequences or by the newer mapping techniques.[6] Chronic myocarditis typically is characterized by the absence of edema on T2-weighted imaging.

Takotsubo cardiomyopathy

CMR has a pivotal role in differentiating takotsubo cardiomyopathy (TCM) from acute myocarditis and acute coronary syndrome, in particular in cases of myocardial infarction with nonobstructed coronary arteries.[41] The presence of significant myocardial edema and absence of myocardial scarring on LGE sequences in TCM is a main differentiating marker from acute coronary syndrome. In the acute phase, edema commonly presents a circumferential pattern with mid to apical predominance and associated regional wall motion abnormalities. Subtle late enhancement, although not often seen, may be present with a patchy appearance; this represents expanded interstitial space due to edema.[42]

Because TCM generally is recognized as a reversible cardiomyopathy, the chronic phase of this pathology should demonstrate a resolution in edema with no evidence of myocardial scarring. Persistent edema extending beyond 3 months, however, has been reported and associated with a more unfavorable outcome, particularly in the context of arrhythmic presentation.[43,44]

Sarcoidosis

CMR has been recognized to aid prognostication and risk stratification in patients with sarcoidosis, with LGE a predictor of mortality.[45] LGE usually is seen in the midmyocardium or subepicardium with a patchy appearance.[46,47] This pattern is observed most commonly in the basal septum or lateral wall. It can, however, mimic an ischemic pattern, not following a coronary distribution, with transmural infiltrations and wall thinning.

Amyloidosis

CMR is the imaging modality of choice clearly identifying structural and physiologic features of cardiac amyloidosis.[48] Tissue characterization from CMR can mitigate the need for high-risk invasive tissue biopsy and has an important role in diagnosis and prognosis in patients with cardiac amyloidosis.

The inability to sufficiently null the myocardium reflects abnormal myocardial and blood-pool gadolinium kinetics due to the accumulation of amyloid in the heart. There usually is a global endocardial LGE although transmural enhancement can be seen. The latter is seen more commonly in hereditary transthyretin (ATTR) amyloid compared with primary amyloidosis and infers a poorer prognosis with higher mortality rates.[49]

Hemochromatosis

CMR is the gold standard for noninvasive measurement of myocardial iron deposition, which preferentially occurs in the subepicardium. Current accepted practice requires a single mid–left ventricular T2*-weighted short axis slice with a region of interest over the septum to reduce susceptibility artifact.[50] Long-term surveillance and serial assessments are important because detection of changes on T2* imaging determine adjustments to ongoing treatment.[51,52]

Storage diseases

Use of CMR is an important tool in storage diseases to identify presence of fibrosis. LGE in Anderson-Fabry disease commonly is seen in the midmyocardial inferolateral wall and corresponding low native T1 values on native T1 mapping in areas of fat deposits without LGE.[53,54]

Transplant disease

Among cardiac transplant patients, 24% have acute rejection within the first year of surgery.[55] Although endomyocardial biopsy remains the gold standard for diagnosing acute rejection in a transplanted heart, it requires an invasive procedure and can be complicated by life-threatening events, such as cardiac tamponade and arrhythmias.

A global subendocardial pattern is observed with LGE imaging post–cardiac transplant but a diffuse patchy LGE pattern is seen in both acute and chronic rejection. Current literature suggests that combination of T1-weighted and T2-weighted imaging techniques, including parametric mapping, can assess and diagnose the presence of acute rejection accurately.[56] Elevated signal on T2-mapping in acute rejection is in keeping with myocardial edema,[57] whereas expansion of the extracellular space, resulting in fibrosis, is reflected by increased T1 and ECV values. The tissue characterization achieved by CMR is invaluable in assessing long-term function in cardiac transplant patients and limiting the need for repeated endomyocardial biopsy.

LIMITATIONS OF IMAGING MYOCARDIAL EDEMA, FIBROSIS, AND INFILTRATES

Although CMR often is considered the imaging modality of choice for many of the conditions discussed, it does, however, have some limitations. Patients with heart failure may present acutely or as part of their chronic management. Depending on the severity of their disease, image acquisition may be limited by their ability to lie supine and relatively still for accurate image quality. CMR techniques require breath-holding and this may be difficult for those who are symptomatic with dyspnea or have significant fluid overload, which may preclude this.

Although techniques can be applied to minimize scanning time, these inadvertently reduce image quality. Heart rate is an important factor that could affect image quality, particularly atrial fibrillation. Free breathing and real time are techniques that can facilitate imaging acquisition in patients with limited breath-holding abilities but image quality and precision of the measurements (in particular, volumes and ejection fraction) are reduced.

Magnetic resonance conditional cardiac devices, in particular pacemakers and implantable cardioverter defibrillators, have expanded the indication of CMR in these patients. Recent evidence suggests that even patients with legacy (the non–magnetic resonance–conditional) devices no longer are contraindications for MRI and that these patients can be scanned safely.[58]

SUMMARY

CMR is an invaluable tool for the diagnosis of heart failure given its noninvasive tissue characterization ability to identify the underlying etiologies of heart failure. It provides specific and sensitive information to allow differentiation between ischemic and nonischemic cardiomyopathies. Novel imaging techniques are improving the ability to image patients with heart failure and improve diagnostic accuracy. Finally, the CMR imaging findings not only facilitate the identification of the underlying diagnosis but allow robust prognostication of patients with heart failure.

FUNDING

C. Bucciarelli-Ducci is in part supported by the NIHR Bristol Biomedical Research Centre at the University of Bristol, United Kingdom; University Hospitals Bristol and Weston NHS Foundation Trust, Bristol, United Kingdom. The views expressed in this publication are those of the author(s) and not necessarily those of the NHS, the National Institute for Health Research or the Department of Health and Social Care.

DISCLOSURE

C. Bucciarelli-Ducci is the CEO of the Society of Cardiovascular Magnetic Resonance (part-time role). The other authors have nothing to disclose.

REFERENCES

1. Francone M, Carbone I, Agati L, et al. Utility of T2-weighted short-tau inversion recovery (STIR) sequences in cardiac MRI: an overview of clinical applications in ischemic and non-ischemic heart disease. Radiol Med 2011;116(1):32–46.

2. Friedrich MG, Abdel-Aty H, Taylor A, et al. The salvaged area at risk in reperfused acute myocardial infarction as visualized by cardiovascular magnetic resonance. J Am Coll Cardiol 2008;51:1581–7.

3. Kitabata H, Imanishi T, Kubo T, et al. Coronary microvascular resistance index immediately after primary percutaneous coronary intervention as a predictor of the transmural extent of infarction in patients with ST segment elevation anterior acute myocardial infarction. JACC Cardiovasc Imaging 2009;2(3):263–72.

4. Aletras AH, Kellman P, Derbyshire JA, et al. ACUT2E TSE-SSFP: a hybrid method for T2-weighted imaging of edema in the heart. Magn Reson Med 2008; 59(2):229–35.

5. Giri S, Chung YC, Merchant A, et al. T2 quantification for improved detection of myocardial edema. J Cardiovasc Magn Reson 2009;11:56.

6. Ferreira VM, Schulz-Menger J, Holmvang G, et al. Cardiovascular magnetic resonance in nonischemic myocardial inflammation. Expert recommendations. J Am Coll Cardiol 2018;72(24):3158–76.

7. Matsumoto H, Matsuda T, Miyamoto K, et al. Peri-infarct zone on early contrast enhanced CMR imaging in patients with acute myocardial infarction. JACC Cardiovasc Imaging 2011;4(6):610–8.

8. Dastidar AG, Rodrigues JCL, Baritussio A, et al. MRI in the assessment of ischemic heart disease. Heart 2016;102(3):239–52.

9. McAlindon EJ, Pufulete M, Harris JM, et al. Measurement of myocardium at risk with cardiovascular MR: comparison of techniques for edema imaging. Radiology 2015;275(1):61–70.

10. Kim RJ, Judd RM, Chen E-L, et al. Relationship of elevated 23Na magnetic resonance image intensity to infarct size after acute reperfused myocardial infarction. Circulation 1999;100:185–92.

11. Hansen ESS, Pedersen S, Pedersen SB, et al. Validation of contrast enhanced cine steady-state free precession and T2-weighted CMR for assessment of ischemic myocardial area-at-risk in the presence of reperfusion injury. Int J Cardiovasc Imaging 2019;35:1039–45.

12. Aletras AH, Tilak GS, Natanzon A, et al. Retrospective determination of the area at risk for reperfused acute myocardial infarction with T2-weighted cardiac magnetic resonance imaging histopathological and displacement encoding with stimulated echoes (DENSE) functional validations. Circulation 2006; 113:1865–70.

13. Carlsson M, Ubachs JFA, Hedström E, et al. Myocardium at risk after acute infarction in humans on cardiac magnetic resonance: quantitative assessment during follow-up and validation with single-photon emission computed tomography. JACC Cardiovasc Imaging 2009;2:569–76.

14. Schlebert EB. Myocardial scar and fibrosis. Heart Fail Clin 2019;15(2):179–89.

15. Mahrholdt H, Wagner A, Judd RM, et al. Delayed enhancement cardiovascular magnetic resonance assessment of non-ischemic cardiomyopathies. Eur Heart J 2005;26(15):1461–74.

16. Jordan JH, Vasu S, Morgan TM, et al. Anthracycline-associated T1 mapping characteristics are elevated independent of the presence of cardiovascular co-morbidities in cancer survivors. Circ Cardiovasc Imaging 2016;9(8):e004325.

17. Dastidar AG, Harries I, Pontecorboli G, et al. Native T1 mapping to detect extent of acute and chronic myocardial infarction: comparison with late gadolinium enhancement technique. Int J Cardiovasc Imaging 2019;35(3):517–27.

18. Messroghli DR, Radjenovic A, Kozerke S, et al. Modified Look-Locker inversion recovery (MOLLI) for high resolution T1 mapping of the heart. Magn Reson Med 2004;52:141–6.

19. Chow K, Flewitt JA, Green JD, et al. Saturation recovery single-shot acquisition (SASHA) for myocardial T1 mapping. Magn Reson Med 2014;71: 2082–95.

20. Piechnik SK, Ferreira VM, Dall'Armellina E, et al. Shortened Modified Look-Locker Inversion recovery (ShMOLLI) for clinical myocardial T1-mapping at 1.5 and 3 T within a 9 heartbeat breathhold. J Cardiovasc Magn Reson 2010;12:69.

21. Miller CA, Naish JH, Bishop P, et al. Comprehensive validation of cardiovascular magnetic resonance techniques for the assessment of myocardial extracellular volume. Circ Cardiovasc Imaging 2013;6: 373–83.

22. Treibel TA, Fontana M, Maestrini V, et al. Automatic measurement of the myocardial interstitium: synthetic extracellular volume quantification without hematocrit sampling. JACC Cardiovasc Imaging 2016; 9:54–63.

23. Biesbroek PS, Amier RP, Teunissen PFA, et al. Changes in remote myocardial tissue after acute myocardial infarction and its relation to cardiac remodeling: a CMR T1 mapping study. PLoS One 2017;12:e0180115.

24. Chavhan GB, Babyn PS, Thomas B, et al. Principles, techniques, and applications of T2*-based MR imaging and its special applications. Radiographics 2009;29:1433–49.

25. Pennell DJ, Udelson JE, Arai AE, et al. Cardiovascular function and treatment in β-thalassemia major: a consensus statement from the American Heart Association. Circulation 2013;128:281–308.

26. Westwood M, Anderson LJ, Firmin DN, et al. A single breath-hold multiecho T2* cardiovascular magnetic resonance technique for diagnosis of myocardial iron overload. J Magn Reson Imaging 2003;18:33–9.

27. Anderson LJ, Holden S, Davis B, et al. Cardiovascular T2-star (T2*) magnetic resonance for the early

diagnosis of myocardial iron overload. Eur Heart J 2001;22:2171–9.

28. Kirk P, Roughton M, Porter JB, et al. Cardiac T2* magnetic resonance for prediction of cardiac complications in thalassemia major. Circulation 2009; 120:1961–8.

29. Ambale-Venkatesh B, Lima JAC. Cardiac MRI: a central prognostic tool in myocardial fibrosis. Nat Rev Cardiol 2015;12(1):18–29.

30. Kim RJ, Fieno DS, Parrish TB, et al. Relationship of MRI delayed contrast enhancement to irreversible injury, infarct age, and contractile function. Circulation 1999;100:1992–2002.

31. Kim RJ, Wu E, Rafael A, et al. The use of contrast-enhanced magnetic resonance imaging to identify reversible myocardial dysfunction. N Engl J Med 2000;343:1445–53.

32. Mahrholdt H, Wagner A, Holly TA, et al. Reproducibility of chronic infarct size measurement by contrast-enhanced magnetic resonance imaging. Circulation 2002;106(18):2322–7.

33. Mewton N, Liu CY, Croisille P, et al. Assessment of myocardial fibrosis with cardiac magnetic resonance. J Am Coll Cardiol 2011;57(8):891–903.

34. Moon JCC, Reed E, Sheppard MN, et al. The histologic basis of late gadolinium enhancement cardiovascular magnetic resonance in hypertrophic cardiomyopathy. J Am Coll Cardiol 2004;43: 2260–4.

35. Bing R, Cavalcante JL, Everett RJ, et al. Imaging and impact of myocardial fibrosis in aortic stenosis. JACC Cardiovasc Imaging 2019;12(2):283–96.

36. Iles L, Pfluger H, Phrommintikul A, et al. Evaluation of diffuse myocardial fibrosis in heart failure with cardiac magnetic resonance contrast-enhanced T1 mapping. J Am Coll Cardiol 2008;52(19):1574–80.

37. Kammerlander AA, Marzluf BA, Zotter-Tufaro C, et al. T1 mapping by CMR imaging: from histological validation to clinical implication. JACC Cardiovasc Imaging 2016;9(1):14–23.

38. Diao KY, Yang ZG, Xu HY, et al. Histologic validation of myocardial fibrosis measure by T1 mapping: a systematic review and meta-analysis. J Cardiovasc Magn Reson 2016;18(1):92.

39. Abdel-Aty H, Zagrosek A, Schulz-Menger J, et al. Delayed enhancement and T2-weighted cardiovascular magnetic resonance imaging differentiate acute from chronic myocardial infarction. Circulation 2004;109:2411–6.

40. Friedrich MG, Sechtem U, Schulz-Menger J, et al, International Consensus Group on Cardiovascular Magnetic Resonance in Myocarditis. Cardiovascular magnetic resonance in myocarditis: a JACC white paper. J Am Coll Cardiol 2009;53:1475–87.

41. Abdel-Aty H, Cocker M, Friedrich MG. Myocardial edema is a feature of Tako-Tsubo cardiomyopathy and is related to the severity of systolic dysfunction:

insights from T2-weighted cardiovascular magnetic resonance. Int J Cardiol 2009;132:291–3.

42. Haghi D, Fluechter S, Suselbeck T, et al. Cardiovascular magnetic resonance findings in typical versus atypical forms of the acute apical ballooning syndrome (Takotsubo cardiomyopathy). Int J Cardiol 2007;120(2):205–11. Elsevier.

43. Neil C, Nguyen TH, Kucia A, et al. Slowly resolving global myocardial inflammation/edema in Tako-Tsubo cardiomyopathy: evidence from T2- weighted cardiac MRI. Heart 2012;98(17):1278–84.

44. Dastidar AG, Frontera A, Palazzuoli A, et al. TakoTsubo cardiomyopathy: unravelling the malignant consequences of a benign disease with cardiac magnetic resonance. Heart Fail Rev 2015;20(4): 415–21.

45. Greulich S1, Deluigi CC, Gloekler S, et al. CMR imaging predicts death and other adverse events in suspected cardiac sarcoidosis. JACC Cardiovasc Imaging 2013;6(4):501–11.

46. Serra JJ, Monte GU, Mello ES, et al. Images in cardiovascular medicine. Cardiac sarcoidosis evaluated by delayed-enhanced magnetic resonance imaging. Circulation 2003;107(20):e188–9.

47. Vignaux O. Cardiac sarcoidosis: spectrum of MRI features. AJR Am J Roentgenol 2005;184(1):249–54.

48. Maceira AM, Joshi J, Prasad SK, et al. Cardiovascular magnetic resonance in cardiac amyloidosis. Circulation 2005;111(2):186–93.

49. Fontana M, Pica S, Reant P, et al. Prognostic value of late gadolinium enhancement cardiovascular magnetic resonance in cardiac amyloidosis. Circulation 2015;132:1570–9.

50. Messroghli DR, Moon JC, Ferreira VM, et al. Clinical recommendations for cardiovascular magnetic resonance mapping of T1, T2, T2* and extracellular volume: a consensus statement by the Society for Cardiovascular Magnetic Resonance (SCMR) endorsed by the European Association for Cardiovascular Imaging (EACVI). J Cardiovasc Magn Reson 2017;19(1):75.

51. Ptaszek LM1, Price ET, Hu MY, et al. Early diagnosis of hemochromatosis-related cardiomyopathy with magnetic resonance imaging. J Cardiovasc Magn Reson 2005;7(4):689–92.

52. Wood JC. History and current impact of cardiac magnetic resonance imaging on the management of iron overload. Circulation 2009;120: 1937–9.

53. Deva DP, Hanneman K, Li Q, et al. Cardiovascular magnetic resonance demonstration of the spectrum of morphological phenotypes and patterns of myocardial scarring in Anderson- Fabry disease. J Cardiovasc Magn Reson 2016;18:14.

54. Sado DM, White SK, Piechnik SK, et al. Identification and assessment of Anderson-Fabry disease by cardiovascular magnetic resonance noncontrast

myocardial T1 mapping. Circ Cardiovasc Imaging 2013;6(3):392–8.

55. Patel JK, Kobashigawa JA. Should we be doing routine biopsy after heart transplantation in a new era of anti-rejection? Curr Opin Cardiol 2006;21: 127–31.

56. Vermes E, Pantaléon C, Auvet A, et al. Cardiovascular magnetic resonance in heart transplant patients: diagnostic value of quantitative tissue markers: T2 mapping and extracellular volume fraction, for acute rejection diagnosis. J Cardiovasc Magn Reson 2018;20(1):59.

57. Olymbios M, Kwiecinski J, Berman DS, et al. Imaging in heart transplant patients. JACC Cardiovasc Imaging 2018;11(10):1514–30.

58. Nazarian S, Hansford R, Rahsepar AA, et al. Safety of magnetic resonance imaging in patients with cardiac devices. N Engl J Med 2017;377:2555–64.

Magnetic Resonance-Based Characterization of Myocardial Architecture

David E. Sosnovik, MD[a,b,c],*

KEYWORDS

- Myocardium • Microstructure • Diffusion tensor • Magnetic resonance • Tractography
- Cellular architecture • Heart

INTRODUCTION

The fractional shortening of an adult cardiomyocyte in vitro is less than 15%. It has been postulated that this value may reflect the loss of normal loading conditions, but similar values have been obtained in vivo.[1] Interestingly, this degree of shortening cannot produce the level of strain seen in the heart if its myocytes are modeled into simple radial, circumferential, or longitudinal patterns. Moreover, although the primary eigenvector (preferred direction) of myocardial strain is radial,[2] there are no radially oriented cardiomyocytes in the heart.[3] Two fundamental questions thus arise: How does the arrangement of cardiomyocytes in the heart amplify the level of their fractional shortening to produce a far greater change in myocardial strain and, in the absence of radial cardiomyocytes, how does their contraction result in yield in the radial direction?[4]

Dissection and histologic examination of the heart have provided important insights. It has been established for over 50 years that the cardiomyocytes in the heart are arranged in a crossing double-helical pattern.[5] Myocytes in the subepicardium have a negative or left-handed helix angle, those in the subendocardium a positive or right-handed helix angle, whereas those in the midmyocardium are circumferential.[3,5] These

observations have been confirmed in numerous studies using diffusion tensor MRI of excised hearts,[6,7] and more recently in the human heart in vivo (**Fig. 1**).[8] Interestingly this microstructural pattern is already present in the human heart by the middle of the second trimester and is highly conserved across mammalian species (**Fig. 2**).[9] Although histology remains of major value, it does not allow the microstructure of the heart to be examined dynamically and under physiologic loading conditions and, unlike MRI, it does not easily support three-dimensional analysis of tissue architecture.

Several tools have been developed to image the 3D microstructure of the heart with microscopic resolution, including phase based x-ray tomography,[10] optical coherence tractography,[11] and microscopy of optically cleared sections of the myocardium.[12] These techniques have confirmed the observations previously made with histology and ex vivo diffusion tensor MRI (DTI), although the physical basis of the techniques is very different. Computed tomography and optical-based approaches exploit the anisotropy of image intensity to create a structure tensor, in which the gradient is lowest along the axis of cardiomyocyte orientation and highest orthogonal to it. Diffusion MRI techniques, in contrast, measure the physical diffusion of water in a tissue.[13] When this is

Funding: Funded in part by the following grants to D.E. Sosnovik from the National Institutes of Health: R01HL141563, R01HL112831.

[a] Cardiology Division, Cardiovascular Research Center, Massachusetts General Hospital, Harvard Medical School, Boston, MA, USA; [b] Department of Radiology, Athinoula A. Martinos Center for Biomedical Imaging, Massachusetts General Hospital, Harvard Medical School, Boston, MA, USA; [c] Division of Health Sciences and Technology, Harvard Medical School and Massachusetts Institute of Technology, Cambridge, MA, USA
* 149 13th Street, Charlestown, MA 02129.
E-mail address: sosnovik@nmr.mgh.harvard.edu

Heart Failure Clin 17 (2021) 85–101
https://doi.org/10.1016/j.hfc.2020.08.007
1551-7136/21/© 2020 The Author. Published by Elsevier Inc. This is an open access article under the CC BY-NC-ND license (http://creativecommons.org/licenses/by-nc-nd/4.0/).

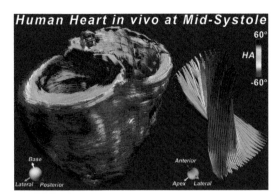

Fig. 1. Cardiomyocyte orientation streamline (COST) tractography of the human heart in vivo. The tracts have been color-coded by the cardiomyocyte helix angle, which ranges from approximately 60° in the subendocardium to −60° in the subepicardium. A magnified view of COST tracts in the lateral wall of the heart is provided in the inset. The COSTs in the midmyocardium are circumferential but in the subendocardium and subepicardium they have a significant longitudinal component and cross over each other with an angle of approximately 120°. (*From* Mekkaoui C, Reese TG, Jackowski MP, et al. Diffusion tractography of the entire left ventricle by using free-breathing accelerated simultaneous multisection imaging. Radiology. 2017;282(3):850–6; with permission.)

unrestricted by the tissue's microstructure the resulting diffusion profile follows a 3D Gaussian pattern. This is not the case in the heart, where diffusion is highly restricted by the cardiomyocyte cell membrane and its intracellular contents. Consequently, diffusion is highest along the long axis of cardiomyocte orientation and lowest orthogonal to it.

The diffusion of water in the heart is detected with motion-sensitizing magnetic gradients (**Fig. 3**).[14,15] When these are applied in the direction of diffusion the signal is attenuated by e^{-bD}, where D is the diffusion coefficient of the tissue and the b value is the strength of diffusion encoding. In the heart a b value of 500 s/mm² is most frequently used. A plot of the natural log (ln) of signal attenuation versus b value is predictably linear with 2 important deviations. At very low b values (<100 s/mm²) the signal is lower than expected due to the effects of intravoxel incoherent motion (IVIM),[16,17] which reflects diffusion and the convective flow of protons in the intravascular compartment of the heart. Conversely, at high b values (>1000 s/mm²) the signal is larger than expected and is best characterized by a diffusion kurtosis model. The description of IVIM and diffusion kurtosis imaging is beyond the scope of this review, where we confine the discussion to the

linear range of the diffusion regime. The interested reader is also referred to previous reviews on diffusion MRI, which complement the present one.[14,15]

TRANSLATIONAL MOTION

The application of diffusion-encoding gradients sensitizes the protons in the heart to motion due to translation, convection/flow, and diffusion. Moreover, the level of physical translation in the beating heart is several orders of magnitude greater than the diffusion coefficient of protons in the heart. In vivo diffusion imaging strategies must therefore be tailored to eliminate the effects of translation and convection, and isolate the effects of diffusion. The impact of convective flow in the capillary compartment can be eliminated by using a reference image with a low, rather than zero, b value and with the IVIM approach mentioned above. It should be noted, however, that capillaries and cardiomyocytes are highly aligned and the motion of protons in a capillary thus likely reflects the orientation of the adjacent cardiomyocytes.

Two strategies have been developed to eliminate the impact of translation on the diffusion signal (see **Fig. 3**). The first involves the use of a diffusion-encoded stimulated echo (STE) sequence,[18,19] which is inherently compensated for all moments of bulk motion. The second strategy involves the design of diffusion-encoding gradients that are compensated specifically for constant velocity (M1)[20,21] and acceleration (M2).[22–24] The M1/M2-compensated diffusion-encoding gradients are used with a spin echo, rather than STE, refocusing scheme. The readout used for in vivo diffusion imaging has to be rapid to minimize motion artifacts as well as the decay of transverse magnetization, which is far more rapid in the heart than the brain. The vast majority of studies have used single-shot echo-planar imaging readouts, although recent data suggest that spiral readouts may hold significant promise as well.[25]

DIFFUSION-ENCODING SCHEME

The STE and spin echo (SE) approaches both have advantages and limitations. The principal advantage of the STE approach lies in the ability to run the sequence on a scanner with standard gradients (40–45 mT/m), including those with wide bores (70 cm). The sequence also has a shorter echo time (TE), which limits distortion in certain segments of the heart, such as the lateral wall. The principal disadvantage of the STE approach lies in its low signal-to-noise ratio and consequent

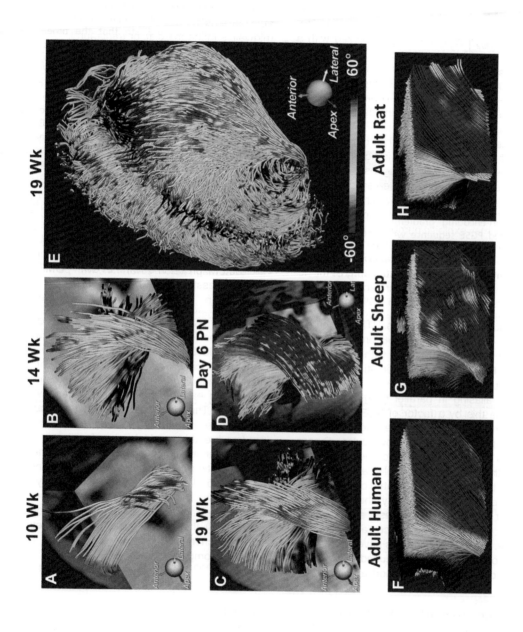

10 Wk

14 Wk

19 Wk

Day 6 PN

19 Wk

Adult Human

Adult Sheep

Adult Rat

Anterior Lateral Apex

60°

-60°

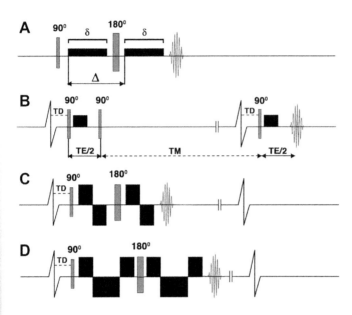

Fig. 3. Pulse sequences for diffusion MRI of the heart. The diffusion-encoding gradients are represented by black rectangles (rise and fall times are ignored), TD is the trigger delay, TE is the echo time, δ is the duration of the diffusion-encoding gradient, and Δ represents the time between diffusion gradients. Breaks in the baseline of the electrocardiogram indicate that the timeline is not drawn to scale. (*A*) The pulsed gradient spin echo (PGSE) or Stejskal-Tanner sequence has monopolar diffusion-encoding gradients on either side of a 180° refocusing pulse. The sequence is extremely sensitive to motion and has a relatively long TE, but supports high-quality ex vivo imaging. (*B*) Dual-gated STE sequence, where the diffusion time equals TE/2 plus the mixing time (TM) and is thus equal to 1 RR interval. (*C*) Velocity- or M1-compensated PGSE sequence with bipolar diffusion-encoding gradients on either side of the 180° refocusing pulse. (*D*) Acceleration or M2-compensated PGSE sequence where the diffusion-encoding gradients on both sides of the refocusing pulse have a 1-2′-1 configuration. The M1 and M2 compensated PGSE sequences require systems with ultra-high gradient strengths, which allow δ and TE to be kept acceptably short. (*From* Sosnovik DE, Wang R, Dai G, Reese TG, Wedeen VJ. Diffusion MR tractography of the heart. J Cardiovasc Magn Reson. 2009;11:47; with permission.)

need for numerous breath-holds. DTI of the human heart, for example, required 96 breath-holds to cover the entire left ventricle without any slice gaps (see **Fig. 1**).[8] The implementation of simultaneous multislice imaging, using the blipped controlled aliasing in parallel imaging approach can reduce this by a factor of 3 (**Fig. 4**),[8,26] but even 32 breath-holds can be beyond the capacity of many patients with cardiovascular disease. Strategies to perform STE DTI of the heart during free-breathing have been implemented but are limited by the STE being generated over 2 successive heartbeats.[27] Consequently, these strategies have met with limited success and the STE approach remains in essence a breath-hold sequence. Most clinical studies have reduced the number of breath-holds required by limiting anatomic coverage to 1 to 3 short-axis slices.

Implementation of the SE approach requires ultra-high-performing gradients (80 mT/m), which are less widely available and also reduce bore size to 60 cm. The long duration (δ) of the diffusion-encoding gradients also lengthens the TE and can lead to distortion in the lateral wall of the heart. The principal advantage of the SE approach lies in the ability to acquire the data during free-breathing, which also facilitates more extensive anatomic coverage. Initial implementations of motion-compensated SE diffusion encoding involved M1 (velocity) compensation only.[20,21] Subsequently more sophisticated M2 (acceleration-compensated) schemes were introduced (see **Fig. 3**) that can be used with a variety of readout schemes.[22–24,28] Several studies have directly compared the STE and SE approaches.[29,30] However, some of these studies

---

Fig. 2. Ex vivo tractography of the developing and adult human heart. (*A–C*) COSTs in the lateral wall of the developing human heart at various stages of gestation. By 19 weeks the characteristic crossing pattern of the COST tracts is clear and the heart's microstructure resembles that of (*D*) a postnatal human heart (PN). (*E*) COST tractography of an entire heart at 19 weeks of gestation shows that its microstructure is maturing. (*F–H*) Ex vivo COST tractography of a small section of the lateral wall in the adult human, sheep, and rat heart, respectively, shows that the architecture of the heart is highly conserved across species. (*From* [*A–E*] Mekkaoui C, Porayette P, Jackowski MP, et al. Diffusion MRI tractography of the developing human fetal heart. PloS One. 2013;8(8):e72795; with permission; and [*F–H*] Mekkaoui C, Huang S, Chen HH, et al. Fiber architecture in remodeled myocardium revealed with a quantitative diffusion CMR tractography framework and histological validation. J Cardiovasc Magn Reson. 2012;14:70; with permission.)

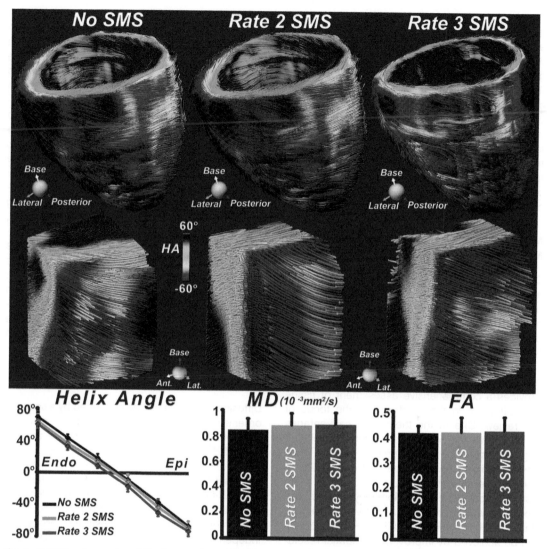

Fig. 4. COST tractography of the human heart in vivo using simultaneous multislice (SMS) excitation. Images of the entire left ventricle and a small section of tissue in the lateral wall are shown. Image quality is well preserved even at an SMS rate of 3, which allows the number of breath-holds to be reduced by a factor of 3. No significant differences are seen in the transmural slope of HA, or the values of MD and FA, between the accelerated and nonaccelerated images. (*From* Mekkaoui C, Reese TG, Jackowski MP, et al. Diffusion tractography of the entire left ventricle by using free-breathing accelerated simultaneous multisection imaging. Radiology. 2017;282(3):850–6; with permission.)

were conducted on scanners with standard gradient systems, which are inherently not suited to the SE technique, and are thus of unclear value. It is important to note that the normal values for mean diffusivity (MD) and fractional anisotropy (FA), which are both important metrics of diffusion, differ between the 2 techniques.[29,30] MD is significantly higher and FA is significantly lower with the SE approach. The reasons for this can be easily understood by examining the mechanism of diffusion sensitization in both sequences.[31]

The STE diffusion sequence consists of three 90° radiofrequency excitation pulses, applied over 2 successive heartbeats. A small diffusion-encoding gradient is applied after the first excitation pulse, and the second excitation pulse is applied TE/2 later. This begins the mixing time (TM) during which physical diffusion of the proton along its random path continues, while it is subject to T1 rather than the far more rapid process of T2 decay. The TM during an STE sequence is extremely long (1RR interval) and provides a major contribution to the b value and diffusion sensitization. In contrast, during an SE sequence diffusion encoding occurs only during the application of the diffusion-encoding gradients. Although the gradient amplitude during this time is far higher than during the STE sequence, the duration of diffusion-encoding is drastically shorter. This likely biases the detection of rapidly diffusing protons, whereas the long mixing time of the STE sequence favors the detection of more slowly diffusing protons also. Values obtained with 1 sequence in patients must, therefore, be reference to values obtained with the same sequence in healthy controls.

METRICS OF DIFFUSION AND MICROSTRUCTURE

Diffusion imaging of the heart is highly quantitative and provides both scalar metrics of tissue properties as well as vector-based indices of tissue microstructure. Several formalisms have been developed to quantify tissue diffusion, including IVIM, diffusion kurtosis imaging, and diffusion tensor imaging (DTI). The most widely used technique in the cardiovascular domain is DTI, which provides a comprehensive assessment of tissue microstructure in the heart and is the focus of this review. One of the theoretic disadvantages of DTI, however, lies in its limited spatial and angular resolution. All the metrics derived from the tensor in each voxel represent a depiction of the average diffusion in that voxel. If 2 or more distinct populations of cardiomyocytes exist in a voxel they will combine into a single average population for that voxel. Mitigation of this problem can be achieved by improving the spatial resolution of DTI, which is currently approximately $2.5 \times 2.5 \times 8 \text{ mm}^3$ in the human heart.[8] This, however, is not easily achieved since DTI is already a highly signal-to-noise constrained technique. Another approach has been to use high angular resolution techniques, such as q-ball and diffusion spectrum imaging (DSI).[32] These approaches are based on a 6-dimensional formalism (3D k-space and 3D q-space) that, with some limitations, is able to resolve multiple cardiomyocyte populations per voxel.[14] DSI may in theory be more suited to resolving highly disordered microstructure, for instance, in the border zone of an infarct (**Fig. 5**),[32] but at present is extremely challenging to perform in vivo. It should also be stressed that several studies using DTI have compared very well with late gadolinium enhancement (LGE) imaging and have provided important insights into the microstructure of the infarct, border, and remote zones (see **Fig. 5**).[6,33,34]

The most widely used scalar metrics of diffusion in the heart are its MD and FA.[13] MD provides an overall metric of the restriction of water diffusion in the heart. In areas of the myocardium with acute injury MD is increased, reflecting the lysis of cells and the increase in tissue edema.[21] Increases in MD, therefore, correlate very strongly with increases in T2 (**Fig. 6**) and further work is needed to determine whether the 2 measures provide independent diagnostic and prognostic information. FA, however, provides a unique measure of tissue microstructure based on its degree of anisotropy. Diffusion in a highly structured and anisotropic tissue, such as the myocardium, shows a strong directional dependence, which is reflected by FA. The destruction of tissue structure by infarction reduces FA,[21] and changes in tissue microstructure in infiltrative and hypertrophic cardiomyopathies can also reduce FA.[35,36] It should be noted that, like MD, FA is affected by edema resulting from acute injury and inflammation. As the edema resolves, MD will decrease and FA will increase (see **Fig. 6**),[21] providing a more accurate depiction of the underlying physical microstructure.

THE DIFFUSION TENSOR

Diffusion in a tissue can be described by a second-order symmetric tensor. Values along the diagonal of the tensor (D_{xx}, D_{yy}, and D_{zz}) describe the degree of diffusion along the principal axes (x, y, z) of the system.[14,15] The off-diagonal elements of the tensor describe the degree of correlation between diffusion in 2 directions and the elements above and below the diagonal are, therefore, equal to each other. The diffusion tensor thus contains 6 independent values and requires diffusion-encoding to be performed in a minimum of 6 independent directions, in addition to a reference image with little/no diffusion encoding. This places a fundamental lower limit on the number of heartbeats needed (and hence breath-hold duration) to acquire a single diffusion tensor dataset, 14 for STE-based sequences, and 7 for SE-based sequences. In practice more than 6 directions (10–12) are frequently acquired to over-specify the tensor, requiring fairly long breath-holds for the STE sequence.

Several key parameters can be derived from the diffusion tensor, including the principal direction of diffusion (primary eigenvector, E1) and its associated eigenvalue ($\lambda 1$). Because water diffuses most readily along the long axis of myocytes, the primary eigenvector describes the average orientation of the cardiomyocytes in that voxel.[3] In the heart, the projection of this vector out of the local radial plane has been used to define the helix angle

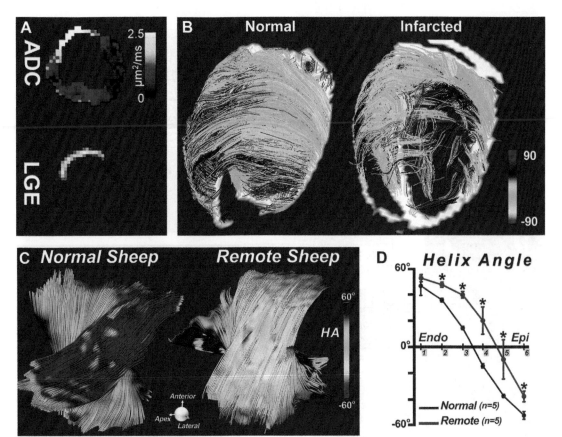

Fig. 5. Detection and characterization of chronic infarction with diffusion MRI. (*A*) Swine with 8-week-old infarct, which is well detected by measuring the apparent diffusion coefficient. (*B*) Ex vivo imaging of a chronic anterior infarct in a rat heart with diffusion spectrum imaging. A complex network of residual myofibers is found in the infarct, particularly at the border zone. (*C, D*) Microstructural remodeling in the remote zone in sheep with large anteroseptal infarcts. The COST tracts in the lateral wall (remote zone) undergo a rightward/positive shift in their orientation or helix angle. * = statistically significant. (*From* [*A*] Nguyen C, Fan Z, Xie Y, et al. In vivo contrast free chronic myocardial infarction characterization using diffusion-weighted cardiovascular magnetic resonance. J Cardiovasc Magn Reson. 2014;16(1):68; with permission; and [*B*] Sosnovik DE, Wang R, Dai G, et al. Diffusion spectrum MRI tractography reveals the presence of a complex network of residual myofibers in infarcted myocardium. Circ Cardiovasc Imaging. 2009;2(3):206–12; with permission; and [*C–D*] Mekkaoui C, Huang S, Chen HH, et al. Fiber architecture in remodeled myocardium revealed with a quantitative diffusion CMR tractography framework and histological validation. J Cardiovasc Magn Reson. 2012;14:70; with permission.)

(HA) of a cardiomyocyte (**Fig. 7**).[6] In most species this angle ranges from approximately 60° in the subendocardium to approximately −60° in the subepicardium. The secondary eigenvector of the tensor (E2) describes the diffusion of water along the surface of myocytes that have been arranged into sheets.[7,37] The myocardium has a highly dynamic sheet structure and it is the movement of these sheets through the cardiac cycle that forms the basis of radial strain.[7,37,38] The angle of the secondary eigenvector with the epicardial tangent plane forms a sheet angle, referred to as E2A. This angle is low in diastole and increases substantially in systole as the sheets of the heart undergo radial reorientation and shearing (**Fig. 8**).[38] Several other angles can be derived from the diffusion tensor but, as of yet, these are not used routinely and have not been shown to have direct pathophysiological correlates.

Dynamic imaging of E2A has been extensively studied over the last few years. In patients with dilated cardiomyopathy the sheets in the heart do not undergo sufficient radial reorientation in systole and E2A thus remains lower than normal.[38] Conversely, in hypertrophic cardiomyopathy (HCM) the sheets retain a more radial configuration in diastole than in normal hearts.[38] It remains unknown whether these changes in sheet dynamics are primary and cause the reduction in

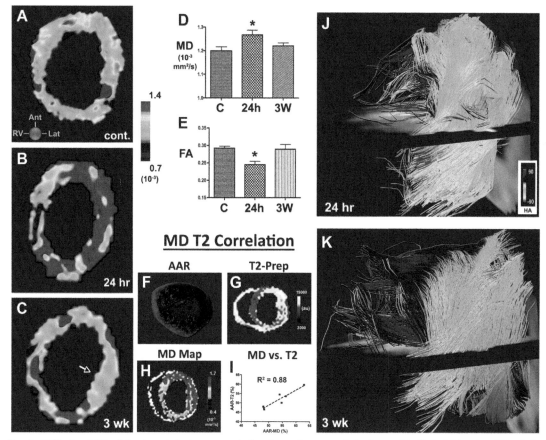

Fig. 6. Diffusion MRI of the heart during acute ischemia and myocardial edema. (*A–E*) Serial in vivo DTI of the murine heart before and after transient ligation of the left coronary artery. MD maps at baseline (*A*), 24 hours postinjury (*B*), and 3 weeks postinjury (*C*) are shown. Acute injury is associated with a transient increase in MD, which resolves within 3 weeks (*arrow*). The transient increase in MD (*D*) is accompanied by a transient decrease in FA (*E*), which also returns toward baseline. (*F–I*) MD and T2 are highly correlated in acute ischemia. (*F*) Microsphere injection showing area-at-risk (AAR). Both T2 (*G*) and MD (*H*) are highly increased in the AAR and (*I*) correlate strongly. (*J, K*) Serial in vivo tractography. (*J*) COST tractography at 24 hours reflects both the loss of microstructure and the presence of edema. (*K*) In vivo tractography of the same mouse 3 weeks later shows the true extent of microstructural damage, without the confounding effects of edema. * = statistically significant. (*From* Sosnovik DE, Mekkaoui C, Huang S, et al. Microstructural impact of ischemia and bone marrow-derived cell therapy revealed with diffusion tensor magnetic resonance imaging tractography of the heart in vivo. Circulation. 2014;129(17):1731–41; with permission.)

contraction/relaxation or whether they are secondary and simply a marker of reduced strain. Much like the relationship between MD and T2, it is unclear whether sheet dynamics by DTI and myocardial strain (by echo or MRI) are independent measurements or correlated measurements of the same phenomenon.

DIFFUSION TRACTOGRAPHY

Tractography refers to the integration of a vector field into streamlines.[14] In the brain and skeletal muscle streamlines of the primary eigenvector field depict nerve tracts and myofibers, respectively. In the heart the situation is more complex. The primary eigenvector field can be integrated into streamlines, which can be thought of as virtual myofibers, and in the past the 2 terms were used interchangeably. It should be stressed, however, that the myocardium has no myofibers in the same physical sense as skeletal muscle. Rather, the myocytes in the heart are arranged in a 3D laminar network with each myocyte making physical connections with numerous neighboring myocytes. As discussed above, whereas the primary direction of contraction occurs along the long axis of a cardiomycyte, the yield of this contraction is ultimately manifested by rotation

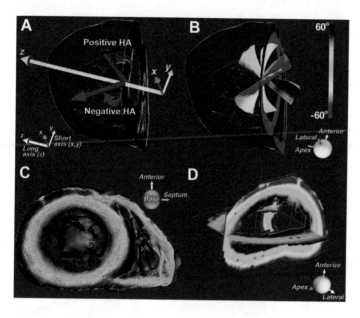

Fig. 7. Definition of the cardiomyocyte orientation or helix angle (HA). Ex vivo tractography of a normal human heart. (*A*) The HA is defined by the angle of the primary eigenvector with the local radial plane. (*B*) The cardiomyocytes in the subendocardium have a positive HA and those in the subepicardium a negative HA. Cardiomyocytes in the midmyocardium have low HA values and are circumferential. (*C, D*) This pattern is highly conserved throughout the heart. It should be stressed that, unlike DNA, the myocytes in the heart are not linked into continuous physical helices. The term HA, although widely used, should be thought of as the cardiomyocyte orientation angle (CAO) at a discrete point. (*From* Mekkaoui C, Huang S, Chen HH, et al. Fiber architecture in remodeled myocardium revealed with a quantitative diffusion CMR tractography framework and histological validation. J Cardiovasc Magn Reson. 2012;14:70; with permission.)

and shearing of the myocyte sheets in the radial plane.[4] The propagation of electrical impulses between myocytes was previously thought to occur across gap junctions in a strict end-to-end configuration, analogous to conduction in nerve fibers, but this too has now been shown to be far more complex in the heart.[39]

Although no physical myofibers exist in the heart, the integration of cardiomyocyte orientation streamlines (COSTs) into tracks is extremely valuable. The angle between adjacent cardiomyocytes in these COSTs describes the tractographic propagation angle (PA).[40] The PA in healthy myocardium, at the standard resolutions used for DTI, is <4°/voxel (**Fig. 9**),[40] and is highly conserved between species. An increase in PA denotes an increase in microstructural disorder and heterogeneity in the heart, and can be used to detect myocardial infarcts with a high degree of accuracy (**Fig. 10**).[40] Moreover, the degree of disorder depicted by PA also correlates strongly with the presence of arrhythmogenic substrate on electro-anatomical mapping. Regions with very high degrees of microstructural disorder (PA > 10°) have very low bipolar voltages,[40] consistent with dense scar, and do not generally support the conduction of electrical impulses. In contrast, areas with moderate degrees of disorder (PA values of 4°–10°) show electrical properties characteristic of arrhythmogenic substrate (**Fig. 11**).[40]

The myocardium is a mechanical continuum and an injury at 1 point may perturb myocyte

architecture at a distal location. COST tractography provides an integrated 3D depiction of myofiber architecture over the entire myocardial continuum and is thus inherently suited to studying the heart. Infarction in the septum, for instance, was shown by tractography to result in a rightward (positive) shift in COSTs in the remote zone of the heart (see **Fig. 5**).[6] DTI and COST tractography are also particularly well suited to detecting the loss or regeneration of microstructurally intact myocardium. In a study of bone marrow-derived stem cell therapy, serial in vivo DTI showed that in most cases MD increased and FA decreased after cell injection.[21] Similar results were obtained when the donor and recipient mice were of the same or different strains (**Fig. 12**). Moreover, COST tractography showed in most cases that bone marrow-derived cells did not regenerate tissue with a coherent microstructure or one that resembled functional myocardium (see **Fig. 12**).[21] DTI has also been used to assess the impact of exosomes secreted by cardiosphere-derived cells (CDCs) on regeneration and remodeling in infarcted swine.[41] In most cases (67%) no evidence of regeneration was seen. However, in a minority, exosome injection was associated with a reduction in infarct size and the restoration of normal microstructure in the border zone of the infarct. Overall, the predominant effect of exosome injection was to reduce infarct expansion and preserve existing myocardial microstructure and function (see **Fig. 12**).[41] These preclinical

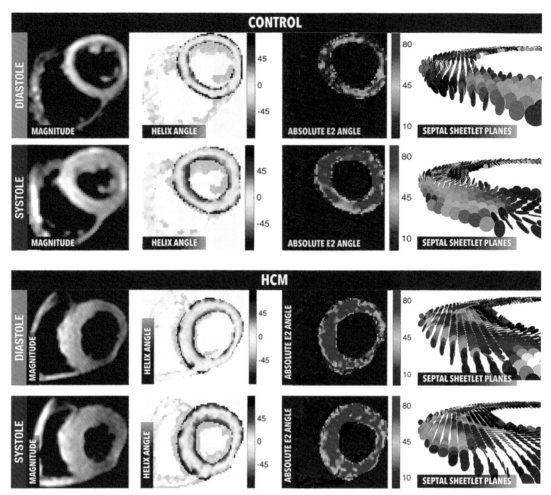

Fig. 8. Imaging of sheet angle dynamics in the heart. Helix and sheet angle (E2A) maps of a healthy subject and subject with HCM are shown. Visual inspection of the HA maps does not reveal any major differences between systole and diastole or between the healthy control and HCM subject. In contrast, the sheet angle (E2A) is low in diastole and increases substantially during systole in the healthy control. In HCM, however, the sheets fail to assume the characteristic diastolic conformation (low E2A) and the diastolic and systolic E2A maps appear similar. (*From* Nielles-Vallespin S, Khalique Z, Ferreira PF, et al. Assessment of myocardial microstructural dynamics by in vivo diffusion tensor cardiac magnetic resonance. J Am Coll Cardiol. 2017;69(6):661–76; with permission.)

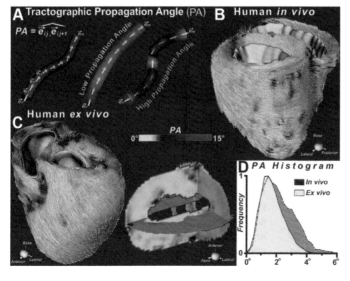

Fig. 9. Tractography of the heart using the COST propagation angle (PA). (*A*) The PA is defined as the angle between 2 adjacent segments (primary eigenvectors) in a COST tract, reflecting the change in cardiomyocyte orientation along the tract. Areas of myocardium with low PA are coherent and have a highly ordered microstructure. PA tractography in a human heart (*B*) in vivo and (*C*) ex vivo. In most areas of the heart the PA is highly uniform and <4°/voxel. PA values are slightly higher at the right ventricular insertion site and apex. (*D*) Histograms of PA in the human heart show that most tract segments have a PA <4°, both in vivo and ex vivo. (*From* Mekkaoui C, Jackowski MP, Kostis WJ, et al. Myocardial scar delineation using diffusion tensor magnetic resonance tractography. J Am Heart Assoc. 2018;7(3); with permission.)

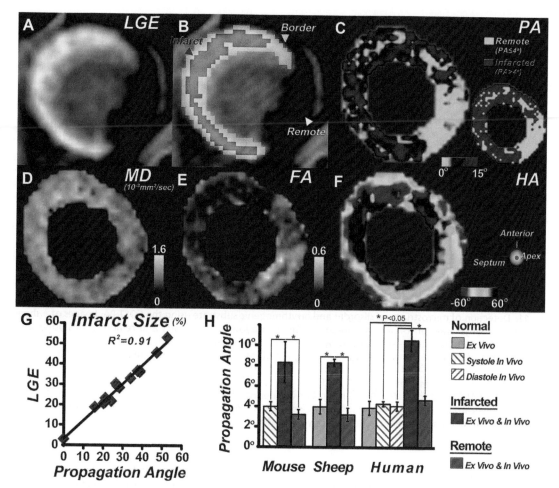

Fig. 10. Detection and characterization of myocardial infarction with diffusion tensor MRI and the COST propagation angle. Short-axis slices of a subject with a large anteroseptal infarct are shown. (*A, B*) LGE of the infarct with segmentation into infarct, border, and remote zones. (*C*) PA map, segmented in the inset into infarct and remote zones using a PA threshold of 4°. (*D–F*) MD in the infarct is increased, FA is decreased, and the transmural distribution of the HA is altered. (*G*) A high correlation is seen between infarct size calculated by PA and LGE. (*H*) A PA threshold of 4° accurately detects myocardial infarction across species, with both ex vivo and in vivo imaging. (*From* Mekkaoui C, Jackowski MP, Kostis WJ, et al. Myocardial scar delineation using diffusion tensor magnetic resonance tractography. J Am Heart Assoc. 2018;7(3); with permission.)

studies predict and match the clinical experience with cell therapy in the heart to date, which has produced moderate, inconsistent and nonsustained results.

CLINICAL STUDIES

The clinical experience with DTI is growing and studies have been performed in patients with myocardial infarction, nonischemic cardiomyopathy, HCM, congenital heart disease, and cardiac amyloidosis. In many of these studies strong correlations have been observed between metrics of diffusion and important parameters of disease pathophysiology.

DTI of patients with cardiac amyloidosis seems to hold significant promise (**Fig. 13**).[35] In a recent study MD in these patients was significantly increased and correlated strongly with native T1 measurements. A corresponding reduction in FA was seen and correlated strongly with increases in the myocardial extracellular volume fraction. The E2A sheet angle retained a more systolic conformation than controls, consistent with findings in patients with HCM.[38] The HA of the cardiomyocytes showed an increase in circumferential orientation and a reduction in the transmural slope of HA (HAT), which correlated strongly with a reduction in longitudinal strain.[35] As tailored therapies for amyloid continue to be developed, DTI

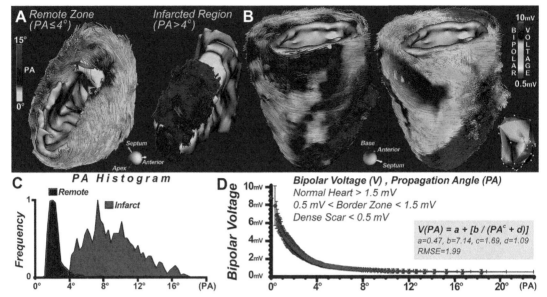

Fig. 11. Detection of microstructural disorder and arrythmogenic substrate using the COST PA. Images of a sheep heart with a large anterior infarct are shown. (*A*) Segmentation of the infarct and remote zones using a PA threshold of 4°. (*B*) COST tracts color-coded by PA and the local endocardial voltage, respectively (see inset for voltage map and measurement locations). (*C*) Histogram of PA in the infarct and remote zones. (*D*) Regions of the myocardium with a PA <4° have voltages ≥1.5 mV (normal myocardium), those with PA values between 4°and 10° have voltages between 0.5 and 1.5 mV (border zone), and those with a PA >10° have voltage ≤0.5 mV (dense scar). The relationship between endocardial voltage and PA is nonlinear, particularly in healthy myocardium. (*From* Mekkaoui C, Jackowski MP, Kostis WJ, et al. Myocardial scar delineation using diffusion tensor magnetic resonance tractography. J Am Heart Assoc. 2018;7(3); with permission.)

may have an important role in guiding their development and, ultimately, their use in the clinical setting.

Microstructural remodeling following myocardial infarction is difficult to study because of the confounding effects of myocardial edema.[21] Early studies of DTI postinfarction showed that MD in the infarct was increased, FA was reduced, and myocyte orientation was highly perturbed in the infarct and infarct-adjacent zones.[42,43] In a subsequent small study of patients with large anteroseptal myocardial infarctions, that were approximately 1 year old, similar findings in MD and FA were seen.[40] HA maps and COST tractography also showed profound perturbations in microstructure in both the infarct and border zones.[40] However, some segments with LGE showed surprisingly mild changes in HA, best detected by measuring its transmural slope or its variance. The entire infarct zone, in contrast, was exquisitely detected with 2D PA maps and COST tractograms classified by PA (see **Figs. 10** and **11**).[40] This replicates the experience in HCM, where foci of LGE are not always detected on HA maps.[44] Microstructural remodeling in ischemic cardiomyopathy may thus be best characterized by changes in PA,

and should ideally be performed once the edema associated with the acute injury has resolved.

Several studies have examined the role of DTI in dilated cardiomyopathy. The proportion of more longitudinally oriented cardiomyocytes normally increases in systole as the heart contracts and its dimensions decrease. In patients with dilated cardiomyopathy, however, little difference in myocyte orientation was seen between systole and diastole.[45] In a subsequent study, however, differences in HA between controls and patients with dilated cardiomyopathy were not significant, and the principal finding related to sheet dynamics (lower E2A values in systole) in these patients (see **Fig. 8**).[38] As mentioned above, it remains unknown whether these phenomena are primary or secondary to a reduction in radial strain. Interestingly, in patients with dilated cardiomyopathy who showed a recovery in systolic function over time, a corresponding improvement in sheet dynamics was seen by DTI.[46]

Studies of DTI in patients with HCM have produced promising results. Initial work did not reveal any systematic changes in HA, even in the presence of LGE.[44] A subsequent study also found no changes in HA but did document

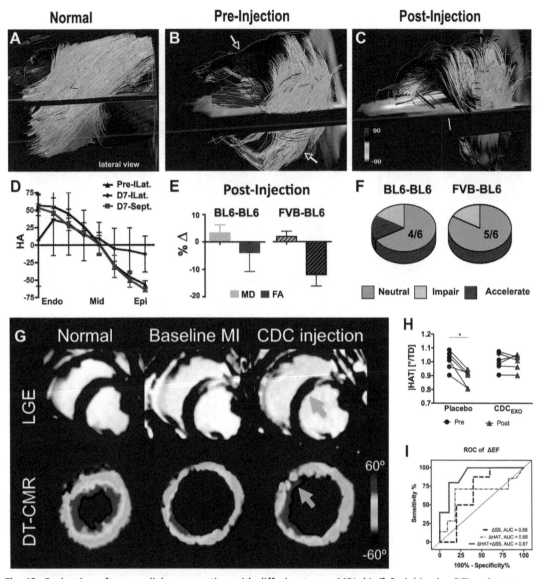

Fig. 12. Evaluation of myocardial regeneration with diffusion tensor MRI. (*A–F*) Serial in vivo DTI and tractography in mice with healed infarcts injected with bone marrow mononuclear cells (BMMCs). COST tracts intersecting a region-of-interest in the lateral wall are shown. (*A*) Normal mouse. (*B*) Infarcted mouse preinjection and (*C*) post-BMMC injection. Note the presence of coherent tracts (*arrows*) in the anterolateral and inferolateral walls, which are lost after injection. (*D*) Transmural HA plot in the inferolateral (ILat) wall preinjection resembles the uninjured septum. Postinjection, however, the HA slope (*black*) is severely perturbed. (*E*) BMMC injection was associated with no change or an increase in MD, a decrease in FA, and the loss of correctly oriented tracts in 11/12 mice. (*F*) No difference was seen when the donor and recipient strains of the BMMCs were matched or mismatched. (*G–I*) Serial in vivo DTI in infarcted swine injected with exosomes secreted by cardiosphere-derived cells (CDCs). Injection of the exosomes reduced scar size (*arrow*) by LGE and in some cases (2/6) resulted in a local restoration of the transmural slope of HA (HAT). (*H*) The overall effect of exosome injection, however, was to preserve HAT in noninfarcted myocardium and limit infarct expansion. (*I*) Changes in scar size and HAT both predicted a change in ejection fraction. * = statistically significant. (*From* [A–F] Sosnovik DE, Mekkaoui C, Huang S, et al. Microstructural impact of ischemia and bone marrow-derived cell therapy revealed with diffusion tensor magnetic resonance imaging tractography of the heart in vivo. Circulation. 2014;129(17):1731–41; with permission; and [G–I] Nguyen CT, Dawkins J, Bi X, Marban E, Li D. Diffusion tensor cardiac magnetic resonance reveals exosomes from cardiosphere-derived cells preserve myocardial fiber architecture after myocardial infarction. JACC Basic Transl Sci. 2018;3(1):97–109; with permission.)

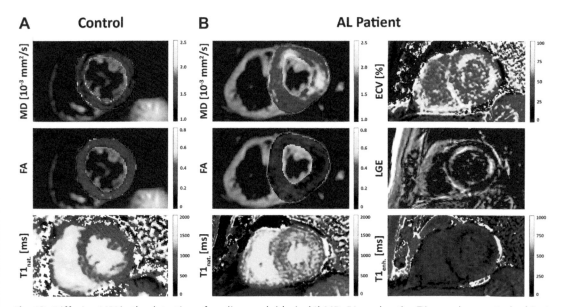

Fig. 13. Diffusion MRI in the detection of cardiac amyloidosis. (*A*) MD, FA, and native T1 maps in a control subject. (*B*) MD, FA, native T1, extracellular volume fraction (ECV), LGE, and postcontrast T1 maps in a patient with amyloid. MD is increased and FA is reduced in the subject with amyloid, particularly in those areas showing LGE and increased ECV. (*From* Gotschy A, von Deuster C, van Gorkum RJH, et al. Characterizing cardiac involvement in amyloidosis using cardiovascular magnetic resonance diffusion tensor imaging. J Cardiovasc Magn Reson. 2019;21(1):56; with permission.)

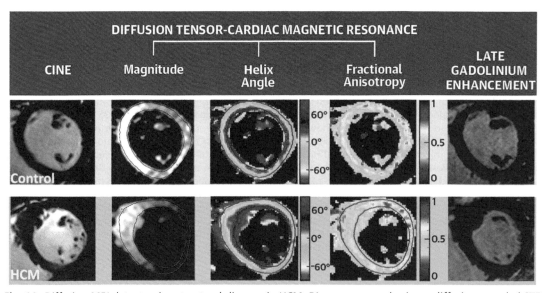

Fig. 14. Diffusion MRI detects microstructural disarray in HCM. FA was measured using a diffusion-encoded STE sequence in diastole. In healthy subjects, FA in the septum is highest in the midmyocardium. In subjects with HCM, FA in the hypertrophied portions of the septum is reduced. (*From* Ariga R, Tunnicliffe EM, Manohar SG, et al. Identification of myocardial disarray in patients with hypertrophic cardiomyopathy and ventricular arrhythmias. J Am Coll Cardiol. 2019;73(20):2493–2502; with permission.)

persistent systolic conformation (high E2A) of the myocardial sheets in diastole (see **Fig. 8**).[38] More recently, FA in the septum in HCM was found to be reduced and a marker for ventricular tachycardia (**Fig. 14**).[36] It is important to note subtle, but important, technical differences between this study and prior studies in HCM, which have all used diffusion-encoded STE sequences. The long mixing time of STE sequences makes them theoretically vulnerable to effects from myocardial strain,[47,48] although the actual impact of this remains unclear and a matter of considerable debate.[38,49] In most earlier studies FA was measured in systole with no strategy to mitigate the theoretic effects of strain,[38,44] whereas in the latter study,[36] FA was measured at a point in diastole designed to minimize the effects of strain.[48,50] Further studies will be needed to replicate the predictive value of reduced FA for ventricular arrhythmias and to determine the optimal approach to image these patients.

SUMMARY

The microstructure of the heart is intricate and plays an important role in optimizing its mechanical and electrical performance. Diffusion MRI provides a technique to probe myocardial microstructure noninvasively and without the need for exogenous contrast agents. The technique, at present, remains experimental but has already provided important insights into the pathophysiology of several conditions. Ongoing improvements in hardware, sequence design and image analysis should further accelerate progress in the field, and it is likely that diffusion MRI will soon become part of the clinical cardiac imaging armamentarium.

DISCLOSURE

The Martinos Center for Biomedical Imaging receives research support from Siemens Medical, Erlangen Germany.

REFERENCES

1. Aguirre AD, Vinegoni C, Sebas M, et al. Intravital imaging of cardiac function at the single-cell level. Proc Natl Acad Sci U S A 2014;111(31):11257–62.
2. Hess AT, Zhong X, Spottiswoode BS, et al. Myocardial 3D strain calculation by combining cine displacement encoding with stimulated echoes (DENSE) and cine strain encoding (SENC) imaging. Magn Reson Med 2009;62(1):77–84.
3. Scollan DF, Holmes A, Winslow R, et al. Histological validation of myocardial microstructure obtained from diffusion tensor magnetic resonance imaging. Am J Physiol 1998;275(6 Pt 2):H2308–18.
4. Axel L, Wedeen VJ, Ennis DB. Probing dynamic myocardial microstructure with cardiac magnetic resonance diffusion tensor imaging. J Cardiovasc Magn Reson 2014;16:89.
5. Streeter DD Jr, Spotnitz HM, Patel DP, et al. Fiber orientation in the canine left ventricle during diastole and systole. Circ Res 1969;24(3):339–47.
6. Mekkaoui C, Huang S, Chen HH, et al. Fiber architecture in remodeled myocardium revealed with a quantitative diffusion CMR tractography framework and histological validation. J Cardiovasc Magn Reson 2012;14:70.
7. Hales PW, Schneider JE, Burton RA, et al. Histoanatomical structure of the living isolated rat heart in two contraction states assessed by diffusion tensor MRI. Prog Biophys Mol Biol 2012;110(2–3):319–30.
8. Mekkaoui C, Reese TG, Jackowski MP, et al. Diffusion tractography of the entire left ventricle by using free-breathing accelerated simultaneous multisection imaging. Radiology 2017;282(3):850–6.
9. Mekkaoui C, Porayette P, Jackowski MP, et al. Diffusion MRI tractography of the developing human fetal heart. PLoS One 2013;8(8):e72795.
10. Teh I, McClymont D, Zdora MC, et al. Validation of diffusion tensor MRI measurements of cardiac microstructure with structure tensor synchrotron radiation imaging. J Cardiovasc Magn Reson 2017;19(1):31.
11. Goergen CJ, Chen HH, Sakadzic S, et al. Microstructural characterization of myocardial infarction with optical coherence tractography and two-photon microscopy. Physiol Rep 2016;4(18):e12894.
12. Lee SE, Nguyen C, Yoon J, et al. Three-dimensional cardiomyocytes structure revealed by diffusion tensor imaging and its validation using a tissue-clearing technique. Sci Rep 2018;8(1):6640.
13. Basser PJ. Inferring microstructural features and the physiological state of tissues from diffusion-weighted images. NMR Biomed 1995;8(7–8):333–44.
14. Sosnovik DE, Wang R, Dai G, et al. Diffusion MR tractography of the heart. J Cardiovasc Magn Reson 2009;11:47.
15. Mekkaoui C, Reese TG, Jackowski MP, et al. Diffusion MRI in the heart. NMR Biomed 2017;30(3).
16. Delattre BM, Viallon M, Wei H, et al. In vivo cardiac diffusion-weighted magnetic resonance imaging: quantification of normal perfusion and diffusion coefficients with intravoxel incoherent motion imaging. Invest Radiol 2012;47(11):662–70.
17. Spinner GR, von Deuster C, Tezcan KC, et al. Bayesian intravoxel incoherent motion parameter mapping in the human heart. J Cardiovasc Magn Reson 2017;19(1):85.

18. Edelman RR, Gaa J, Wedeen VJ, et al. In vivo measurement of water diffusion in the human heart. Magn Reson Med 1994;32(3):423–8.

19. Reese TG, Weisskoff RM, Smith RN, et al. Imaging myocardial fiber architecture in vivo with magnetic resonance. Magn Reson Med 1995;34(6):786–91.

20. Gamper U, Boesiger P, Kozerke S. Diffusion imaging of the in vivo heart using spin echoes—considerations on bulk motion sensitivity. Magn Reson Med 2007;57(2):331–7.

21. Sosnovik DE, Mekkaoui C, Huang S, et al. Microstructural impact of ischemia and bone marrow-derived cell therapy revealed with diffusion tensor magnetic resonance imaging tractography of the heart in vivo. Circulation 2014;129(17):1731–41.

22. Nguyen C, Fan Z, Sharif B, et al. In vivo three-dimensional high resolution cardiac diffusion-weighted MRI: a motion compensated diffusion-prepared balanced steady-state free precession approach. Magn Reson Med 2014;72(5):1257–67.

23. Stoeck CT, von Deuster C, Genet M, et al. Second-order motion-compensated spin echo diffusion tensor imaging of the human heart. Magn Reson Med 2016;75(4):1669–76.

24. Nguyen C, Fan Z, Xie Y, et al. In vivo diffusion-tensor MRI of the human heart on a 3 tesla clinical scanner: an optimized second order (M2) motion compensated diffusion-preparation approach. Magn Reson Med 2016;76(5):1354–63.

25. Gorodezky M, Scott AD, Ferreira PF, et al. Diffusion tensor cardiovascular magnetic resonance with a spiral trajectory: an in vivo comparison of echo planar and spiral stimulated echo sequences. Magn Reson Med 2018;80(2):648–54.

26. Setsompop K, Gagoski BA, Polimeni JR, et al. Blipped-controlled aliasing in parallel imaging for simultaneous multislice echo planar imaging with reduced g-factor penalty. Magn Reson Med 2012; 67(5):1210–24.

27. Nielles-Vallespin S, Mekkaoui C, Gatehouse P, et al. In vivo diffusion tensor MRI of the human heart: reproducibility of breath-hold and navigator-based approaches. Magn Reson Med 2013;70(2):454–65.

28. Aliotta E, Wu HH, Ennis DB. Convex optimized diffusion encoding (CODE) gradient waveforms for minimum echo time and bulk motion-compensated diffusion-weighted MRI. Magn Reson Med 2017; 77(2):717–29.

29. Scott AD, Nielles-Vallespin S, Ferreira PF, et al. An in-vivo comparison of stimulated-echo and motion compensated spin-echo sequences for 3 T diffusion tensor cardiovascular magnetic resonance at multiple cardiac phases. J Cardiovasc Magn Reson 2018;20(1):1.

30. von Deuster C, Stoeck CT, Genet M, et al. Spin echo versus stimulated echo diffusion tensor imaging of the in vivo human heart. Magn Reson Med 2016; 76(3):862–72.

31. Rose JN, Nielles-Vallespin S, Ferreira PF, et al. Novel insights into in-vivo diffusion tensor cardiovascular magnetic resonance using computational modeling and a histology-based virtual microstructure. Magn Reson Med 2019;81(4):2759–73.

32. Sosnovik DE, Wang R, Dai G, et al. Diffusion spectrum MRI tractography reveals the presence of a complex network of residual myofibers in infarcted myocardium. Circ Cardiovasc Imaging 2009;2(3): 206–12.

33. Nguyen C, Fan Z, Xie Y, et al. In vivo contrast free chronic myocardial infarction characterization using diffusion-weighted cardiovascular magnetic resonance. J Cardiovasc Magn Reson 2014;16(1):68.

34. Kung GL, Vaseghi M, Gahm JK, et al. Microstructural infarct border zone remodeling in the post-infarct swine heart measured by diffusion tensor MRI. Front Physiol 2018;9:826.

35. Gotschy A, von Deuster C, van Gorkum RJH, et al. Characterizing cardiac involvement in amyloidosis using cardiovascular magnetic resonance diffusion tensor imaging. J Cardiovasc Magn Reson 2019; 21(1):56.

36. Ariga R, Tunnicliffe EM, Manohar SG, et al. Identification of myocardial disarray in patients with hypertrophic cardiomyopathy and ventricular arrhythmias. J Am Coll Cardiol 2019;73(20):2493–502.

37. Dou J, Tseng WY, Reese TG, et al. Combined diffusion and strain MRI reveals structure and function of human myocardial laminar sheets in vivo. Magn Reson Med 2003;50(1):107–13.

38. Nielles-Vallespin S, Khalique Z, Ferreira PF, et al. Assessment of myocardial microstructural dynamics by in vivo diffusion tensor cardiac magnetic resonance. J Am Coll Cardiol 2017;69(6):661–76.

39. Hulsmans M, Clauss S, Xiao L, et al. Macrophages facilitate electrical conduction in the heart. Cell 2017;169(3):510–22.e20.

40. Mekkaoui C, Jackowski MP, Kostis WJ, et al. Myocardial scar delineation using diffusion tensor magnetic resonance tractography. J Am Heart Assoc 2018;7(3):e007834.

41. Nguyen CT, Dawkins J, Bi X, et al. Diffusion tensor cardiac magnetic resonance reveals exosomes from cardiosphere-derived cells preserve myocardial fiber architecture after myocardial infarction. JACC Basic Transl Sci 2018;3(1):97–109.

42. Wu MT, Tseng WY, Su MY, et al. Diffusion tensor magnetic resonance imaging mapping the fiber architecture remodeling in human myocardium after infarction: correlation with viability and wall motion. Circulation 2006;114(10):1036–45.

43. Wu MT, Su MY, Huang YL, et al. Sequential changes of myocardial microstructure in patients postmyocardial infarction by diffusion-tensor cardiac MR:

correlation with left ventricular structure and function. Circ Cardiovasc Imaging 2009;2(1):32–40.

44. McGill LA, Ismail TF, Nielles-Vallespin S, et al. Reproducibility of in-vivo diffusion tensor cardiovascular magnetic resonance in hypertrophic cardiomyopathy. J Cardiovasc Magn Reson 2012;14:86.

45. von Deuster C, Sammut E, Asner L, et al. Studying dynamic myofiber aggregate reorientation in dilated cardiomyopathy using in vivo magnetic resonance diffusion tensor imaging. Circ Cardiovasc Imaging 2016;9(10):e005018.

46. Khalique Z, Ferreira PF, Scott AD, et al. Diffusion tensor cardiovascular magnetic resonance of microstructural recovery in dilated cardiomyopathy. JACC Cardiovasc Imaging 2018;11(10):1548–50.

47. Reese TG, Wedeen VJ, Weisskoff RM. Measuring diffusion in the presence of material strain. J Magn Reson B 1996;112(3):253–8.

48. Stoeck CT, Kalinowska A, von Deuster C, et al. Dualphase cardiac diffusion tensor imaging with strain correction. PLoS One 2014;9(9):e107159.

49. Ferreira PF, Nielles-Vallespin S, Scott AD, et al. Evaluation of the impact of strain correction on the orientation of cardiac diffusion tensors with in vivo and ex vivo porcine hearts. Magn Reson Med 2018; 79(4):2205–15.

50. Tseng WY, Reese TG, Weisskoff RM, et al. Cardiac diffusion tensor MRI in vivo without strain correction. Magn Reson Med 1999;42(2):393–403.

Cardiovascular Magnetic Resonance in Valvular Heart Disease–Related Heart Failure

Seth Uretsky, MD, FACC[a], Steven D. Wolff, MD, PhD, FACR[b],*

KEYWORDS

- Valvular heart disease • Heart failure • Magnetic resonance imaging

KEY POINTS

- MRI has an important clinical role in assessing the severity of valvular heart disease.
- It is the gold standard for assessing ventricular size and function.
- It is integral to the accurate assessment of valvular disease in patients with heart failure.

VALVULAR DISEASE AND HEART FAILURE

Chronic valvular heart disease can lead to heart failure and death after a long phase during which there is compensatory adaptation of the ventricles and atria.[1] This long compensatory phase may last years and makes the timing of intervention a difficult clinical decision. Gaasch and Meyer[1] highlighted 3 stages in the adaptation left ventricular (LV) structure and function in chronic mitral regurgitation, which can be adapted with slight variation to other regurgitant lesions. The first stage, chronic compensated mitral regurgitation, is marked by LV enlargement, eccentric hypertrophy, and normal systolic function. The second stage, the transitional stage, is marked by mild LV systolic dysfunction, which is still reversible with correction of the valvular disease. Stage 3, the decompensated phase, is marked by progressive and irreversible ventricular changes. This highlights the need for accurate assessment of the severity of valvular heart disease and ventricular function. A full assessment in a patient with valvular heart disease includes evaluating whether the patient is symptomatic from the valvular disease, quantifying the severity of the valvular disease, and quantifying the hemodynamic effects on the atria and ventricles from the valve disease. Although symptom assessment is best done with a clinical evaluation and/or treadmill testing, MRI is well suited to assess the severity of the valve disease and the hemodynamic effects on the atria and ventricles. The initial adaptation to chronic aortic, mitral, tricuspid, or pulmonic regurgitation is the dilatation of the ventricle that receives the regurgitant volume (LV for mitral and aortic and right ventricle [RV] for tricuspid and pulmonic). This adaptation can be measured by an increase in the end-diastolic volume (EDV). Uretsky and colleagues[2] showed a tight correlation between aortic ($r^2 = 0.8$) and mitral ($r^2 = 0.8$) regurgitant volume and LV EDV. As the regurgitant volume increased so did the EDV. For a given amount of regurgitation, the LV EDV increased in size more in aortic regurgitation than mitral regurgitation owing to the fact that mitral regurgitation is a pure volume overload and aortic regurgitation is both a volume and pressure overload. This study highlights that the regurgitant volume quantified by MRI is consistent with the hemodynamic effects on the

[a] Department of Cardiovascular Medicine, Gagnon Administration, Meade B, Morristown Medical Center/Atlantic Health System, 100 Madison Avenue, Morristown, New Jersey 07960, USA; [b] NeoSoft, LLC, N27 W23910A Paul Road, Pewaukee, WI 53072, USA
* Corresponding author.
E-mail address: swolff@neosoftmedical.com

Heart Failure Clin 17 (2021) 103–108
https://doi.org/10.1016/j.hfc.2020.09.002
1551-7136/21/© 2020 Elsevier Inc. All rights reserved.

ventricle. In another study, Uretsky and colleagues[3] showed that mitral regurgitant volume presurgery quantified by MRI had an excellent correlation to the postsurgical decrease in LV EDV (r = 0.85;P<.0001). In that study, there was no correlation between the regurgitant volume quantified by echocardiography and the postsurgical decrease in LV EDV. These 2 studies highlight the relationship between the regurgitant volume quantified by MRI and the hemodynamic effects on the LV. Two studies looked at longitudinal follow-up in patients with asymptomatic mitral regurgitation. Myerson and colleagues[4] followed 109 asymptomatic patients with mitral regurgitation for a mean of 2.5 years ± 1.9 years. Indications for surgery were development of symptoms, an end-systolic dimension greater than 4.0 cm, or pulmonary hypertension with a repairable valve. Twenty-five patients had an indication for surgery, including 19 who developed symptoms. MRI-based mitral regurgitant volume of greater than 55 mL was the best predictor of patients who had an indication for surgery. There was no echocardiographic parameter that was predictive of outcomes in this study. Similarly, Penicka and colleagues[5] followed 258 asymptomatic patients with mitral regurgitation for a median of 5 years for clinical indications for mitral valve surgery, including development of symptoms, an LV end-systolic dimension greater than or equal to 45 mm or an LV ejection fraction (EF) less than or equal to 60%, new onset of atrial fibrillation, or pulmonary hypertension. The investigators found that mitral regurgitant volume by MRI was the most predictive of outcomes and that echocardiography was not predictive of outcomes. In a cohort of 109 asymptomatic patients with aortic regurgitation, Myerson and colleagues[6] found that over a mean follow-up of 2.6 years ± 2.1 years, aortic regurgitant volume was the best predictor of development of symptoms or other indications for surgery. Harris and colleagues[7] studied 29 patients with aortic regurgitation and found that aortic regurgitant volume and fraction quantified by MRI were the most predictive of all MRI and echocardiographic parameters for outcomes.

Other promising techniques for assessing patients with valvular heart disease include the use of tissue characterization. Late gadolinium enhancement and more recently T1 mapping afford MRI the unique ability to quantify myocardial fibrosis, which may be helpful in determining the timing for valve surgery. A recent study by Kitkungvan and colleagues[8] followed 144 asymptomatic patients with mitral regurgitation followed for a mean of 33 months ± 23 months. Among the 59 patients who had an endpoint requiring

mitral valve surgery (90% due to decompensated heart failure), there was a synergistic effect between mitral regurgitant fraction and extracellular volume. Patients with mitral regurgitant fraction of greater than or equal to 40% and an ECV greater than or equal to 30% had the worst outcomes.

MAGNETIC RESONANCE IMAGING QUANTIFICATION OF VALVULAR HEART DISEASE
Aortic Regurgitation

Aortic regurgitation often can be visualized on bright-blood cine images in diastole as a dark jet originating at the closed aortic cusps and extending into the LV outflow tract. It is difficult to accurately assess the severity of the regurgitation by the appearance of the jet because the jet may not be entirely captured within the imaging slice, and its size and appearance depend on a variety of parameters, such as the type of imaging sequence, echo time (TE), and image spatial resolution.

The severity of aortic regurgitation can be quantified reliably by evaluating diastolic blood flow in the proximal ascending aorta. Breath-held, gated phase-contrast images are best acquired perpendicular to the proximal ascending aorta near the sinotubular junction. Diastolic flow typically is minimal but becomes progressively negative with increasing aortic regurgitation. Because aortic regurgitation is a holodiastolic phenomenon, total diastolic blood flow (and not a temporal fraction of diastole) should be used to quantify aortic regurgitant volume.

Aortic regurgitation can be graded as mild (regurgitant volume <30 mL), moderate (regurgitant volume 30 mL–<60 mL), or severe (regurgitant volume ≥60 mL).[9] MRI is a reliable tool for serially assessing the severity of aortic regurgitation. When comparing regurgitant volume in serial studies, it is important to consider the effect of potential differences in heart rate on regurgitant volume. Aortic regurgitation varies with the duration of diastole, which varies with heart rate. So, a patient with no change in aortic valve pathology has a greater regurgitant volume at a lower heart rate and vice versa.

To normalize for the size of the heart, aortic regurgitation also can be graded in terms of regurgitant fraction (mild <30%, moderate 30%–<50%, and severe ≥50%).[9] There are 2 schools of thought for determining regurgitant fraction. Regurgitant volume can either be divided by the LV stroke volume or the forward aortic flow. These values are identical in the case of isolated aortic regurgitation but may be substantially different if there is concomitant mitral regurgitation (or, less commonly, a ventricular septal defect). The advantage of normalizing regurgitant volume to the LV stroke volume is that regurgitant volume is expressed as a percentage of total LV output. Because surgical therapy is predicated on protecting the LV from excessive volume overload, the authors believe that this method makes the most sense. A potential drawback of this method is that on serial studies, however, a patient with no change in aortic valve pathology can have a lower aortic regurgitant fraction if the patient develops increasing mitral regurgitation.

Pitfalls in quantifying aortic regurgitation generally relate to accurately determining the regurgitant volume. For a variety of reasons, regurgitant volume may vary temporally, during an MRI examination. Examples include heart rate variability from an irregular cardiac rhythm, changes in anxiety, or sinus arrhythmia during breath-holding. As a result, the authors recommend that flow in the proximal ascending aorta be assessed multiple times during an examination to determine the reproducibility of the results. Breath-holding is preferred to free-breathing because images have less motion artifact and because it allows better comparison to the LV stroke volume that is obtained from cine acquisitions that typically are breath-held.

The regurgitant volume may be underestimated if the phase-contrast images are not acquired correctly near the sinotubular junction. For example, if the imaging slice is located in the middle or distal ascending aorta, diastolic flow underestimates the regurgitant volume. Similarly, if the phase-contrast image is located at the level of the regurgitant jet, regurgitant flow is underestimated due to turbulent flow and intravoxel dephasing. It is important that the phase-contrast images be acquired truly perpendicular to the aorta. If they are not, diastolic regurgitant flow may be underestimated.

A unique technical problem with MRI flow quantification relates to baseline error. This error, which is thought to be due to eddy currents, causes a velocity and flow offset that causes overestimation or underestimation of blood flow. It is especially pronounced in enlarged blood vessels, such as an enlarged aorta in a patient with aortic regurgitation. To minimize this error, software can be used that corrects for this error. Because the error is dependent on the imaging plane, measuring flow in both the pulmonary artery and the aorta is helpful to have 2 separate independent measures that can be used to calculate aortic regurgitation.

Patients with aortic regurgitation sometimes have concomitant aortic stenosis. Elevated blood velocities may result in aliasing during systole. Phase-contrast images with velocity aliasing in systole still can be used to accurately determine regurgitant volume as long as there is no aliasing in diastole. Although most phase-contrast images are acquired with ECG gating, some are acquired with peripheral pulse gating when ECG gating is not robust. Images acquired with peripheral pulse gating allow for accurate determination of aortic regurgitant volume.

In patients with isolated aortic regurgitation, there are alternative, indirect methods for quantifying regurgitant severity. For example, aortic regurgitant volume can be calculated as the difference between LV stroke volume and total aortic flow. In patients where the aortic flow values are questionable, aortic regurgitant volume can be calculated as the difference between LV stroke volume and total pulmonary artery flow or as the difference between LV stroke volume and RV stroke volume.

Mitral Regurgitation

Mitral regurgitation often can be visualized on bright-blood cine images in systole as a dark jet originating at the closed mitral leaflets and extending into the left atrium. It is difficult to accurately assess the severity of the regurgitation by the appearance of the jet because the jet may not be entirely captured within the imaging slice, and its size and appearance depend on a variety of parameters, such as the type of imaging sequence, TE, and image spatial resolution.

The severity of mitral regurgitation can be quantified reliably by subtracting the forward flow in the ascending aorta or main pulmonary artery from the LV stroke volume.[10] Breath-held, gated phase-contrast images are best acquired perpendicular to the ascending aorta or main pulmonary artery.

Mitral regurgitation can be graded as mild (regurgitant volume <30 mL), moderate (regurgitant volume 30 mL–<60 mL), or severe (regurgitant volume ≥60 mL).[9] MRI is a reliable tool for serially assessing the severity of mitral regurgitation. When comparing regurgitant volume in serial studies, it is important to consider the effect of potential differences in systolic blood pressure on regurgitant volume. A patient with no change in mitral valve pathology has a greater regurgitant volume with higher systolic blood pressures and vice versa.

To normalize for the size of the heart, mitral regurgitation also can be graded in terms of regurgitant fraction (mild <30%, moderate 30%–<50%, and severe $\geq$50%).[9] There are 2 schools of thought for determining regurgitant fraction. Regurgitant volume can be divided either by the LV stroke volume or by the forward aortic flow. These values are identical in cases of isolated mitral regurgitation but may be substantially different if there is concomitant aortic regurgitation (or, less commonly, a ventricular septal defect). The advantage of normalizing regurgitant volume to the LV stroke volume is that regurgitant volume is expressed as a percentage of total LV output. Because surgical therapy is predicated on protecting the LV from excessive volume overload, the authors believe that this method makes the most sense. A potential drawback of this method, however, is that on serial studies, a patient with no change in mitral valve pathology can have a lower mitral regurgitant fraction if the patient develops increasing aortic regurgitation.

Pitfalls in quantifying mitral regurgitation generally relate to accurately determining the regurgitant volume. For a variety of reasons, regurgitant volume may vary temporally, during an MRI examination. Examples include heart rate variability from an irregular cardiac rhythm, changes in anxiety, or sinus arrhythmia during breath-holding. As a result, the authors recommend that flow in the ascending aorta and/or main pulmonary artery be assessed multiple times during an examination to determine the reproducibility of the results. Breath-holding is preferred to free-breathing because images have less motion artifact and because it allows better comparison to the LV stroke volume that is obtained from cine acquisitions that typically are breath-held.

Aortic and Mitral Regurgitation

The quantitative nature of MRI lends itself well to the quantification of multivalve disease. For example, in a patient with both aortic and mitral regurgitation, the diastolic flow of the proximal ascending aorta still can be used to quantify the severity of the aortic regurgitation. To calculate mitral regurgitation, the regurgitant volume is simply the LV stroke volume minus the sum of the net forward flow and the aortic regurgitant volume. The net forward flow can be determined by integrating the flow in the aorta or the main pulmonary artery over the entire cardiac cycle, because these values are identical in the absence of an intracardiac shunt.

Aortic Stenosis

Aortic stenosis can be visualized on bright-blood MRIs as a systolic jet of dark blood that originate at the aortic cusps and which extends into the proximal ascending aorta. Quantification of stenosis severity cannot be based reliably on the appearance of the jet because its appearance may vary, depending on the image sequence type, and imaging parameters, such as TE and spatial resolution. In addition, the jet may be incompletely visualized on a single slice if the jet passes out of the imaging plane.

The severity of aortic stenosis can be quantified using a few methods. The easiest method is to determine the aortic valve area by planimetry. In this technique, bright-blood, steady-state free precession (SSFP) images are acquired perpendicular to the stenotic jet. Typically, several thin ($\leq$5 mm) contiguous SSFP cine image slices are acquired originating at the aortic annulus and extending into the proximal ascending aorta. Aortic valve planimetry is performed on a systolic image, when the cusps are maximally open, and at a slice location where the cusps maximally narrow the aortic valve lumen (typically, this occurs at the tips of the cusps). The aortic valve area is determined by the area of a region of interest that includes the bright blood passing through the narrowest part of the valve and excludes adjacent dark regions that represent aortic cusp calcifications and intravoxel dephasing from high shear stress blood adjacent to the aortic cusps.

The planimetered valve area and the LV volume–versus–time curve can be used to calculate the instantaneous transvalvular pressure gradient. This method has been named the cardiac output valve area (COVA) method. The LV volume–versus–time curve is obtained by segmenting the endocardium on short-axis, bright-blood cine images for all systolic phases. The phase-to-phase change in the LV volume represents the instantaneous blood flow across the aortic valve, provided there is no significant aortic regurgitation or ventricular septal defect. Formulae, such as the Gorlin equation or the Hakki equation, can be used to determine the instantaneous transvalvular pressure gradient, given the planimetered aortic valve area and the instantaneous flow across the aortic valve.

Alternatively, a series of phase-contrast cine images acquired through the LV outflow tract and proximal ascending aorta can be used to determine the aortic valve area. This technique is analogous to the echocardiographic techniques that use the continuity equation. For example, from these images, the area of the LV outflow tract at peak systole can be planimetered and also the peak systolic velocity in the LV outflow tract and at the aortic valve cusps determined. Using the principle of continuity, the aortic valve area is calculated as the product of the LV outflow tract area and the peak velocity of blood (v) in the LV outflow tract divided by the peak velocity of blood at the aortic cusps. A simplified Bernoulli equation also can be used to estimate the transvalvular pressure gradient from the peak velocity of blood at the aortic cusps (peak pressure gradient = 4 v^2; mean pressure gradient = 2.4 v^2).

A potential artifact to beware of when using phase-contrast techniques on high-velocity jets has to do with signal loss due to high blood velocities and intravoxel dephasing. When the MRI signal is insufficient, the phase value is dominated by noise, resulting in a velocity value that can vary over the complete velocity encoding range and which could be substantially different from the true value. In other words, when there is signal loss, the reported pixel's velocity can be underestimated or overestimated. A mask can be applied to the velocity image to remove unreliable data from pixels whose signal is low. Although this helps by eliminating velocity values from unreliably noisy pixels, there still is the risk of not reporting peak velocities from pixels with little or no signal that may have represented high velocity values. An advantage of the COVA method is that it does not suffer from this potential problem because it does not use phase-velocity data.

Mitral Stenosis

Mitral stenosis sometimes can be visualized on cine images as a bright diastolic jet on bright-blood cine images that originates at the mitral valve leaflet tips and extends into the LV. The jet often is better appreciated on gradient-echo images because the background blood signal is not as high as it is on the SSFP images. The pressure gradient between the left atrium and LV generally is not high enough to generate velocities that would make the jet dark, as in the case of aortic stenosis.

Quantifying mitral stenosis can be done by planimetry. Typically, a series of bright-blood cine images is acquired perpendicular to the jet from the mitral annulus through the leaflet tips. Mitral valve planimetry is performed on an early diastolic image, when the leaflets are maximally open, and at a slice location where the leaflets maximally narrow the mitral valve lumen (typically, this occurs near the tips of the leaflets). The mitral valve area is determined by the area of a region of interest that includes the bright blood passing through the narrowest part of the valve.

An alternative MRI method for determining the mitral valve area uses pressure half-time in a manner analogous to echocardiography. In this case, a series of phase-contrast cine images are acquired perpendicular to the jet from the mitral annulus through the leaflet tips. A small region of interest is placed so as to show blood velocities where the mitral valve is at its most narrow. The early diastolic velocities are interrogated and the pressure half-time is calculated. The mitral valve area is then estimated as 220/pressure half-time.

Pulmonic and Tricuspid Regurgitation and Stenosis

The right-sided valve lesions, pulmonic stenosis/regurgitation, and tricuspid stenosis/regurgitation can be quantified in a manner analogous to the left-sided valve lesions, described previously. Multivalve disease (ie, pulmonic and tricuspid regurgitation) also is quantified in an analogous manner.

SUMMARY

MRI is a noninvasive method to accurately quantify the severity of valvular heart disease and the hemodynamic consequences of valvular heart disease, including the advent of heart failure.

CLINICS CARE POINTS

- Cardiac MRI can assess valvular stenosis and regurgitation.
- It is more accurate than echocardiography in assessing valvular regurgitant severity and its effect on left ventricular size and function.
- Echocardiography often overestimates the severity of mitral regurgitation and results in inappropriate surgery.

DISCLOSURE

Steven D. Wolff is the owner of NeoSoft, LLC.

REFERENCES

1. Gaasch WH, Meyer TE. Left ventricular response to mitral regurgitation: implications for management. Circulation 2008;118:2298–303.
2. Uretsky S, Supariwala A, Nidadovolu P, et al. Quantification of left ventricular remodeling in response to isolated aortic or mitral regurgitation. J Cardiovasc Magn Reson 2010;12:32.
3. Uretsky S, Gillam L, Lang R, et al. Discordance between echocardiography and MRI in the assessment of mitral regurgitation severity: a prospective multicenter trial. J Am Coll Cardiol 2015;65:1078–88.
4. Myerson SG, d'Arcy J, Christiansen JP, et al. Determination of clinical outcome in mitral regurgitation with cardiovascular magnetic resonance quantitation. Circulation 2016;133:2287–96.

5. Penicka M, Vecera J, Mirica DC, et al. Prognostic implications of magnetic resonance-derived quantification in asymptomatic patients with organic mitral regurgitation: comparison with doppler echocardiography-derived integrative approach. Circulation 2018;137:1349–60.

6. Myerson SG, d'Arcy J, Mohiaddin R, et al. Aortic regurgitation quantification using cardiovascular magnetic resonance: association with clinical outcome. Circulation 2012;126:1452–60.

7. Harris AW, Krieger EV, Kim M, et al. Cardiac magnetic resonance imaging versus transthoracic echocardiography for prediction of outcomes in chronic aortic or mitral regurgitation. Am J Cardiol 2017; 119:1074–81.

8. Kitkungvan D, Yang EY, El Tallawi KC, et al. Prognostic implications of diffuse interstitial fibrosis in asymptomatic primary mitral regurgitation. Circulation 2019;140:2122–4.

9. Nishimura RA, Otto CM, Bonow RO, et al. 2014 AHA/ACC guideline for the management of patients with valvular heart disease: a report of the American college of cardiology/American heart association task force on practice guidelines. J Am Coll Cardiol 2014;63:e57–185.

10. Uretsky S, Argulian E, Narula J, et al. Use of cardiac magnetic resonance imaging in assessing mitral regurgitation: current evidence. J Am Coll Cardiol 2018;71:547–63.

Assessment of Pericardial Disease with Cardiovascular MRI

Natalie Ho, MD[a], Gillian Nesbitt, MD[b], Kate Hanneman, MD, MPH, FRCPC[c,d], Paaladinesh Thavendiranathan, MD, SM, FRCPC[c,e,f],*

KEYWORDS

- Pericarditis • Constrictive pericarditis • Pericardial effusion • Pericardial masses
- Cardiovascular magnetic resonance

KEY POINTS

- Cardiovascular MRI (CMR) plays a complementary role to other imaging modalities in the diagnosis of pericardial disease.
- CMR can help determine the extent and degree of pericardial involvement in pericardial disease.
- CMR tissue characterization techniques enable identification of pericardial inflammation and differentiating pericardial masses.
- CMR can provide a robust assessment of the hemodynamic changes associated with pericardial constriction.
- CMR can guide treatment decisions and response to treatment in pericardial diseases.

INTRODUCTION

Pericardial diseases can contribute to significant morbidity and mortality. Patients can present with a range of symptoms, from pleuritic chest pain to shortness of breath, volume overload, and a low cardiac output. Pericardial disease can be grouped into clinical syndromes including pericarditis, pericardial effusion, constrictive pericarditis, pericardial masses, and congenital diseases of the pericardium. The causes of pericardial diseases are broad and include infectious, autoimmune, postmyocardial infarction, and malignant diseases.[1,2]

The diagnosis and management of pericardial diseases rely heavily on clinical suspicion followed by detailed clinical history and noninvasive, multimodality imaging. Among imaging modalities, cardiovascular MRI (CMR) is uniquely suited for the assessment of pericardial disease due to its ability to define pericardial anatomy, evaluate tissue characteristics, and assess the associated functional consequences. This review aims to (1) help the general cardiologist understand the utility of CMR in the diagnosis and management of pericardial disease; (2) review different CMR sequences for characterizing pericardial disease; and (3) understand how CMR can guide management of pericardial disease.

[a] Division of Cardiology, Scarborough Health Network, Scarborough General Hospital, 3050 Lawrence Avenue, Toronto, Ontario M1P 2V5, Canada; [b] Division of Cardiology, Mount Sinai Hospital, Suite 1609, 600 University Avenue, Toronto, Ontario M5G 1X5, Canada; [c] Department of Medical Imaging, University Health Network, University of Toronto, Toronto, Ontario, Canada; [d] Department of Medical Imaging, Toronto General Hospital, 585 University Avenue, Toronto, Ontario M5G 2N2, Canada; [e] Division of Cardiology, Peter Munk Cardiac Centre, University Health Network, University of Toronto, Toronto, Ontario, Canada; [f] Division of Cardiology and Radiology, Toronto General Hospital, 4N-490, 585 University Avenue, Toronto, Ontario M5G 2N2, Canada
* Corresponding author. Division of Cardiology, Peter Munk Cardiac Center, Toronto General Hospital, 4N-490, 200 Elizabeth Street, Toronto, Ontario M5G 2C4, Canada.
E-mail address: dinesh.thavendiranathan@uhn.ca

Heart Failure Clin 17 (2021) 109–120
https://doi.org/10.1016/j.hfc.2020.08.008
1551-7136/21/© 2020 Elsevier Inc. All rights reserved.

NORMAL ANATOMY AND PHYSIOLOGY OF THE PERICARDIUM

The pericardium is a multilayered sac made of serosal and fibrous components and is conventionally divided into the visceral and parietal pericardium. A serosal layer composed of a single, continuous layer of mesothelial cells reflects on itself and drapes around the entire surface of the heart and roots of the great vessels, forming a pericardial space that normally contains less than 50 mL of serous fluid and lubricates the heart as it beats.[1,3] External to the serosal layer is a fibrous layer composed of collagen fibers interspersed with elastic fibrils. The fibrous sac surrounds the heart and is contiguous with the adventitia of the great vessels superiorly, the central tendon of the diaphragm inferiorly, the sternopericardial ligaments anteriorly, and the parietal pleura laterally.[4] The fibrous sac, together with the parietal layer of serosa that lines its inner surface, comprises the parietal pericardium. The pericardium is often thought to be avascular; however, the parietal pericardium does contain a few small blood vessels.[3] The inner serosal layer surrounding the surface of the heart is referred to as the visceral pericardium or epicardium.

Anatomically, the pericardium partitions the heart and proximal great vessels from the remaining thoracic space, providing structural support and limiting the contiguous spread of infection and malignancy. Hemodynamically, it exerts pressure on the heart, thereby limiting the acute distension of the cardiac chambers and facilitating interventricular/ventriculoatrial interaction.[5] The pericardium maintains the cylindrical shape of the left and right ventricles and likely contributes more to the internal pressure of the thinner walled right atrium and right ventricle than the thicker walled left ventricle.[6]

MULTIMODALITY IMAGING IN PERICARDIAL DISEASE

The main imaging modalities used in the assessment of pericardial disease include chest radiography, echocardiography, cardiac computed tomography, and CMR. Each imaging modality has strengths and limitations in the evaluation of the pericardium as outlined in **Table 1**. CMR has the unique strength of providing both morphologic and functional assessment of the pericardium in addition to tissue characterization. CMR provides adequate spatial and temporal resolution, high inherent tissue contrast, and a wide field of view. The limitations of CMR include its high cost, limited availability, and dependence on patient factors, including patient ability to follow breathing instructions and presence of arrhythmias. However, respiratory gated sequences or real-time sequences can be used to maximize image quality in these situations.

GENERAL ASSESSMENT OF THE PERICARDIUM BY CARDIOVASCULAR MRI

CMR studies for pericardial disease typically begin with assessment of pericardial anatomy, and this is often accomplished using black-blood T1-weighted spin echo sequences with breath hold in select imaging planes or a single-shot fast spin-echo sequence covering the entire chest in an axial plane. These sequences provide high spatial resolution allowing for the measurement of pericardial thickness. On these sequences, the pericardium is a circumferential layer with low signal intensity, typically best seen in the right atrioventricular groove and adjacent to the right ventricular (RV) free wall. The pericardium is usually not well seen along the left ventricular (LV) free wall due to the relative lack of pericardial fat and the low signal intensity of adjacent lung parenchyma and myocardium.[7] CMR evaluation of the pericardium can be limited by partial volume averaging, cardiac motion, inclusion of pericardial fluid, and chemical shift artifacts. Therefore, normal pericardium on CMR can measure up to 4 mm in thickness, despite normal pericardium by autopsy being 0.5 to 1 mm in thickness.[8] After pericardial anatomy has been assessed, additional sequences can be performed based on the specific clinical question (**Box 1**, **Table 2**).

CONGENITAL ABNORMALITIES OF THE PERICARDIUM

Congenital abnormalities of the pericardium include pericardial cysts, diverticula, and partial or complete absence of the pericardium. Pericardial cysts are encapsulated, fluid-filled structures surrounded by a single layer of mesothelial cells connected to the pericardium, although only a few cases demonstrate visible communication with the pericardial sac on surgical specimens.[9] The most common location for a pericardial cyst is on the right side (70%) at the cardiophrenic angle (90%) (**Fig. 1**).[1,7] They are usually asymptomatic and are often initially detected incidentally on chest radiography, where they appear as a masslike density (most commonly at the right cardiophrenic angle). On CMR, they appear as well-defined structures of fluid signal intensity adjacent to the pericardial space. The signal intensity of pericardial cysts on T1- and T2-

Table 1
Strengths and limitations of multimodality imaging in pericardial disease

Imaging Modality	Strengths	Limitations
Chest radiograph	• Widely available • Identifies pericardial calcification • Recognition of pericardial/pleural effusion	• No hemodynamic information
Echocardiography	• Widely available • Relatively low cost • Portable and can be done at the bedside • Provides structural and hemodynamic information • Allows real-time assessment of hemodynamic consequences of pericardial disease • Excellent temporal resolution	• Limited field of view • Limited tissue characterization • Operator dependent • Dependent on patient factors
Cardiac CT	• High spatial resolution • Complete anatomic assessment of the pericardium and surrounding mediastinum/pleura • Allows for the evaluation of extracardiac abnormalities • Can define the presence and extent of pericardial calcium • Useful for preoperative assessment • Calcification clearly visualized on non-contrast imaging	• Ionizing radiation • Iodinated contrast • Limited dynamic imaging • Affected by arrhythmias
Cardiovascular MRI	• Excellent for tissue characterization • Allows assessment of ventricular global and regional function and morphology • Allows quantification of flow and dynamic imaging to assess interventricular dependence	• Time consuming • High cost • Limited by arrhythmias or difficulty with breath-hold • Contraindicated in the setting of certain cardiac devices • Calcifications not clearly seen • Not feasible if the patient is hemodynamically unstable

weighted imaging is typically similar to water. On the other hand, pericardial diverticula are focal outpouchings of the pericardial sac in direct communication with the pericardial space, as evidenced by change in size with change in patient positioning.[10]

Congenital absence of the pericardium is rare (Fig. 2), with a reported incidence of less than 1/10,000.[11] Complete left-sided defects are the most common and comprise 70% of all cases followed by right-sided defects (17%) with the most rare being complete bilateral absence of the pericardium (9%).[12] Typical imaging findings in the setting of complete pericardial absence include a "teardrop" shape of the heart, elongation of the atria, leftward displacement of the heart, and cardiac hypermobility. Partial absence of the pericardium can result in herniation of part of the heart, including the left atrium and left atrial appendage.[11]

PERICARDIAL MASSES

Pericardial masses are uncommon and can be divided broadly into benign and malignant masses. Pericardial malignancies account for 6.7% to 12.8% of all cardiac tumors arising from the heart.[13] Primary pericardial malignancies are rare, with a prevalence less than 0.01% in large autopsy series, with secondary involvement being 100 to 1000 times more prevalent.[13–15] Signs of malignant disease include invasion into the epicardial fat, myocardium or cardiac chambers, associated complex/hemorrhagic effusion, mediastinal/hilar

---

Box 1
Cardiovascular MRI sequences and planes in the assessment of pericardial disease

Sequence

Scouts

- Acquired in the axial, sagittal, and coronal planes
- Used for localization and planning

Black-blood fast spin echo/turbo spine echo sequences

- Typically acquired in the axial plane covering the entire chest
- Used to define pericardial anatomy and measure pericardial thickness

Cine bSSFP

- Acquired in standard cardiac imaging planes
- Allows for quantification of ventricular volumes and ejection fraction
- Allows qualitative assessment of ventricular shape and motion

Myocardial tagging

- Typically 3 short-axis slices acquired (basal, mid, and apical)
- Long-axis views can also be useful
- Used to evaluate adherence and immobility of the pericardium over the myocardium

Real-time cine sequences

- Usually acquired in short-axis plane at the level of the papillary muscles and including the diaphragm
- Allows assessment of respirophasic interventricular septal shift where the interventricular septum bows toward the LV during inspiration (diaphragm moves downward)

T2-weighted fast spin echo sequences (eg, STIR or SPAIR)

- May be acquired in the vertical long axis, 4-chamber, LVOT, or short-axis views
- Allows evaluation of pericardial edema and inflammation

Phase contrast images

- Acquired in cross-section, perpendicular to the flow of blood
- Assess tricuspid and mitral inflow patterns throughout the respiratory cycle

Postcontrast dynamic cardiac perfusion

- Acquired in select planes that include pericardial mass
- Used to assess vascularization of pericardial masses

Late gadolinium enhancement

- Often acquired in the vertical long axis, 4-chamber, LVOT, and short-axis views
- Allows evaluation of pericardial neovascularization/inflammation
- Fat saturation can be used to help distinguish pericardial delayed enhancement from epicardial fat

Abbreviations: bSSFP, balanced stead state free precession; LVOT, left ventricular outflow tract; SPAIR, spectral attenuated inversion recovery; STIR, short tau inversion recovery.

---

lymphadenopathy, and ill-defined margins.[4,16] Metastatic involvement of the pericardium can occur through direct invasion, lymphatic spread, or hematogenous dissemination. Common primary malignancies that can metastasize to the pericardium include breast, lung, esophageal, kidney, or melanoma. On CMR, malignant masses/nodules will commonly have heterogeneous signal intensity on T1- and T2-weighted imaging, reflecting areas of edema, hemorrhage, and or necrosis. First-pass perfusion imaging can help define vascularity of masses. The appearance on late gadolinium enhancement (LGE) imaging can be variable and is often heterogeneous.[4]

Table 2
Summary of cardiovascular MRI sequences for the assessment of congenital abnormalities of the pericardium and pericardial neoplasms

	MRI Sequence	Imaging Planes	Findings
Congenital absence of the pericardium	• T1 TSE/FSE (eg, HASTE) • bSSFP axial stack/cines	• Axial/coronal/sagittal stack of the chest • Vertical long axis, 4-chamber, LVOT, and short-axis views	• Lack of pericardium, seen best in the AV groove and adjacent to the RV free wall • Varying degrees of leftward and posterior deviation of the heart
Pericardial cyst	• T1 TSE/FSE • Black-blood T2-weighted FSE images (eg, STIR/SPAIR) • LGE • bSSFP cines	• Axial/coronal/sagittal stack of the chest • Vertical long-axis, 4-chamber, LVOT, and short-axis views	• Low signal on T1-weighted images (unless fluid is proteinaceous) • High signal intensity on T2-weight images • Lack of contrast enhancement on DHE
Pericardial masses	• T1 TSE/FSE • Black-blood T2-weighted FSE images (with and without fat suppression) • Postcontrast dynamic cardiac perfusion • LGE • bSSFP cines focused on the mass	• Axial/coronal/sagittal stack of the chest • Vertical long-axis, 4-chamber, LVOT, and short-axis views • Off-axis views focused on the mass	• Well-defined mass with varying degrees of perfusion and T1/T2 signal intensity, depending on mass composition • Lipomas are hyperintense on T1, intermediate in signal intensity on T2, and demonstrate signal drop out on fat suppressed imaging
Acute pericarditis	• T1 TSE/FSE • Black-blood T2-weighted FSE images • LGE	• Axial/coronal/sagittal stack of the chest • Vertical long-axis, 4-chamber, LVOT, and short-axis views	• Allows assessment of pericardial effusion, edema and inflammation suggestive of vascularized granulation tissue, fibrin etc. • Identify myocardial involvement
Pericardial constriction	• T1 TSE/FSE • Black-blood T2-weighted FSE images • Free breathing real-time cine • LGE	• Axial/coronal/sagittal stack of the chest • Vertical long-axis, 4-chamber, LVOT, and short-axis views • Free-breathing sequences done in SAX including the diaphragm	• Allows assessment of pericardial thickness and constrictive physiology • Allows identification of on-going inflammation, pericardial enhancement • Can help rule out myocardial pathology (ie, causes of restrictive cardiomyopathy)

(continued on next page)

Table 2
(continued)

	MRI Sequence	Imaging Planes	Findings
Pericardial effusion	• T1 TSE/FSE • Black-blood T2-weighted FSE images • LGE	• Axial/coronal/sagittal stack of the chest • Vertical long-axis, 4-chamber, LVOT, and short axis views	• Effusion is bright on bSSFP, dark on black-blood T1-weighted spin echo sequences and has signal void in PSIR images

Abbreviations: AV, atrioventricular; bSSFP, balanced stead state free precession; FSE, fast-spin echo; HASTE, half fourier acquisition single-shot turbo spin echo imaging; LGE, late gadolinium enhancement; LVOT, left ventricular outflow tract; SPAIR, spectral attenuated inversion recovery; STIR, short tau inversion recovery; TSE, turbo spin echo.

Primary pericardial malignancies are rare and include mesothelioma, sarcomas, lymphomas, and primitive neuroendocrine tumors. Primary malignant mesothelioma of the pericardium is extremely rare, with a reported incidence of 0.022% in autopsy series, but accounts for approximately half of primary pericardial malignancies.[13] Mesothelioma can originate from the pericardium or spread from the adjacent pleura. On CMR, mesothelioma typically appears as nodular pericardial masses and is often associated with complex pericardial effusions. Pericardial sarcomas are rare and can include angiosarcoma, fibrosarcoma, and liposarcoma. On CMR, sarcomas appear as nodular masses with heterogeneous T1 and T2 signal intensity, depending on the degree of necrosis and hemorrhage.[17] Pericardial lymphoma usually presents as an ill-defined, diffuse mass commonly affecting the right atrium, epicardial fat, and atrioventricular groove. Lymphoma is usually hypointense on T1-weighted imaging and iso-to hyperintense on T2-weighted imaging and is often associated with a hemorrhagic pericardial effusion.[18]

Benign primary neoplasms of the pericardium include angiomas, lymphangiomas, fibromas, teratomas, and lipomas. Lipomas are neoplasms of mature fat cells and usually grow insidiously, only resulting in symptoms due to compressive effects or arrhythmias.[13,19] Lipomas have hyperintense signal on T1-weighted images, intermediate to high signal on T2-weighted images and signal drop out with fat suppression. Lipomas usually do not visibly enhance postcontrast administration. Hemangiomas of the pericardium usually arise from the visceral pericardium and histologically are most commonly cavernous. They typically have heterogeneous intermediate-to-high T1 signal intensity due to slow flow and high signal

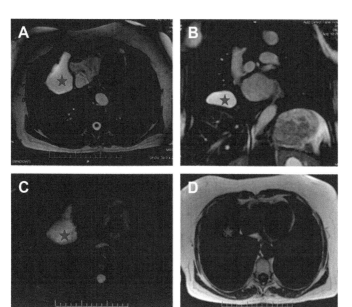

Fig. 1. Pericardial cyst in the right cardiophrenic angle that measured 7.8 × 5.8 × 3 cm (AP × TR × CC). (*A*) bSSFP images in axial orientation and (*B*) bSSFP image in a coronal orientation demonstrates the location of the cyst in the anterior right cardiophrenic angle. (*C*) The cyst is homogenously hyperintense on T2-weighted imaging (T2 SPAIR) and (*D*) homogenously hypointense on T1-weighted imaging (T1 TSE). Star demonstrates the cyst. bSSFP, balanced steady-state free precession; SPAIR, spectrally adiabatic inversion recovery; TSE, turbo spin echo.

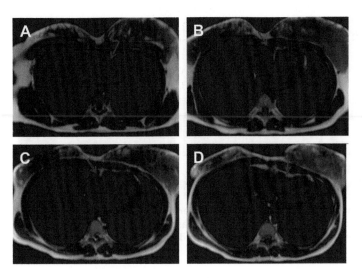

Fig. 2. Complete congenital absence of the pericardium. Multiple axial slices demonstrate absence of the pericardium. (*A*) Most cranial axial slice demonstrating a portion of the left upper lobe of the lung extending into the space between the ascending aorta and main pulmonary artery (*arrow*) supporting absence of the pericardium. (*B–D*) More caudal axial slices, all demonstrating absence of the pericardium (*arrows*).

intensity on T2-weighted images.[4,20] Contrast enhancement is heterogeneous.

ACUTE PERICARDITIS

Acute pericarditis is an inflammatory process of the pericardium characterized by vascularized granulation tissue, fibrin, and fluid accumulation.[4,21] Diagnostic criteria include (1) acute onset pleuritic chest pain, (2) classic concave upward ST elevation with PR depression on electrocardiography, (3) a pericardial friction rub on cardiac auscultation, and (4) a new or worsening pericardial effusion. A diagnosis is made by the presence of 2 or more of these criteria. However, in the absence of meeting this criteria, a diagnosis can still be made by the presence of ancillary findings such as increased inflammatory markers, white blood cell count, fever, and/or troponin elevation.[22,23] The cause of acute pericarditis includes infections, connective tissue disorders, drug reactions, radiation, uremia, myocardial infarction, and pericardial trauma. However, 30% of cases are idiopathic, with no clear inciting factor.[23] CMR is generally not required for evaluation of uncomplicated acute pericarditis meeting classic diagnostic criteria and responding appropriately to therapy. However, it can be useful for those with incessant (ongoing symptoms >4–6 weeks, but <3 months), recurrent (symptom recurrence after 4–6 weeks of quiescence), or chronic (>3 months of ongoing symptoms) pericarditis.[2]

Acute pericarditis presents with varying degrees of pericardial thickening, ranging from normal to mildly thickened, with an average pericardial thickness of 4.8 ± 2.9 mm reported in some series.[21,24] Pericardial edema and inflammation can be

evaluated using both T2-weighted and LGE imaging (**Fig. 3**). Acutely inflamed pericardium is usually hyperintense on T2-weighted imaging (eg, T2-STIR/SPAIR) and correlates with findings of edema, neovascularization, and granulation tissue.[1,21,25] Care must be taken to differentiate intense pericardial signal on T2-weighted imaging from pericardial effusion.

Typically, given its relatively low vascularity, the normal pericardium does not take up gadolinium. In response to injury, there is increased vascularity of the pericardium and resultant infiltration of neutrophils and deposition of fibrin.[26] Enhancement of the pericardium on LGE imaging suggests pericardial inflammation or fibrosis.[21,25] This process can extend into adjacent epicardial fat or myocardium, in cases of myopericarditis, which occurs in approximately 15% of cases.[2] High signal intensity of the pericardium on LGE imaging can sometimes be confused with pericardial fat. Fat suppression helps distinguish pericardial enhancement from fat and may increase specificity for true pericardial edema and fibrosis/inflammation.[2] A retrospective, observational study in patients with established recurrent pericarditis found that quantification of pericardial LGE can predict patients who develop ongoing recurrent pericarditis.[27] However, in current clinical practice, enhancement of the pericardium is typically evaluated qualitatively.

Although CMR can be used to assess acute pericarditis, it adds greater value in patients with complicated pericarditis, such as those whose pain does not respond appropriately to therapy or those with recurrent pain after appropriately tapered antiinflammatory treatment.[2,23] This scenario can be challenging, especially when patients

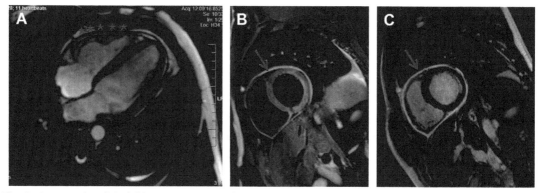

Fig. 3. Acute pericarditis. (*A*) bSSFP cine image demonstrating prominent pericardium along the anterior lateral wall of the RV (*stars*). (*B*) T2-weighted imaging (SPAIR) demonstrates increase in diffuse pericardial edema (*arrow*). (*C*) Late gadolinium enhancement imaging suggesting diffuse pericardial enhancement.

do not meet clinical criteria for recurrent pericarditis.[28] In these patients, CMR may be helpful to differentiate those with ongoing pericardial inflammation who may benefit from intensified antiinflammatory treatment from those who have no ongoing inflammation and in whom alternative causes of chest pain should be sought. In the context of recurrent pericarditis, a retrospective, single-center observational study demonstrated that patients who underwent CMR-guided treatment had overall less glucocorticoid use without an increase in constrictive pericarditis, pericardial window, or pericardiectomy. These findings suggest that clinicians may be more comfortable tapering therapy when CMR demonstrates no active inflammation on LGE imaging.[29]

PERICARDIAL CONSTRICTION

Pericardial constriction is characterized by an inelastic pericardium that restricts diastolic filling of the heart. This can occur as a result of advanced fibrosis or calcification of the pericardium following pericardial injury (ie, pericarditis, prior radiation, or postpericardiectomy) or from malignant infiltration of the pericardium. Pericardial constriction as a cause of heart failure is an important diagnosis to make, as traditional heart failure therapies are often unhelpful and directed therapies (eg, pericardiectomy) may be curative.[8,30] Although echocardiography and right heart catheterization have historically been pivotal in establishing the diagnosis, assessment can be limited by technical factors and operator expertise and can occasionally be inconclusive. CMR is well suited for the assessment of pericardial constriction, as it allows complete anatomic assessment of the pericardium, hemodynamic evaluation, and tissue characterization.

Pericardial constriction often presents with thickening of the pericardium, usually best appreciated on black-blood T1-weighted imaging, although up to 20% of patients have normal pericardial thickness[24] (**Fig. 4**). The pericardium will appear as a low signal intensity structure. Very low signal intensity areas suggest calcification. Short- and long-axis balanced steady-state free precession (bSSFP) cine images allow for the assessment of myocardial function and typical features of pericardial constriction, including a diastolic septal bounce (**Fig. 5**), conical and tubular deformity of the right and left ventricles respectively, rapid early diastolic filling with diastolic restraint, and qualitative tethering of the pericardium. The latter can also be assessed more objectively with tagged cine images, where tag lines are superimposed on the myocardium at the beginning of a cine sequence and subsequent deformation of these lines due to sliding of the myocardium along the pericardium can be measured.[31]

Real-time bSSFP cine imaging in the mid-short axis plane during approximately 10 seconds of free breathing can be used to visually assess respirophasic septal shift during inspiration,[32] marked by downward motion of the diaphragm. In patients with constrictive physiology, the interventricular septum bows toward the LV during inspiration (a marker of ventricular interdependence) (see **Fig. 5**). Early diastolic inversion or septal flattening at the onset of inspiration distinguishes patients with pericardial constriction from normal controls and patients with restrictive cardiomyopathy,[5] which can be quantified by dividing the RV free wall to septum distance by the overall biventricular distance during inspiration and expiration, a ratio called the "relative septal excursion." In a study looking at the hierarchical

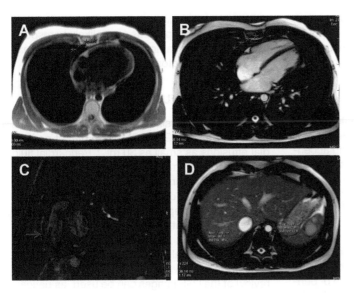

Fig. 4. Constrictive pericarditis. (*A*) HASTE image demonstrating significant pericardial thickening, which is confirmed on bSSFP cine image (*B*). (*C*) There is pericardial enhancement on LGE. (*D*) The IVC is dilated with an increased IVC to aorta area ratio. HASTE, half fourier single-shot turbo spin echo; IVC, inferior vena cava.

relationship among various CMR criteria for the diagnosis of pericardial constriction, with surgical confirmation, a relative septal excursion greater than or equal to 12% combined with increased pericardial thickness was the best discriminator of pericardial constriction with a sensitivity and specificity of 100% and 90%, respectively.[33]

Inferior vena cava (IVC) plethora, measured by taking the cross-sectional area of the suprahepatic IVC and dividing by the abdominal aorta cross-sectional area, can also support the diagnosis of constrictive pericarditis by demonstrating the presence of elevated right atrial pressures[34] (see **Fig. 4**).

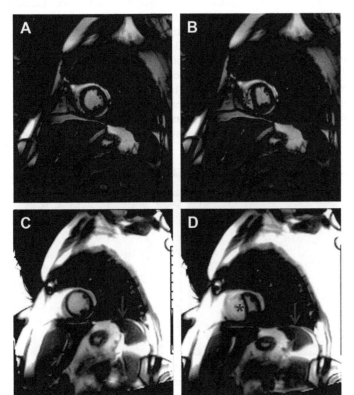

Fig. 5. Pericardial constriction. (*A, B*) Diastolic septal bounce based on segmented bSSFP cine images. The star demonstrates the septal flattening in diastole. (*C, D*) Respirophasic septal shift demonstrated based on real-time cine acquisition. Arrow demonstrates flatting of the diaphragm with inspiration, whereas the star demonstrates the septal flattening.

Although these findings can be very suggestive, they are only indirect signs of constrictive physiology. Classically, echocardiography has been pivotal in demonstrating dissociation between intracardiac and intrathoracic pressures through discordant respirophasic variation in diastolic inflow across the mitral valve (MV) and tricuspid valve (TV). CMR real-time phase contrast flow measurement of simultaneous TV and MV inflow velocities is a novel method of establishing accentuated and discordant respirophasic changes in mitral and tricuspid inflow velocities and supports the diagnosis of constrictive pericarditis.[35] However, further validation of this application of real-time phase contrast imaging is pending.

CMR has led to the identification of a subset of cases of pericardial constriction in which there is ongoing acute or subacute inflammation in the pericardium as evidenced by the presence of pericardial LGE. Histopathologic correlation with CMR has demonstrated that the presence of pericardial LGE correlates with greater fibroblastic proliferation, chronic inflammation, and neovascularization, which indicates ongoing active inflammation, whereas patients without LGE demonstrate more pericardial fibrosis and calcification ("burnt out" phase).[26] The reported sensitivity of LGE for identifying pericardial inflammation has been reported at 94% to 100%.[36] Treatment of patients with constrictive pericarditis and evidence of LGE on CMR with antiinflammatory medical therapy has resulted in reduced LGE and overall clinical improvement, which suggests that at least some of the LGE is due to active inflammation,[21] and this has given rise to the term "transient constriction," which describes the distinct subtype of constrictive pericarditis where diastolic filling is impaired due to acute or subacute pericardial inflammation that is reversible with antiinflammatory therapy.[37] In the "burnt out" phase, patients are unlikely to respond to further antiinflammatory therapy and may require pericardiectomy to relieve symptoms.

PERICARDIAL EFFUSION

The presence and size of a pericardial effusion is well delineated on CMR. CMR can detect pericardial effusions as small as 30 mL.[7] Pericardial fluid appears dark on black-blood spin echo sequences. However, nonlinear motion of fluid during the cardiac cycle can occasionally cause higher signal on spin echo sequences. Effusions will appear bright on SSFP/gradient echo sequences (**Fig. 6**); however, pericardial fat may have similar signal intensity, making it difficult to distinguish from pericardial fluid.[38] When in doubt, review of the LGE images can be used, as pericardial fluid does not take up gadolinium and will appear dark on PSIR images (see **Fig. 6**). Furthermore, pericardial effusions on cine bSSFP images will demonstrate typical fluidlike motion that gets displaced in diastole, as opposed to pericardial fat that moves with the ventricle throughout the cardiac cycle.

Pericardial effusions are defined as physiologic if fluid is only seen in the pericardial recesses or if only seen during systole and get displaced during diastole. Pericardial effusions that persist throughout the cardiac cycle are defined based on the width of adjacent fluid as small (<1.0 cm), moderate (1.0–2.0 cm), or large (>2.0 cm).[1] However, this definition is somewhat arbitrary, and a more qualitative description of the location and extent of fluid is often more helpful. Loculated pericardial effusions can occur, usually after the pericardium has been previously instrumented. The signal characteristics of the effusion can help

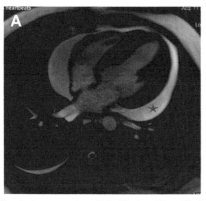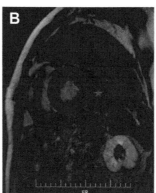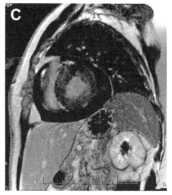

Fig. 6. Large pericardial effusion identified on 4-chamber bSSFP image (*A*). (*B*) Delayed enhancement magnitude image in short axis demonstrates pericardial effusion, which appears (*C*) black on phase sensitive inversion recover images.

with predicting the composition and cause of the fluid. An effusion with signal characteristics similar to water suggest a transudative effusion, whereas exudates with higher protein content and cell count tend to have shorter T1 relaxation (higher signal on T1-weighted images) and shorter T2 relaxation (lower signal on T2-weighted images).[39] A pericardial effusion associated with grossly thickened pericardium and high signal intensity on T2-weighted images associated with enhancement on LGE images should raise the possibility of tuberculous pericarditis in the right clinical context.[40]

Although CMR is not the imaging modality of choice in assessing the hemodynamic significance of pericardial effusions, signs of pericardial constraint and impending tamponade are occasionally seen. Significantly elevated pericardial pressures can result in chamber compression or collapse, typically the lowest pressure chambers first, such as the right atrium (during ventricular systole) followed by the right ventricle (during diastole); this can be masked in the setting of severe pulmonary hypertension, evidenced by pulmonary artery dilation, RV hypertrophy, and interventricular septal flattening, in which case the left atrium may be the lowest pressure chamber and may experience collapse first.[6] Dilation of the superior vena cava and IVC can also be seen, reflective of the increased central venous pressures. Exaggerated respirophasic variation of the interventricular septum and abnormal septal motion are also signs of a hemodynamically significant pericardial effusion. These signs of increased ventricular interdependence in the setting of a pericardial effusion can also suggest the presence of an effusive-constrictive pericardial effusion, defined as the persistence of pericardial constraint after the removal of pericardial fluid.[4] The presence of signs of increased intrapericardial pressure in the context of pericardial effusion should warrant further clinical assessment.

SUMMARY

Diseases of the pericardium can pose a significant diagnostic challenge. Multimodality imaging has revolutionized our understanding of pericardial pathology and allowed for accurate, noninvasive diagnosis of pericardial disease that can directly guide treatment. CMR is a comprehensive imaging modality allowing not only complete anatomic characterization of the pericardium but also hemodynamic assessment and tissue characterization, making it a key imaging modality in the assessment and management of patients with pericardial disease.

DISCLOSURE

Dr. Thavendiranathan (147814) is supported by the Canadian Institutes of Health Research New Investigator Award and a Canada Research Chair in Cardiooncology.

REFERENCES

1. Klein AL, Abbara S, Agler DA, et al. American society of echocardiography clinical recommendations for multimodality cardiovascular imaging of patients with pericardial disease: endorsed by the society for cardiovascular magnetic resonance and society of cardiovascular computed tomography. J Am Soc Echocardiogr 2013;26(9):965–1012.e15.
2. Cremer PC, Kumar A, Kontzias A, et al. Complicated pericarditis: understanding risk factors and pathophysiology to inform imaging and treatment. J Am Coll Cardiol 2016;68(21):2311–28.
3. Rodriguez ER, Tan CD. Structure and anatomy of the human pericardium. Prog Cardiovasc Dis 2017; 59(4):327–40.
4. Rajiah P. Cardiac MRI: part 2, pericardial diseases. AJR Am J Roentgenol 2011;197(4):W621–34.
5. Francone M, Dymarkowski S, Kalantzi M, et al. Real-time cine MRI of ventricular motion: a novel approach to assess ventricular coupling. J Magn Reson Imaging 2005;21(3):305–9.
6. Borlaug BA, Reddy YNV. The role of the pericardium in heart failure. JACC Heart Fail 2019;7(7):574–85.
7. Bogaert J, Francone M. Cardiovascular magnetic resonance in pericardial diseases. J Cardiovasc Magn Reson 2009;11(1):1–14.
8. Ariyarajah V, Jassal DS, Kirkpatrick I, et al. The utility of cardiovascular magnetic resonance in constrictive pericardial disease. Cardiol Rev 2009;17(2): 77–82.
9. Jeung MY, Gasser B, Gangi A, et al. Imaging of cystic masses of the mediastinum. Radiographics 2002;22(SPEC. ISS):79–93.
10. Bogaert J, Francone M. Pericardial disease: value of CT and MR imaging. Radiology 2013;267(2):340–56.
11. Yamano T, Sawada T, Sakamoto K, et al. Magnetic resonance imaging differentiated partial from complete absence of the left pericardimn in a case of leftward displacement of the heart. Circ J 2004; 68(4):385–8.
12. Shah AB, Kronzon I. Congenital defects of the pericardium : a review. Eur Heart J Cardiovasc Imaging 2015;16(8):821–7.
13. Restrepo CS, Vargas D, Ocazionez D, et al. Primary pericardial tumors. Radiographics 2013;33(6): 1613–30.
14. Butany J, Leong SW, Carmichael K, et al. A 30-year analysis of cardiac neoplasms at autopsy. Can J Cardiol 2005;21(8):675–80.

15. MacGee W. Metastatic and invasive tumours involving the heart in a geriatric population: a necropsy study. Virchows Arch A Pathol Anat Histopathol 1991;419(3):183–9.

16. Hoey ETD, Shahid M, Ganeshan A, et al. MRI assessment of cardiac tumours: part 2 , spectrum of appearances of histologically malignant lesions and tumour mimics. Quant Imaging Med Surg 2014;4(6):489–97.

17. Araoz PA, Eklund HE, Welch TJ, et al. CT and MR imaging of primary cardiac malignancies. Radiographics 1999;19(6):1421–34.

18. Jeudy J, Kirsch J, Tavora F, et al. From the radiologic pathology archives: cardiac lymphoma: radiologic-pathologic correlation. Radiographics 2012;32(5):1369–80.

19. Noly PE, Mongeon FP, Rochon A, et al. Pericardial constriction caused by a giant lipoma. Circulation 2016;133(17):1709–12.

20. Sparrow PJ, Kurian JB, Jones TR, et al. MR imaging of cardiac tumors. Radiographics 2005;25(5):1255–76.

21. Young PM, Glockner JF, Williamson EE, et al. MR imaging findings in 76 consecutive surgically proven cases of pericardial disease with CT and pathologic correlation. Int J Cardiovasc Imaging 2012;28(5):1099–109.

22. Adler Y, Charron P, Imazio M, et al. 2015 ESC guidelines for the diagnosis and management of pericardial diseases the task force for the diagnosis and management of pericardial diseases of the European society of cardiology (ESC) endorsed by : the European association for cardio-thoracic surgery. Eur Heart J 2015;36(42):2921–64.

23. Imazio M, Spodick DH, Brucato A, et al. Controversial issues in the management of pericardial diseases. Circulation 2010;121(7):916–28.

24. Talreja DR, Edwards WD, Danielson GK, et al. Constrictive pericarditis in 26 patients with histologically normal pericardial thickness. Circulation 2003;108(15):1852–7.

25. Taylor AM, Dymarkowski S, Verbeken EK, et al. Detection of pericardial inflammation with late-enhancement cardiac magnetic resonance imaging: initial results. Eur Radiol 2006;16(3):569–74.

26. Zurick AO, Bolen MA, Kwon DH, et al. Pericardial delayed hyperenhancement with CMR imaging in patients with constrictive pericarditis undergoing surgical pericardiectomy: a case series with histopathological correlation. JACC Cardiovasc Imaging 2011;4(11):1180–91.

27. Kumar A, Sato K, Verma BR, et al. Quantitative assessment of pericardial delayed hyperenhancement helps identify patients with ongoing recurrences of pericarditis. Open Heart 2018;5(2):1–9.

28. Imazio M, Demichelis B, Parrini I, et al. Recurrent pain without objective evidence of disease in patients with previous idiopathic or viral acute pericarditis. Am J Cardiol 2004;94(7):973–5.

29. Alraies MC, AlJaroudi W, Yarmohammadi H, et al. Usefulness of cardiac magnetic resonance-guided management in patients with recurrent pericarditis. Am J Cardiol 2015;115(4):542–7.

30. Khandaker MH, Espinosa RE, Nishimura RA, et al. Pericardial disease: diagnosis and management. Mayo Clin Proc 2010;85(6):572–93.

31. Jeung M-Y, Germain P, Croisille P, et al. Myocardial tagging with MR imaging : overview of normal and pathologic findings. Radiographics 2012;32(5):1381–98.

32. Geske JB, Anavekar NS, Nishimura RA, et al. Differentiation of constriction and restriction. J Am Coll Cardiol 2016;68(21):2329–47.

33. Bolen MA, Rajiah P, Kusunose K, et al. Cardiac MR imaging in constrictive pericarditis: multiparametric assessment in patients with surgically proven constriction. Int J Cardiovasc Imaging 2015;31(4):859–66.

34. Hanneman K, Thavendiranathan P, Nguyen ET, et al. Use of cardiac magnetic resonance imaging based measurements of inferior vena cava cross-sectional area in the diagnosis of pericardial constriction. Can Assoc Radiol J 2015;66(3):231–7.

35. Thavendiranathan P, Verhaert D, Walls MC, et al. Simultaneous right and left heart real-time, free-breathing CMR flow quantification identifies constrictive physiology. JACC Cardiovasc Imaging 2012;5(1):15–24.

36. Xu B, Harb SC, Klein AL. Utility of multimodality cardiac imaging in disorders of the pericardium. Echo Res Pract 2018;5(2):R37–48.

37. Gentry J, Klein AL, Jellis CL. Transient constrictive pericarditis: current diagnostic and therapeutic strategies. Curr Cardiol Rep 2016;18(5):41.

38. Vakamudi S, Ho N, Cremer PC. Pericardial effusions: causes, diagnosis, and management. Prog Cardiovasc Dis 2017;59(4):380–8.

39. Rienmüller R, Gröll R, Lipton MJ. CT and MR imaging of pericardial disease. Radiol Clin North Am 2004;42(3):587–601.

40. Tse G, Ali A, Francisco A, et al. Tuberculous constrictive pericarditis. Belg Tijdschr Geneesk 1960;16(4):1209–15.

The Role of Cardiovascular MRI in Cardio-Oncology

Wendy Bottinor, MD, MSCI[a,b,]*, Cory R. Trankle, MD[a], W. Gregory Hundley, MD[a]

KEYWORDS

- Cardio-oncology • Cardiovascular MRI • Cardiotoxicity • Tissue characterization

KEY POINTS

- The accuracy and reproducibility of cardiovascular MRI (CMR) makes it an ideal method for noninvasive assessment in settings where precise quantification of left or right ventricular function is required.
- CMR can be particularly useful in individuals with poor acoustic windows, discordant clinical data, or when tissue characterization is required.
- Tissue characterization is particularly useful in the diagnosis of deposition diseases, inflammatory diseases, and for understanding the pathophysiology of early cardiotoxicity.
- As CMR becomes more widely used, further investigation will be required to define the role of CMR in the screening, diagnosis, and prevention of cancer therapy–related cardiotoxicity.

With cardiovascular disease emerging as a leading cause of morbidity and mortality among individuals undergoing treatment of cancer and cancer survivors, cardiovascular MRI (CMR) is increasingly used to identify those at risk for or with evolving cardiac or vascular injury.[1,2] Within the field of cardio-oncology, the role of CMR has not been fully defined; however, CMR is suggested for individuals with poor echocardiographic windows, a borderline left ventricular ejection fraction (LVEF), or discrepant clinical values.[3–5] In addition, CMR may be particularly useful in detecting subclinical cardiovascular disease.

Here the authors review current data guiding the role of CMR in cardio-oncology. They discuss the value of CMR in a variety of clinical scenarios including left and right ventricular systolic dysfunction that promotes both clinical and subclinical disease, myocyte atrophy, immune check point inhibitor (ICI) mediated myocarditis, cardiac amyloidosis, myocardial fibrosis, hypovolemia, and the identification of early myocellular injury (**Table 1**). The authors describe CMR techniques that can be useful in these clinical scenarios (**Fig. 1**). Lastly, they evaluate current and future investigative efforts using CMR to further our

Funding: This publication is supported in part by the To-morrow's Research Fund St. Baldrick's Scholar Award (Award Number 636214). The content is solely the responsibility of the authors and does not necessarily represent the official views of St. Baldrick's Foundation. This publication is supported in part by the American Heart Association (Award Number (19CDA34760181). The content is solely the responsibility of the authors and does not necessarily represent the official views of the American Heart Association. This publication is supported in part by the National Institutes of Health (Award Number (1R01HL118740-01, 1R01CA199167-01, R21CA226960-01A1). The content is solely the responsibility of the authors and does not necessarily represent the official views of the National Institutes of Health.

[a] Department of Internal Medicine, Division of Cardiovascular Medicine, Pauley Heart Center, Virginia Commonwealth University, Gateway Building, 1200 East Marshall Street, Richmond, VA 23298, USA; [b] Division of Cardiovascular Medicine, Department of Medicine, Vanderbilt University School of Medicine, 2220 Pierce Avenue, 383 Preston Research Building, Nashville, TN 37232-6300, USA
* Corresponding author. Virginia Commonwealth University, Gateway Building, 1200 East Marshall Street, Richmond, VA 23298.
E-mail address: bottinorw@mymail.vcu.edu

Heart Failure Clin 17 (2021) 121–133
https://doi.org/10.1016/j.hfc.2020.08.009

Table 1
Summary of select clinical cardio-oncology conditions and potential cardiovascular MRI features

Clinical Conditions in Cardio-Oncology	CMR Features
Left ventricular systolic dysfunction	Reduced LVEF Abnormal GLS/GCS Abnormal segmental intramyocardial strain +/− LGE +/− Abnormal T1 and T2 mapping
RV dysfunction	Reduced RVEF Abnormal GLS/GCS
Myocyte atrophy	Reduced LV mass Increased end systolic wall stress
ICI myocarditis	LGE Elevated T2 inversion recovery times
Amyloid deposition	Difficulty nulling LV myocardium Global subendocardial LGE RV LGE
Myocardial fibrosis	Elevated ECVF LGE Increased myocardial T1
Hypovolemia	Reduced LV volumes Reduced LVEF Abnormal GLS/GCS Reduced LV mass
Early myocellular injury	Elevated T2 relaxation times Increased ECVF Increased native T1

Abbreviations: ECVF, extracellular volume fraction; GCS, global circumferential strain; GLS, global longitudinal strain; LGE, late gadolinium enhancement; RVEF, right ventricular ejection fraction.

understanding of cardiovascular disease as a result of cancer or its treatment.

VENTRICULAR VOLUMES AND EJECTION FRACTION

A decrease in LVEF is most frequently used to identify early evidence of LV myocardial injury as a result of treatment of cancer.[3,6] LVEF can be measured by a variety of imaging techniques including a multigated acquisition (MUGA) scan, transthoracic echocardiography, or CMR.

Although the first clinical noninvasive cardiovascular assessments of LVEF were performed primarily with MUGA scanning, this technique is now used less frequently due to its dependence on the administration of ionizing radiation and limited ability to provide assessment of additional cardiac structures.[7] Today, transthoracic echocardiography is often used to assess LVEF because it is widely available and portable, does not expose patients to ionizing radiation, and provides information regarding cardiac structures.

There are however some limitations to the use of transthoracic echocardiography in patients with or having received treatment of cancer. These include (1) poor acoustic windows, (2) the potential for foreshortening the LV or using imprecise geometric assumptions, and (3) suboptimal endocardial definition, all of which can impair the ability to assess ventricular volumes and LVEF. Consequently, the range of detectable changes in LVEF for an individual patient can be quite large. In patients with cancer, the minimum change in LVEF detectable with 95% confidence by 2-dimensional echocardiography–based volumetric quantification techniques is approximately 10 LVEF units.[8,9] Data in adult survivors of childhood onset malignancy have shown that 2-dimensional echocardiography overestimates LVEF by approximately 5% in this population.[10]

CMR does not incorporate ionizing radiation, does not exhibit window or geometric limitations, and provides precise ventricular endocardial definition. These features result in highly reproducible accurate assessments of right or LV measurements of end systolic and end diastolic ventricular volumes necessary for the determination of right ventricular ejection fraction or LVEF. The superior imaging ability of CMR was highlighted by a study from Bellenger and colleagues,[11] in which only 69% of echo images were of adequate quality for 2-dimensional LVEF measurement; however, all CMR studies were analyzable. Several studies have demonstrated higher accuracy and interstudy reproducibility with CMR, suggesting the minimal detectable change in LVEF is approximately 5% (**Table 2**).[12–17] In a direct comparison of interstudy reproducibility between CMR and transthoracic echocardiography, Grothues and colleagues[18] demonstrated a superior reproducibility of LVEF quantified by CMR techniques relative to transthoracic echocardiography.

The accurate measurement of end systolic and end diastolic ventricular volumes by CMR can also be beneficial for assessing the cause for changes in LVEF. LVEF and right ventricular ejection fraction measurements are preload dependent. This is of particular importance in cardiooncology, as individuals undergoing cancer therapy often develop hypovolemia related to

Standard Cinematic Sequences

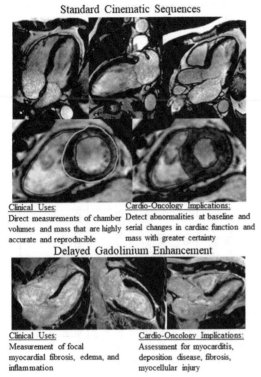

Strain Analysis

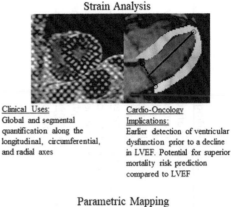

Clinical Uses:
Global and segmental
quantification along the
longitudinal, circumferential,
and radial axes

Cardio-Oncology
Implications:
Earlier detection of ventricular
dysfunction prior to a decline
in LVEF. Potential for superior
mortality risk prediction
compared to LVEF

Clinical Uses:
Direct measurements of chamber
volumes and mass that are highly
accurate and reproducible

Cardio-Oncology Implications:
Detect abnormalities at baseline and
serial changes in cardiac function and
mass with greater certainty

Delayed Gadolinium Enhancement

Clinical Uses:
Measurement of focal
myocardial fibrosis, edema, and
inflammation

Cardio-Oncology Implications:
Assessment for myocarditis,
deposition disease, fibrosis,
myocellular injury

Parametric Mapping

Native T1 Map   Post-Contrast T1 Map   Native T2 Map

Clinical Uses:
Global/regional T1 and T2 values
Extracellular volume calculation
Measurement of myocardial
fibrosis, edema, and inflammation

Cardio-Oncology Implications:
Characterize tissue changes which
may predict functional loss or
treatment toxicity

Fig. 1. The role of CMR imaging techniques in clinical cardio-oncology.

treatment effects such as decreased oral intake and emesis. Changes in LVEF due to decreases in LV end-diastolic volume are common, and changes in volume should be accounted for when comparing serial LVEF measurements.[19]

An additional advantage of CMR relates to its 3-dimensional method of acquisition. Two-dimensional echocardiography relies on geometric assumptions regarding ventricular morphology that becomes less certain in many pathologic states. Grouthes and colleagues[18] have shown significantly superior reproducibility of measurements of LVEF in individuals with heart failure or LV hypertrophy when comparing CMR and echocardiography. Semelka and colleagues[17] have determined the percent variability between studies of LVEF, and end-diastolic volume measurements in individuals with heart failure or LV hypertrophy are less than 5%. Therefore, the 3-dimensional approach of CMR can be particularly advantageous when analyzing individuals with morphologically abnormal ventricles.

Right ventricular dysfunction has been observed in approximately one-third of individuals receiving trastuzumab for breast cancer treatment and one-third of childhood cancer survivors.[20,21] Because of the complex morphology of the right ventricle, and the three-dimensional approach of CMR, this

remains the gold standard for right ventricular volumes and ejection fraction assessments. Although lower than the reproducibility for the LV, CMR measurements of right ventricular mass, volumes, and ejection fraction remain highly reproducible both in healthy individuals and those with cardiovascular pathology.[22]

STRAIN IMAGING

CMR can also be used to assess myocardial strain, a measurement of myocardial tissue deformation that is assessed along all 3 dimensions of contraction in the longitudinal, circumferential, and radial directions. In individuals with cancer, a decrease in transthoracic echocardiography–derived measures of longitudinal strain along multiple LV segments (termed global longitudinal strain [GLS]) of 10% to 15% during chemotherapy treatment is predictive of early cardiotoxicity defined as a decline in LVEF or the development of heart failure.[23] Myocardial strain is also a volume-dependent measurement, and changes in LV volume may cause declines in myocardial strain due to reductions in LV end-diastolic volume.[24]

CMR-derived myocardial strain has demonstrated superiority over echocardiography to

Table 2
Summary of studies evaluating the accuracy and reproducibility of cardiovascular MRI

Author and Year	Study Design	Study Population	N	Study Objectives	Study Findings
Longmore et al,[12] 1985	Prospective Cohort Study	Angina pectoris	20	Determine accuracy of CMR volumetric measurements	Accuracy of volumetric measurements determined by comparing left and right ventricular stroke volumes. Approximately 2% error in measurements
Rehr et al,[13] 1985	Cohort Study	Ventricular casts	15	Determine correlation between directly measured and CMR-calculated cast volumes	Correlation coefficient 0.993–0.997 for normal resolution CMR. Absolute error in volume measurement 1%–11%
Sechtem et al,[14] 1987	Prospective Cohort Study	Healthy volunteers	10	Determine variability of interobserver and intraobserver ventricular measurements	Correlation coefficient for left and right ventricular stroke volumes 0.95. Interobserver variability of left and right ventricular volumes 0.99 and 0.95, respectively
Mogelvang et al,[15] 1992	Prospective Cohort Study	Angina pectoris	22	Quantitate left ventricular volumes by CMR and to compare a short axis multislice and transversal contiguous multislice method	No statistically significant difference between stroke volumes measured by CMR and MUGA
Semelka et al,[16] 1990	Prospective Cohort Study	Healthy volunteers	11	Determine interobserver and interstudy variability of measurements of LV mass, volume, LVEF, and systolic wall stress	Interstudy variability of LVEF approximately 2.5%–5%. Interobserver variability in LVEF 2.5%
Semelka et al,[17] 1990	Prospective Cohort Study	Dilated cardiomyopathy/LV hypertrophy	19	Assess interstudy reproducibility in the morphologically abnormal left ventricle	Between studies LVEF varied <5%
Grothues et al,[18] 2002	Prospective Cohort Study	Normal volunteers/heart failure/LV hypertrophy	60	Provide direct comparison of the interstudy reproducibility between CMR and echocardiography	Interstudy reproducibility coefficient of variability was superior for CMR in all patient groups for LV volumes, LVEF, and LV mass

| Bellenger et al,[19] 2000 | Prospective Cohort Study | Chronic heart failure | 52 | Compare the agreement of LV volumes and LVEF by M-mode and 2D echocardiography, radionuclide ventriculography, and cardiovascular MRIe | Correlation coefficient for CMR and 2-dimensional LVEF and LV volumes 0.4 and 0.8, respectively |

Abbreviation: MUGA, multigated acquisition scan.

detect decreased circumferential and longitudinal strain in subjects with preserved systolic function.[25] Automated strain analysis is becoming more readily available and correlates well with subclinical changes in LVEF.[26]

Abnormal GLS has demonstrated a superior long-term prognostic potential to LVEF in determining mortality in populations without cancer, and current data suggest that changes in global circumferential strain in the absence of a decrease in LV end-systolic volume can help predict declines in LVEF at least 2 years after treatment in cancer survivors.[27–29] Abnormal strain has been observed in late survivors of both pediatric and adult onset malignancies.[23,30] The ongoing SUCCOUR trial and CARDIOTOX registry may help further clarify the clinical significance of abnormal strain during cancer therapy.[31,32] Segmental strain measured using fast-strain–encoded segmental intramyocardial strain (fSENC) is also an area of investigation with recent data indicating fSENC may detect LV dysfunction earlier than other imaging techniques.[33]

LEFT VENTRICULAR MASS

A progressive reduction in LV mass and ventricular cavity size with resultant increases in end systolic wall stress, a phenomena termed Grinch syndrome, has been described in late survivors of pediatric onset malignancies.[34] Similar findings have also been described in survivors of adult onset malignancies treated with anthracyclines.[35,36] Jordan and colleagues[36] have demonstrated that a 5% decline in LV mass occurs within 6 months of treatment with anthracycline-based chemotherapy, whereas changes in LV mass do not occur in individuals who receive nonanthracycline-based chemotherapy. Willis and colleagues[37] have detected reductions in LV mass as early as 1 month after anthracycline treatment.

The clinical significance of these declines in LV mass are becoming evident. Jordan and colleagues[36] have correlated reduced LV mass with symptoms of heart failure, even in individuals with preserved LVEF. In a pivotal study of 91 late survivors with anthracycline-mediated reductions in LVEF after cancer therapy, Neilan and colleagues[35] determined that a CMR-derived indexed LV mass less than 57 g/m^2 is predictor of adverse cardiovascular events with a sensitivity of 100% and specificity of 85%. Interestingly, changes in LV mass during cancer therapy have also been observed. These changes may be partly mediated by hypovolemia; therefore, volume status should

likely be considered when interpreting these measurements.[19]

INFLAMMATORY CARDIOMYOPATHY

ICIs modulate the immune system by blocking T-cell inhibition and have revolutionized cancer treatment. Significant cardiotoxicity including pericardial disease, vasculitis, cardiomyopathy, and fulminant myocarditis can occur with ICI therapy.[38–40]

In individuals with ICI-mediated myocarditis, myocardial fibrosis and edema have been observed using late gadolinium enhancement as has elevated T2-weighted short tau inversion recovery (STIR).[41] Although CMR may be helpful in detecting myocarditis, in a recent study, LGE was present in less than half of individuals, and elevated T2-weighted STIR were present in less than one-third of individuals diagnosed with ICI-mediated myocarditis.[41] The ideal role for CMR in the diagnosis of ICI-mediated myocarditis requires further investigation.

AMYLOID DEPOSITION DISEASE

Cardiac involvement is an important prognostic marker for long-term survival in amyloid deposition disease.[42] Although endomyocardial biopsy is the gold standard for diagnosis of cardiac amyloid, CMR has excellent sensitivity and specificity at approximately 85% and 92%, respectively.[43]

Characteristics of cardiac amyloidosis on CMR include abnormal myocardial and blood-pool gadolinium kinetics, resulting in difficulty in nulling LV myocardium.[44] Global subendocardial late enhancement can also be a distinctive feature of cardiac amyloidosis.[45] Distinguishing between light chain (AL) and transthyretin-related (ATTR) amyloidosis is imperative, given the vastly different treatments. Distinctive features that may help distinguish ATTR and AL include the presence of more extensive LGE, transmural LGE, and right ventricular LGE in ATTR compared with that in AL.[46]

MYOCARDIAL FIBROSIS

Myocardial fibrosis can be assessed by a variety of CMR techniques. Late gadolinium enhancement is a standard technique used to identify reactive myocardial fibrosis. Although fibrosis is known to occur as a result of anthracycline treatment, late gadolinium enhancement is not commonly observed, which is thought to be due to the diffuse nature of anthracycline-mediated fibrosis that may be interstitial in nature and therefore not well visualized with LGE-based methods.[47]

LV myocardial extracellular volume fraction (ECVF) measures the relative ratio of myocytes to other tissue within the LV and can be determined by using T1 measurements. In healthy individuals the ratio of the LV myocardial extra—as opposed to myocellular volume—approximates 25%. Although this method appreciates reactive fibrosis, it also reveals interstitial fibrosis.[48] Increases in LV myocardial ECVF have been observed in individuals treated with anthracyclines and may occur as early as the first few months after treatment.[49–51]

Not all increases in LV myocardial ECVF are necessarily related to interstitial fibrosis, as other processes may occupy the interstitial space between the cardiomyocytes. LV myocardial edema resulting from myocellular injury can expand the LV myocardial interstitial space and contribute to elevated CMR measures of LV myocardial ECVF.[48] In addition, cardiomyocyte loss and cardiomyocyte atrophy may play a role in increases in ECVF.[48,49]

Clinically, increases in ECVF have been associated with diastolic dysfunction, larger atrial volumes, and elevated short-term mortality.[47,52] Jordan and colleagues[53] have demonstrated elevations in native T1 in individuals with cancer both pre- and posttreatment compared with

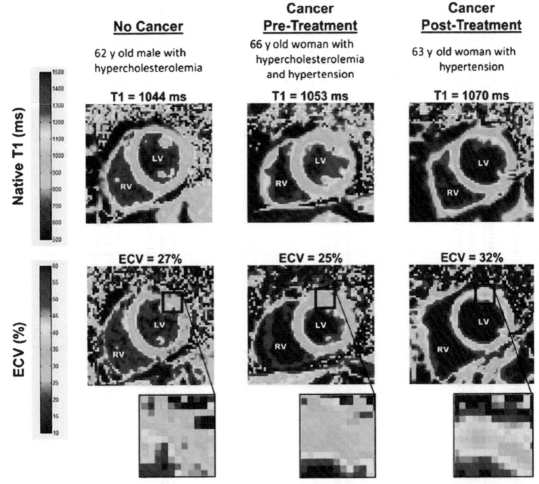

Fig. 2. Comparison of T1 and extracellular volume (ECV) map images. Representative LV short-axis native T1 (*top row*) and ECV (*bottom row*) maps are shown in similarly aged participants. The LV and right ventricular (RV) blood pool cavities are noted. On each image, the color of pixels in the images (color scales on left) identifies the native T1 (milliseconds) and ECV (%). Insets on the ECV maps demonstrate the change in color intensity within the anterorolateral wall of each ventricle. As shown, ECV is elevated in the cancer survivor previously treated with anthracycline-based chemotherapy. (*From* Jordan JH, Vasu S, Morgan TM, et al. Anthracycline-associated T1 mapping characteristics are elevated independent of the presence of cardiovascular comorbidities in cancer survivors. Circ Cardiovascular Imaging. 2016;9(8):e004325; with permission.)

Table 3
Summary of studies evaluating cardiovascular MRI for the tissue characterization of cardiotoxicity

Author and Year	Study Design	Study Population	N	Study Objectives	Study Findings
Neilan et al,[47] 2013	Prospective Cohort Study	Long-term survivors treated with anthracycline	42	Evaluate ECVF in patients treated with anthracyclines	ECVF was increased in patients treated with anthracyclines compared with controls ECVF correlated with left atrial volume and diastolic function
Meléndez et al,[48] 2020	Basic Study	African green monkeys	5	Determine the cause of increased LV ECVF after receipt of anthracyclines	Anthracycline-induced ECVF increases are associated with accumulation of interstitial cardiac fibrosis
Ferreira de Souza et al,[49] 2018	Prospective Cohort Study	Women receiving anthracyclines for breast cancer	27	Use novel CMR markers of myocardial tissue remodeling to investigate anthracycline-induced tissue remodeling	Anthracycline exposure is associated with a reduction in cardiomyocyte size, indicating mechanisms other than interstitial fibrosis and edema can raise ECVF
Farhad et al,[50] 2016	Basic Study	Wild-type male mice	45	Characterize anthracycline-induced cardiotoxicity in mice	Anthracycline-induced cardiotoxicity is associated with an early increase in cardiac edema and a subsequent increase in myocardial fibrosis
Meléndez et al,[51] 2017	Prospective Cohort Study	Patients treated with anthracyclines	56	Determine whether LV myocardial ECVF increases during the initial receipt of anthracyclines	ECVF was elevated 3 mo posttreatment with anthracyclines
Wong et al,[52] 2012	Cohort Study	Consecutive patients undergoing CMR	793	Asses the relationship between ECVF and cardiovascular outcomes	Increased ECVF related to all-cause mortality (hazard ratio, 1.55)

Jordan et al,[53] 2016	Cohort Study	Patients with cancer but no prior therapy/cancer survivors/normal controls	327	Assess whether elevations in ECVF and T2 mapping measures are related to cancer treatment, comorbidities, or the presence of cancer	Elevations in ECVF occur independently of underlying cancer or cardiovascular comorbidities and are related to prior receipt of cardiotoxic cancer treatment
Meléndez et al,[54] 2018	Basic Study	Spontaneously hypertensive rats/wild-type controls	33	Investigate whether LV myocardial fibrosis in the setting of anthracycline exposure is accelerated by the presence of hypertension	During anthracycline treatment hypertensive animals experience more collagen deposition
Tham et al,[55] 2013	Cohort Study	Childhood cancer survivors	30	Investigate CMR tissue characteristics and their association with LV function and structure, exercise capacity, and chemotherapy dose in pediatric cancer survivors	Myocardial T_1 and ECVF are markers of ventricular remodeling and are related to cumulative anthracycline dose, exercise capacity, and myocardial wall thinning
Galán-Arriola et al,[60] 2019	Basic Study	Male large white pigs	20	Identify early anthracycline cardiotoxicity by CMR and its pathologic correlates in a large animal model	T_2 mapping during treatment identifies intracardiomyocyte edema generation as the earliest marker of anthracycline-induced cardiotoxicity

Abbreviation: ECVF, extracellular volume fraction.

controls without cancer. In addition, ECVF has been shown to be elevated in survivors treated with anthracyclines, and these elevations in myocardial T1 and ECVF have been found independent of cardiovascular comorbidities (**Fig. 2**).[53] Basic models, however, have shown that baseline hypertension results in increased myocardial fibrosis during anthracycline exposure.[54]

In early childhood cancer survivors, myocardial T_1 and ECVF are early markers of tissue remodeling. ECVF has been shown to correlate with anthracycline dose and exercise capacity.[55] In addition, both ECVF and T1 mapping correspond with LV mass and wall thickness.[55]

Several clinical studies have demonstrated a strong association between the presence of cardiovascular risk factors, particularly hypertension, and the late development of cardiac disease in childhood cancer survivors.[56–59] Whether increased myocardial fibrosis in the setting of hypertension after anthracycline exposure may contribute to this relationship has yet to be determined.

EARLY CARDIOTOXICITY

Elevated LV myocardial T2 relaxation times may be the earliest noninvasive marker of anthracycline-mediated cardiotoxicity. Murine studies have demonstrated an increase in cardiac edema with subsequent development of myocardial fibrosis after anthracycline exposure.[50] In this model both edema and fibrosis predicted late mortality.[50] In a porcine model, elevated T2 relaxation times correlated with histopathologic evidence of increased myocardial and extracellular water content and cardiomyocyte vacuolization.[60] If anthracycline exposure was halted immediately after an elevation in T2 relaxation time, T2 relaxation time normalized, suggesting potential role for CMR in identifying reversible disease.[60] CMR-based tissue characterization of cancer treatment–related cardiotoxicity is further summarized in **Table 3**.

SUMMARY AND FUTURE DIRECTIONS

CMR is unique among noninvasive imaging techniques due to its ability to provide accurate, reproducible assessments of cardiac function without the need for ionizing radiation. In addition, CMR allows for noninvasive tissue characterization. This is particularly useful in identifying deposition and inflammatory diseases, for understanding subclinical changes in tissue composition, and to further

our understanding of the underlying pathophysiology of cardiotoxicity related to cancer therapy.

As CMR becomes more ubiquitous within the field of cardio-oncology, further research will be required to develop specific criteria for the use of CMR in the diagnosis and screening of cancer therapy–related cardiotoxicity. In addition, CMR will be used to understand the pathophysiology, treatment, and prevention of cancer treatment–related cardiotoxicity. Multiinstitutional collaborations are already underway to investigate imaging and exercise capacity changes early after cancer treatment (UPBEAT), and to investigate the role of statins in preventing cardiotoxicity (PREVENT).[61,62] These current studies and future multiinstitutional collaborations will use the benefits of CMR to further define the role of CMR in the field of cardio-oncology.

DISCLOSURE

The authors have nothing to disclose.

REFERENCES

1. Sturgeon KM, Deng L, Bluethmann SM, et al. A population-based study of cardiovascular disease mortality risk in US cancer patients. Eur Heart J 2019;40(48):3889–97.
2. Armstrong GT, Liu Q, Yasui Y, et al. Late mortality among 5-year survivors of childhood cancer: a summary from the Childhood Cancer Survivor Study. J Clin Oncol 2009;27(14):2328–38.
3. Plana JC, Galderisi M, Barac A, et al. Expert consensus for multimodality imaging evaluation of adult patients during and after cancer therapy: a report from the American Society of Echocardiography and the European Association of Cardiovascular Imaging. Eur Heart J Cardiovasc Imaging 2014; 15(10):1063–93.
4. Armenian SH, Hudson MM, Mulder RL, et al. Recommendations for cardiomyopathy surveillance for survivors of childhood cancer: a report from the International Late Effects of Childhood Cancer Guideline Harmonization Group. Lancet Oncol 2015;16(3):e123–36.
5. Zamorano JL, Lancellotti P, Rodriguez Munoz D, et al. 2016 ESC Position Paper on cancer treatments and cardiovascular toxicity developed under the auspices of the ESC Committee for Practice Guidelines: The Task Force for cancer treatments and cardiovascular toxicity of the European Society of Cardiology (ESC). Eur Heart J 2016;37(36): 2768–801.
6. Seidman A, Hudis C, Pierri MK, et al. Cardiac dysfunction in the trastuzumab clinical trials experience. J Clin Oncol 2002;20(5):1215–21.

7. Schwartz RG, McKenzie WB, Alexander J, et al. Congestive heart failure and left ventricular dysfunction complicating doxorubicin therapy. Seven-year experience using serial radionuclide angiocardiography. Am J Med 1987;82(6):1109–18.

8. Thavendiranathan P, Grant AD, Negishi T, et al. Reproducibility of echocardiographic techniques for sequential assessment of left ventricular ejection fraction and volumes: application to patients undergoing cancer chemotherapy. J Am Coll Cardiol 2013;61(1):77–84.

9. Otterstad JE, Froeland G, St John Sutton M, et al. Accuracy and reproducibility of biplane two-dimensional echocardiographic measurements of left ventricular dimensions and function. Eur Heart J 1997;18(3):507–13.

10. Armstrong GT, Plana JC, Zhang N, et al. Screening adult survivors of childhood cancer for cardiomyopathy: comparison of echocardiography and cardiac magnetic resonance imaging. J Clin Oncol 2012; 30(23):2876–84.

11. Bellenger NG, Burgess MI, Ray SG, et al. Comparison of left ventricular ejection fraction and volumes in heart failure by echocardiography, radionuclide ventriculography and cardiovascular magnetic resonance; are they interchangeable? Eur Heart J 2000; 21(16):1387–96.

12. Longmore DB, Klipstein RH, Underwood SR, et al. Dimensional accuracy of magnetic resonance in studies of the heart. Lancet 1985;1(8442):1360–2.

13. Rehr RB, Malloy CR, Filipchuk NG, et al. Left ventricular volumes measured by MR imaging. Radiology 1985;156(3):717–9.

14. Sechtem U, Pflugfelder PW, Gould RG, et al. Measurement of right and left ventricular volumes in healthy individuals with cine MR imaging. Radiology 1987;163(3):697–702.

15. Mogelvang J, Stokholm KH, Saunamaki K, et al. Assessment of left ventricular volumes by magnetic resonance in comparison with radionuclide angiography, contrast angiography and echocardiography. Eur Heart J 1992;13(12):1677–83.

16. Semelka RC, Tomei E, Wagner S, et al. Normal left ventricular dimensions and function: interstudy reproducibility of measurements with cine MR imaging. Radiology 1990;174(3 Pt 1):763–8.

17. Semelka RC, Tomei E, Wagner S, et al. Interstudy reproducibility of dimensional and functional measurements between cine magnetic resonance studies in the morphologically abnormal left ventricle. Am Heart J 1990;119(6):1367–73.

18. Grothues F, Smith GC, Moon JC, et al. Comparison of interstudy reproducibility of cardiovascular magnetic resonance with two-dimensional echocardiography in normal subjects and in patients with heart failure or left ventricular hypertrophy. Am J Cardiol 2002;90(1):29–34.

19. Melendez GC, Sukpraphrute B, D'Agostino RB Jr, et al. Frequency of Left Ventricular End-Diastolic Volume-Mediated Declines in Ejection Fraction in Patients Receiving Potentially Cardiotoxic Cancer Treatment. Am J Cardiol 2017;119(10):1637–42.

20. Christiansen JR, Massey R, Dalen H, et al. Utility of Global Longitudinal Strain by Echocardiography to Detect Left Ventricular Dysfunction in Long-Term Adult Survivors of Childhood Lymphoma and Acute Lymphoblastic Leukemia. Am J Cardiol 2016; 118(3):446–52.

21. Grover S, Leong DP, Chakrabarty A, et al. Left and right ventricular effects of anthracycline and trastuzumab chemotherapy: a prospective study using novel cardiac imaging and biochemical markers. Int J Cardiol 2013;168(6):5465–7.

22. Grothues F, Moon JC, Bellenger NG, et al. Interstudy reproducibility of right ventricular volumes, function, and mass with cardiovascular magnetic resonance. Am Heart J 2004;147(2):218–23.

23. Thavendiranathan P, Poulin F, Lim KD, et al. Use of myocardial strain imaging by echocardiography for the early detection of cardiotoxicity in patients during and after cancer chemotherapy: a systematic review. J Am Coll Cardiol 2014;63(25 Pt A):2751–68.

24. Jordan JH, Sukpraphrute B, Melendez GC, et al. Early Myocardial Strain Changes During Potentially Cardiotoxic Chemotherapy May Occur as a Result of Reductions in Left Ventricular End-Diastolic Volume: The Need to Interpret Left Ventricular Strain With Volumes. Circulation 2017;135(25):2575–7.

25. Toro-Salazar OH, Gillan E, O'Loughlin MT, et al. Occult cardiotoxicity in childhood cancer survivors exposed to anthracycline therapy. Circ Cardiovasc Imaging 2013;6(6):873–80.

26. Jolly MP, Jordan JH, Melendez GC, et al. Automated assessments of circumferential strain from cine CMR correlate with LVEF declines in cancer patients early after receipt of cardio-toxic chemotherapy. J Cardiovasc Magn Reson 2017;19(1):59.

27. Park JJ, Park JB, Park JH, et al. Global Longitudinal Strain to Predict Mortality in Patients With Acute Heart Failure. J Am Coll Cardiol 2018;71(18): 1947–57.

28. Yadlapati A, Maher TR, Thomas JD, et al. Global longitudinal strain from resting echocardiogram is associated with long-term adverse cardiac outcomes in patients with suspected coronary artery disease. Perfusion 2017;32(7):529–37.

29. Suerken CK, D'Agostino RB Jr, Jordan JH, et al. Simultaneous Left Ventricular Volume and Strain Changes During Chemotherapy Associate With 2-Year Postchemotherapy Measures of Left Ventricular Ejection Fraction. J Am Heart Assoc 2020;9(2): e015400.

30. Tuzovic M, Wu PT, Kianmahd S, et al. Natural history of myocardial deformation in children, adolescents,

and young adults exposed to anthracyclines: Systematic review and meta-analysis. Echocardiography 2018;35(7):922–34.

31. Negishi T, Thavendiranathan P, Negishi K, et al. Rationale and Design of the Strain Surveillance of Chemotherapy for Improving Cardiovascular Outcomes: The SUCCOUR Trial. JACC Cardiovasc Imaging 2018;11(8):1098–105.

32. Lopez-Sendon J, Alvarez-Ortega C, Zamora Aunon P, et al. Classification, prevalence, and outcomes of anticancer therapy-induced cardiotoxicity: the CARDIOTOX registry. Eur Heart J 2020;41(18):1720–9.

33. Steen H, Montenbruck M, Wuelfing P, et al. P3118CMR Fast-SENC intramyocardial LV & RV segmental strain detects cardiotoxicity during oncology treatment and impact of cardioprotection therapy before echocardiography. European Heart Journal 2019;40(Supplement_1). ehz745.0193, https://doi.org/10.1093/eurheartj/ehz745.0193.

34. Lipshultz SE, Scully RE, Stevenson KE, et al. Hearts too small for body size after doxorubicin for childhood ALL: Grinch syndrome. J Clin Oncol 2014;32(15_suppl):10021.

35. Neilan TG, Coelho-Filho OR, Pena-Herrera D, et al. Left ventricular mass in patients with a cardiomyopathy after treatment with anthracyclines. Am J Cardiol 2012;110(11):1679–86.

36. Jordan JH, Castellino SM, Melendez GC, et al. Left Ventricular Mass Change After Anthracycline Chemotherapy. Circ Heart Fail 2018;11(7):e004560.

37. Willis MS, Parry TL, Brown DI, et al. Doxorubicin Exposure Causes Subacute Cardiac Atrophy Dependent on the Striated Muscle-Specific Ubiquitin Ligase MuRF1. Circ Heart Fail 2019;12(3):e005234.

38. Salem JE, Manouchehri A, Moey M, et al. Cardiovascular toxicities associated with immune checkpoint inhibitors: an observational, retrospective, pharmacovigilance study. Lancet Oncol 2018;19(12):1579–89.

39. Johnson DB, Balko JM, Compton ML, et al. Fulminant Myocarditis with Combination Immune Checkpoint Blockade. N Engl J Med 2016;375(18):1749–55.

40. Escudier M, Cautela J, Malissen N, et al. Clinical Features, Management, and Outcomes of Immune Checkpoint Inhibitor-Related Cardiotoxicity. Circulation 2017;136(21):2085–7.

41. Zhang L, Awadalla M, Mahmood SS, et al. Cardiovascular magnetic resonance in immune checkpoint inhibitor-associated myocarditis. Eur Heart J 2020;41(18):1733–43.

42. Gertz MA. Immunoglobulin light chain amyloidosis: 2016 update on diagnosis, prognosis, and treatment. Am J Hematol 2016;91(9):947–56.

43. Zhao L, Tian Z, Fang Q. Diagnostic accuracy of cardiovascular magnetic resonance for patients with suspected cardiac amyloidosis: a systematic review and meta-analysis. BMC Cardiovasc Disord 2016;16:129.

44. Maceira AM, Joshi J, Prasad SK, et al. Cardiovascular magnetic resonance in cardiac amyloidosis. Circulation 2005;111(2):186–93.

45. Vogelsberg H, Mahrholdt H, Deluigi CC, et al. Cardiovascular magnetic resonance in clinically suspected cardiac amyloidosis: noninvasive imaging compared to endomyocardial biopsy. J Am Coll Cardiol 2008;51(10):1022–30.

46. Dungu JN, Valencia O, Pinney JH, et al. CMR-based differentiation of AL and ATTR cardiac amyloidosis. JACC Cardiovasc Imaging 2014;7(2):133–42.

47. Neilan TG, Coelho-Filho OR, Shah RV, et al. Myocardial extracellular volume by cardiac magnetic resonance imaging in patients treated with anthracycline-based chemotherapy. Am J Cardiol 2013;111(5):717–22.

48. Meléndez GC, Vasu S, Lesnefsky EJ, et al. Myocardial Extracellular and Cardiomyocyte Volume Expand After Doxorubicin Treatment Similar to Adjuvant Breast Cancer Therapy. JACC Cardiovasc Imaging 2020;13(4):1084–5.

49. Ferreira de Souza T, Quinaglia ACST, Osorio Costa F, et al. Anthracycline Therapy Is Associated With Cardiomyocyte Atrophy and Preclinical Manifestations of Heart Disease. JACC Cardiovasc Imaging 2018;11(8):1045–55.

50. Farhad H, Staziaki PV, Addison D, et al. Characterization of the Changes in Cardiac Structure and Function in Mice Treated With Anthracyclines Using Serial Cardiac Magnetic Resonance Imaging. Circ Cardiovasc Imaging 2016;9(12):e003584.

51. Meléndez GC, Jordan JH, D'Agostino RB Jr, et al. Progressive 3-Month Increase in LV Myocardial ECV After Anthracycline-Based Chemotherapy. JACC Cardiovasc Imaging 2017;10(6):708–9.

52. Wong TC, Piehler K, Meier CG, et al. Association between extracellular matrix expansion quantified by cardiovascular magnetic resonance and short-term mortality. Circulation 2012;126(10):1206–16.

53. Jordan JH, Vasu S, Morgan TM, et al. Anthracycline-Associated T1 Mapping Characteristics Are Elevated Independent of the Presence of Cardiovascular Comorbidities in Cancer Survivors. Circ Cardiovasc Imaging 2016;9(8). Available at: https://www.ahajournals.org/doi/10.1161/CIRCIMAGING.115.004325.

54. Meléndez GC, Jordan JH, D'Agostino RB Jr, et al. Accelerated Left Ventricular Interstitial Collagen Deposition After Receiving Doxorubicin in Hypertension. J Am Coll Cardiol 2018;72(13):1555–7.

55. Tham EB, Haykowsky MJ, Chow K, et al. Diffuse myocardial fibrosis by T1-mapping in children with subclinical anthracycline cardiotoxicity: relationship

to exercise capacity, cumulative dose and remodeling. J Cardiovasc Magn Reson 2013;15:48.

56. Mulrooney DA, Armstrong GT, Huang S, et al. Cardiac Outcomes in Adult Survivors of Childhood Cancer Exposed to Cardiotoxic Therapy: A Cross-sectional Study. Ann Intern Med 2016;164(2):93–101.

57. Gibson TM, Li Z, Green DM, et al. Blood Pressure Status in Adult Survivors of Childhood Cancer: A Report from the St. Jude Lifetime Cohort Study. Cancer Epidemiol Biomarkers Prev 2017;26(12):1705–13.

58. Armstrong GT, Oeffinger KC, Chen Y, et al. Modifiable risk factors and major cardiac events among adult survivors of childhood cancer. J Clin Oncol 2013;31(29):3673–80.

59. Chow EJ, Baker KS, Lee SJ, et al. Influence of conventional cardiovascular risk factors and lifestyle characteristics on cardiovascular disease after hematopoietic cell transplantation. J Clin Oncol 2014; 32(3):191–8.

60. Galan-Arriola C, Lobo M, Vilchez-Tschischke JP, et al. Serial Magnetic Resonance Imaging to Identify Early Stages of Anthracycline-Induced Cardiotoxicity. J Am Coll Cardiol 2019;73(7): 779–91.

61. Preventing Anthracycline Cardiovascular Toxicity With Statins (PREVENT). 2020. Available at: https:// clinicaltrials.gov/ct2/show/NCT01988571. Accessed May 22, 2020.

62. Understanding and Predicting Breast Cancer Events After Treatment (UPBEAT). 2020. Available at: https://clinicaltrials.gov/ct2/show/NCT02791581. Accessed May 22, 2020.

Intracardiac and Vascular Hemodynamics with Cardiovascular Magnetic Resonance in Heart Failure

Aakash N. Gupta, BS[a], Michael Markl, PhD[a,b],
Mohammed S.M. Elbaz, PhD[a,*]

KEYWORDS

- Heart failure • Intracardiac flow • Intravascular flow • Hemodynamics • 4-D flow MRI

KEY POINTS

- Four-dimensional (4-D) flow magnetic resonance imaging (MRI) has emerged as a potential novel imaging technique for a comprehensive evaluation of the complex, 3-dimensional intracardiac and intravascular flow alterations over the cardiac cycle in heart failure (HF) patients.
- Quantitative 4-D flow MRI-derived hemodynamic markers can assess various, previously unattainable, flow details and may help unravel new insights into the role of flow alterations in the complex cardiac remodeling in HF.
- This article provides a review of emerging applications of 4-D flow MRI-derived intracardiac and intravascular hemodynamic markers for assessing HF and various cardiac pathologies at risk of progressing to HF.

INTRODUCTION

At the epicenter of cardiovascular function is the ability to maintain sufficient and efficient blood flow throughout the body.[1] To achieve this, the heart relies on rhythmic electrical pacing, healthy cardiac and vascular tissue, and optimized chamber configuration to generate pressure gradients that transport blood through the heart.[2] Various disease processes can adversely affect cardiac structure and function and eventually may progress to heart failure (HF), that is, the impaired ventricular capacity to fill with blood or eject blood out of the heart.[3] Standard imaging techniques like echocardiography have limited capability of studying intracardiac hemodynamics because of predominant reliance on 2-dimensional (2-D) planar

flow information. Due to the complex 3-dimensional (3-D) geometry of the heart and the organization of flow within the heart, intracardiac flow is complex and inherently multidirectional. Thus, time-resolved 3-D 3-directional flow imaging is needed to study intracardiac and intravascular hemodynamics efficiently. Recent advances in cardiac magnetic resonance imaging (CMR) have enabled the comprehensive assessment of intracardiac and intravascular flow changes through the development of 4-D flow magnetic resonance imaging (MRI).[4,5] This article reviews emerging applications of 4-D flow MRI-derived hemodynamic markers in the assessment of adult HF populations and various cardiac pathologies that can progress to HF.

[a] Department of Radiology, Feinberg School of Medicine, Northwestern University, 737 North Michigan, Suite 1600, Chicago, IL 60611, USA; [b] Department of Biomedical Engineering, McCormick School of Engineering, Northwestern University, 737 North Michigan, Suite 1600, Chicago, IL 60611, USA
* Corresponding author.
E-mail address: mohammed.elbaz@northwestern.edu

Heart Failure Clin 17 (2021) 135–147
https://doi.org/10.1016/j.hfc.2020.08.010
1551-7136/21/© 2020 Elsevier Inc. All rights reserved.

FOUR-DIMENSIONAL FLOW MAGNETIC RESONANCE IMAGING

Phase-contrast (PC) imaging is a CMR sequence that has long been used to noninvasively measure blood flow velocities.[6] The most commonly used PC technique is 2-D PC with single-direction velocity encoding to measure through-plane flow. However, 2-D PC is inherently limited by the 2-D planar coverage that can be insufficient for assessing the intrinsically 3-D flow, as in the presence of eccentric flow patterns, dynamic regurgitant jets, or complex shunts. Advances in PC imaging have led to 4-D flow MRI, which provides 3-directional velocity encoding with full volumetric (3-D) coverage over the cardiac cycle (**Fig. 1**).[4,7] Visualization of 4-D flow data conventionally is achieved through velocity maximal intensity projections, vector fields (glyphs), pathlines, or streamlines.[8] Given its full 3-D coverage, 4-D flow MRI enables retrospective flow analysis post-acquisition, allowing flexibility and the possibility of ensuring accurate plane repositioning to match patient-specific flow behavior (see **Fig. 1**).[5] For example, multiple planes can be placed at the level of the cardiac valves over the cardiac cycle to allow for simultaneous synchronized flow measurements through all 4 valves.[9] In addition to retrospective plane placement and positioning, 4-D flow MRI permits the 3-D visualization of flow patterns and quantification of hemodynamic parameters in atria, ventricles, and vasculatures (see **Fig. 1**).[10] **Table 1** summarizes key 4-D flow MRI scanning parameters for intracardiac applications. A complete and detailed list of scanning parameters can be found in the 2015 4-D flow MRI consensus statement.[11]

The comprehensive nature of 4-D flow MRI (3-D and 3-directional velocity vectors and time) paved the way for investigating novel 4-D flow-derived hemodynamic parameters. Such parameters can characterize various, previously unattainable, hemodynamic details of intracardiac and intravascular flow (see **Fig. 1**). Hence, they may provide incremental value in the assessment of complex cardiac remodeling and HF severity. **Table 2** summarizes definitions and potential applications of 4-D flow MRI hemodynamic parameters that have been studied in various HF populations. Such markers are versatile and can be measured over various volumes of interest (eg, ventricles, pulmonary, and atria) during a portion (eg, systole or diastole) or the full cardiac cycle. **Fig. 1** depicts a typical analysis pipeline to derive such parameters from 4-D flow MRI. Further descriptions, clinical applications, and uncertainties of these parameters can be found in this systematic review of intracardiac 4-D flow MRI.[10] The following sections provide a review of investigated applications of intracardiac and intravascular 4-D flow MRI-derived hemodynamic parameters in HF and various cardiovascular pathologies at risk of progressing to HF.

HEART FAILURE APPLICATIONS

Initial studies focused on investigating intracardiac kinetic energy (KE) in HF patients (see **Table 2**). A study of 29 HF patients demonstrated higher systolic left ventricular (LV) KE but no significantly different diastolic LV KE compared with healthy controls.[12] Additionally, analysis of LV KE time curves, KE progression over the cardiac cycle, identified altered patterns from healthy controls that were related to LV diastolic dysfunction.[12] Flow components analysis (**Fig. 2**; see **Table 2**) in HF patients has demonstrated reduced direct flow component and direct flow KE but elevated residual flow component and residual flow KE.[13] In a cohort of 34 dilated cardiomyopathy (DCM) patients and 40 ischemic cardiomyopathy patients, direct flow average KE was the only independent predictor of a patient's functional capacity, as measured by the 6-minute walk test; whereas, LV ejection fraction and volumes were not independently predictive.[14]

Vortex formation (see **Table 2**) in the intra-LV blood flow during early and late diastole has been suggested as a potential energy-minimizing blood transportation mechanism. That is, such diastolic vortex formation helps to direct the blood inflow toward the outflow tract minimizing the mechanical energy required to eject blood during systole.[15] It was hypothesized that LV dysfunction and changes to LV geometry may alter the vortex formation and its geometric properties. In a population of 35 patients with heterogeneous HF etiologies, the distance to vortex core and vortex area both were correlated significantly with LV ejection fraction, end-diastolic volume, and peak filling rate.[16] Furthermore, HF patients with reduced ejection fraction demonstrated the presence of vortical blood flow at the apex, whereas HF patients with preserved ejection fraction demonstrated the movement of apical blood toward the ascending aorta with higher flow velocities.[16]

In HF patients with left bundle branch block (LBBB), the LBBB creates a conduction system delay leading to dyssynchronous LV contraction and relaxation. Hemodynamic forces (see **Table 2**) estimated from 4-D flow MRI demonstrated that LV filling forces are more perpendicular to LV inflow direction in the presence of a LBBB.[17]

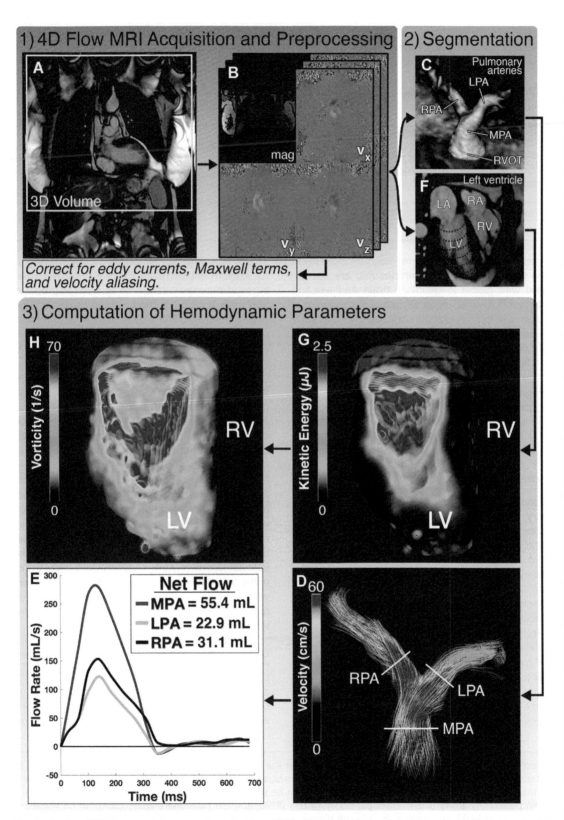

Fig. 1. 4D flow MRI data analysis processing pipeline. (*A*) Three-dimensional volume placed over the heart for 4D flow MRI acquisition. (*B*) Raw 4D flow data consists of three-dimensional anatomical data (mag) and three-

Table 1
Recommendations for 4-dimensional flow magnetic resonance imaging scan parameters for intracardiac applications

Acquisition Parameter	Recommended Value	Comments
Field of view	Maximum	Coverage of cardiac structures of interest
Spatial resolution	2.5–3.0 mm^3 × 2.5–3.0 mm^3 × 2.5–3.0 mm^3	
Temporal resolution	<40 ms	
Velocity sensitivity (venc)	150–200 cm/s	May be increased in presence of valvular stenosis or regurgitation
Electrocardiogram synchronization	Retrospective	Necessary for full diastolic coverage
Scan time	<15 min	

These altered filling forces revealed an increase in the transverse force magnitudes that are associated with global longitudinal strain and ejection fraction.[18] Overall, such abnormal hemodynamic forces are hypothesized to oppose the natural LV geometry and might contribute to pathologic LV remodeling and ultimately HF.[17,18]

These studies explored 4-D flow MRI hemodynamic markers in groups of HF patients with heterogeneous etiologies. Given that HF is the endpoint of many cardiac pathologies, the following sections present studies on the potential of 4-D flow MRI for evaluating various cardiovascular diseases at the risk of progressing to HF.

Ischemic Heart Disease

Ischemic heart disease (IHD), also known as coronary heart disease, arises from inadequate myocardial perfusion typically due to atherosclerotic obstruction of the coronary arteries. In current HF guidelines, CMR plays a vital role in differentiating ischemic and nonischemic etiologies through the assessment of LV anatomy, function, tissue characterization, perfusion, and viability.[19] In particular, 4-D flow MRI-derived KE parameters have been of interest to capture the alterations in intraventricular blood flow arising from LV myocardial dysfunction. In a cohort of 48 patients with a mixture of acute myocardial infarction (MI) and chronic MI, LV blood flow KE parameters were globally reduced compared with controls and were associated with the presence of MI and

infarct size (**Fig. 3**).[20] Importantly, the severity of LV impairment correlated with KE-derived measures of impaired diastolic filling, such as propagation time of KE from the LV base to midventricle during E-wave.[20] The presence of an LV thrombus disturbed normal LV blood flow patterns and demonstrated significantly delayed wash-in of blood to the apical LV.[21]

KE-based parameters also may play a role in the assessment of subtle LV remodeling. In a population of 26 patients with chronic IHD and New York Heart Association class I and class II HF, flow component analysis and KE biomarkers revealed diminished direct flow volume and KE as LV end-diastolic volume increases.[22]

As per conventional diastolic function parameters, filling parameters, such as E/A ratio, E-wave and A-wave acceleration and deceleration times, and flow rates, are crucial echocardiographic parameters to assess and classify LV diastolic dysfunction. These filling parameters can be calculated similarly from 4-D flow MRI using transmitral flow curves and have shown high agreement with echocardiography in classifying patterns of diastolic dysfunction in a study of 47 patients with ischemic HF.[23]

Dilated Cardiomyopathy

DCM is diagnosed based on evidence of LV dilation and impaired systolic contraction.[24] Diagnosis of DCM early in the disease course is challenging with current echocardiographic techniques alone,

directional velocity encoding data (vx, vy, and vz) over the cardiac cycle. Raw data is routinely preprocessed to filter noise and correct for eddy currents, Maxwell terms, and velocity aliasing. From a single acquisition, data in the pulmonary arteries (C) and left ventricle (F) can be segmented for analysis, for example. (D) Flow in the main pulmonary artery (MPA), right pulmonary artery (RPA), and left pulmonary artery (LPA) can be visualized and (E) quantified by retrospectively placing planes (white lines) anywhere in the pulmonary vasculature. These flow volumes are examples of intravascular hemodynamic parameters. (G) Intra-LV kinetic energy and (H) vorticity are examples of intracardiac hemodynamic parameters that can be derived from the left ventricle segmentation.

Table 2
Summary of 4-dimensional flow magnetic resonance imaging hemodynamic parameters, definitions, and clinical applications in heart failure populations

Hemodynamic Parameter	Definition	Heart Failure Clinical Applications
Peak velocity (m/s)	Maximum absolute velocity within flow profile	HCM,[29,67] PH[41]
Flow volume (mL)	Total blood flow volume through a plane over the cardiac cycle (see **Fig. 1**)	PH[41]
Regurgitant volume and fraction (mL and %)	Blood that flows backward across a valve and measured as a volume or fraction of stroke volume (see **Fig. 4**)	Valvular disease[36,40]
E/A filling ratio	The ratio of the peak early filling to peak late filling flow from transmitral flow rate curve	IHD[23]
Simplified pressure gradient (mm Hg)	Pressure gradient calculated from peak velocity using the simplified Bernoulli equation	HCM[29,67]
KE (J)	Energy that drives blood motion (see **Fig. 1**)[60]	IHD,[14,20] DCM,[14] valvular disease[43]
Turbulent KE (J)	KE contained within the turbulent blood flow[42]	Valvular disease,[42] DCM[25]
Viscous energy loss (W)	KE that is lost due to frictional forces induced by viscosity within the blood flow[60,68]	HCM[29]
Helicity (m/s^2)	A measure of the alignment between flow velocity and flow vorticity that drives helical flow[52]	PH[52]
Vorticity (1/s)	The curl of velocity—a measure of vortical flow strength (see **Fig. 1**)[52]	PH[52]
Vortical blood flow duration (s)	Percentage of cardiac time frames, of the cardiac cycle, during which a vortex is present[46]	PH[46,47]
Vortex (size [mL] or area [cm^2])	Group of fluid particles with rotational motion around a common axis[15]	Mixed etiologies[16]
Hemodynamic forces (N)	The force the LV myocardium exerts on intracardiac blood derived from Newton's third law by measuring blood flow acceleration and deceleration[26]	DCM,[17,18] IHD[17,18]
WSS (Pa)	Viscous shear forces exerted tangentially to the vessel wall by flowing blood[69]	PH[41]
Flow components (mL or %)	Decomposition of intraventricular blood flow into 4 quantitative flow components (see **Fig. 2**)[70,71] 1. Direct flow—blood that enters and exits the LV in one cardiac cycle 2. Retained inflow—blood that enters but does not exit the LV in 1 cardiac cycle 3. Delayed ejection flow—blood that resides in the LV and exits in 1 cardiac cycle 4. Residual volume—blood that remains in the LV over 2 cardiac cycles	DCM,[13,14] IHD[14,22]

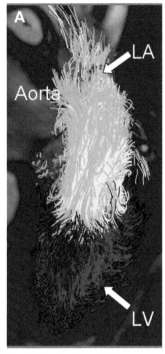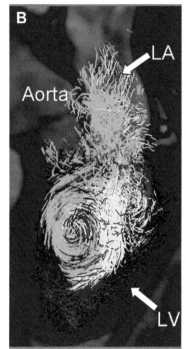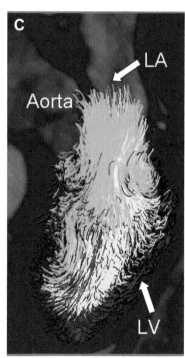

Fig. 2. Illustration of flow components analysis in an example healthy control. Pathline visualization of blood flow over 1 cardiac cycle in the LV at peak early LV filling (*A*), diastasis (*B*), and peak atrial filling (*C*). The pathlines are color-coded to 4 colors according to the corresponding flow component: direct flow, green; retained inflow, yellow; delayed ejection flow, blue; and residual volume, red. LA, left atrium. (*From* Eriksson J, Carlhall CJ, Dyverfeldt P, et al. Semi-automatic quantification of 4D left ventricular blood flow. J Cardiovasc Magn Reson. 2010;12:9.)

because the heart often is normal in size with normal systolic function.[24] Thus, various 4-D flow MRI flow markers have been investigated in this population. Flow component analysis in a small cohort of 10 DCM patients revealed reduced direct flow volume and increased end-diastolic KE compared with controls (see **Table 2**).[13] Analysis of ventricular turbulent KE (TKE) (see **Table 2**) during diastolic filling showed elevated TKE in DCM patients in the basal LV compared with healthy controls.[25]

Although 4-D flow-derived LV hemodynamic forces (see **Table 2**) showed a consistent temporal progression in healthy controls, patients with DCM showed increased variation in the direction and magnitude of these forces during diastole.[26] Taken together, 4-D flow MRI hemodynamic parameters may permit a more detailed understanding of intraventricular flow and association to cardiac function and LV remolding in DCM, but larger studies with longitudinal data remain required.

Hypertrophic Cardiomyopathy

Hypertrophic cardiomyopathy (HCM) arises from pathologic hypertrophy of the myocardium that influences intracardiac flow directly. Most commonly, the interventricular septum hypertrophies leading to LV outflow tract (LVOT) obstruction, high LVOT pressure gradients, mitral regurgitation, and impaired LV diastolic function (**Fig. 4**).[27] Peak LVOT pressure gradient, an important marker of HCM disease severity, has been linked to increased qualitative helical flow patterns in the ascending aorta.[28] Furthermore, the assessment of deranged LVOT flow has been linked to adverse myocardial remodeling in the LV. Studies of 4-D flow MRI suggest a structure-function relationship between increased LVOT pressure gradients and peak systolic viscous energy loss and adverse LV scarring.[29] Importantly, in this cohort of 35 HCM patients, LVOT hemodynamics assessed by 4-D flow MRI showed better correlation with LV scar formation than other conventional metrics of HCM disease severity.[29] The 3-D relative pressure gradient mapping is a promising 4-D flow MRI analysis that utilizes complete flow data (3-D vector field) to noninvasively estimate more complete pressure gradients based on full Bernoulli or Poisson equations.[30,31] This could be used to estimate more accurate maps of transstenotic pressure differences and may play a

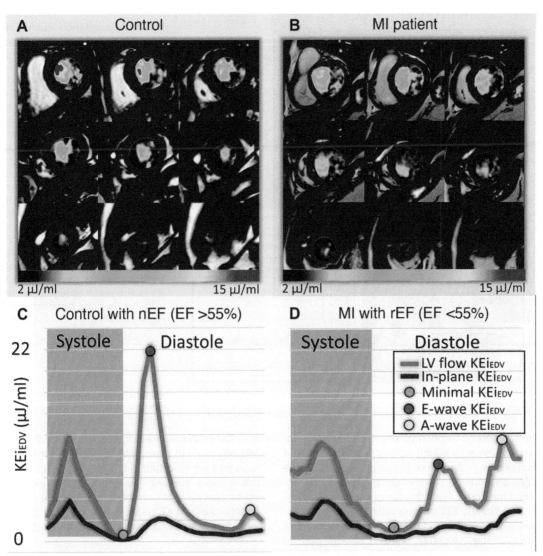

Fig. 3. LV blood flow KE mapping in ischemic heart disease. Short-axis whole LV blood flow KE maps are represented here during peak systole for a control (*A*) and a myocardial infarction (MI) patient (*B*). LV KE over the cardiac cycle is shown for an example control with ejection fraction (EF) that is normal (nEF) (*C*) and an MI patient with reduced ejection fraction (rEF) (*D*). (*Adapted from* Garg P, Crandon S, Swoboda PP, et al. Left ventricular blood flow kinetic energy after myocardial infarction - insights from 4D flow cardiovascular magnetic resonance. J *Cardiovasc Magn Reson* 20, 61 (2018); with permission. (Figures 3 and 4 in original).)

role in the more advanced characterization of LVOT hemodynamics in HCM patients.[32]

Valvular Heart Disease

Current guidelines highlight regurgitation severity as a key parameter in the clinical evaluation and management of patients with valvular heart disease.[33] Although conventional CMR can be employed for the noninvasive assessment of regurgitation severity, it largely relies on indirect measurements of regurgitant volumes and is limited in cases of multivalvular diseases.[34] Conventional CMR techniques depend on an indirect quantification of regurgitation as the difference between LV stroke volume, from multislice cine short-axis images, and forward flow on 2-D PC MRI. Additionally, the placement of the 2-D PC MRI plane requires prospective planning (ie, during the scan) with careful attention to achieve orthogonal placement to the flow direction. This can be challenging in cases of eccentric flow (eg, regurgitant or vortex flow) and hinders multivalvular flow analysis. Use of 4-D flow MRI has addressed many of these challenges by enabling direct regurgitant flow quantification by the retrospective placement of planes anywhere within

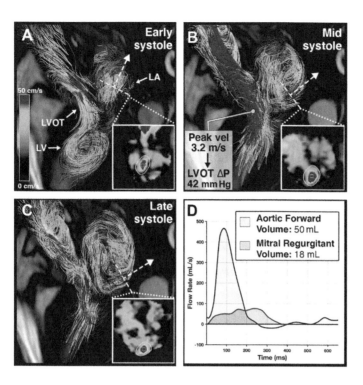

Fig. 4. Regurgitation quantification in hypertrophic cardiomyopathy. Streamline visualization of intracardiac blood flow in the left atrium (LA), left ventricle (LV), and LV outflow tract (LVOT) during early (*A*), mid (*B*), and late systole (*C*). Peak velocity in the LVOT can be extracted from 4D flow data and used to calculate the LVOT pressure gradient by the simplified Bernoulli's equation (*B*). Mitral regurgitation can be quantified by placing a reformatted plane (*white dashed line*) at the level of the mitral regurgitant jet for each time frame, orienting the plane perpendicular (*white dashed arrow*) to the jet, and contouring the regurgitant jet in the plane (*inset*).[38] This results in a flow rate curve for mitral regurgitation (*D*).

the 4-D flow acquisition volume (see **Fig. 4**).[35] For example, valve tracking consists of generating a multiplanar reformatted plane positioned at the valve and oriented perpendicular to the flow for each time frame. From this set of multiplanar reformatted planes, the transvalvular flow can be acquired to calculate both forward and regurgitant flow volumes. Notably, valve tracking permits simultaneous flow quantification through all 4 valves based on a single 4-D flow MRI acquisition and has shown good agreement with both echocardiography and conventional CMR measurements of regurgitation.[9,23,36–39] Translation of valve tracking into clinical practice has been limited primarily by long analysis times. Recent advances have led to automated valve tracking with a reduction in analysis time and improved reliability, as shown in a large study of 114 patients.[40] Furthermore, 4-D flow-derived flow rate, flow volumes, peak flow, and relative pressure fields all may provide further assessment of valvular regurgitation, stenosis, and multivalvular disease.[10,11,32,41]

Few studies also have explored the application of intracardiac energetics to patients with valvular regurgitation. In a cohort of 5 patients with moderate to severe mitral regurgitation (MR), high-velocity MR jets led to elevated left atrial TKE

(see **Table 2**) that was significantly related to the MR volume.[42] In a group of 10 patients with mitral regurgitation who had 4-D flow before and after mitral valve surgery, the preoperative elevated ventricular KE was corrected after surgery except for late-diastolic KE peak, suggesting that physiologic flow conditions were not fully restored.[43]

Pulmonary Hypertension

Pulmonary hypertension (PH) is defined as mean pulmonary arterial pressure (mPAP) greater than or equal to 25 mm Hg and is diagnosed invasively with a right heart catheterization (RHC).[44] Current noninvasive imaging tools, such as echocardiography and CMR, are imperfect in their estimations of mPAP and focus primarily on characterizing the secondary effects of PH on right ventricular (RV) function.[44] Hence, RHC remains the gold standard for definitive PH diagnosis despite its invasiveness.

The use of 4-D flow MRI has permitted visualization and quantification of PH-mediated 3-D vortical blood flow in the pulmonary arteries.[45] Importantly, the duration of vortical blood flow in the main pulmonary artery (**Fig. 5**) evaluated with 4-D flow MRI correlated well with mPAP measured by RHC.[46,47] In a cohort of 145 patients with suspected PH, vortical flow duration-based estimates

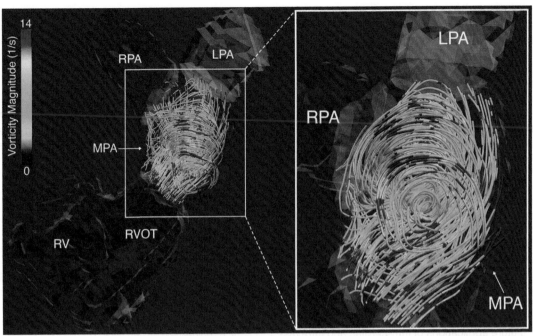

Fig. 5. Vortical blood flow in pulmonary hypertension (PH). Streamline visualization of blood flow in the MPA helps to identify the presence of vortical flow at peak systole (*inset*).[45] RV, right ventricle; RVOT, RV outflow tract; MPA, main pulmonary artery; RPA, right pulmonary artery; LPA, left pulmonary artery.

of mPAP have demonstrated high sensitivity and specificity for the noninvasive diagnosis of PH. These findings now have been replicated at several other centers, indicating its potential as a noninvasive marker of PH.[47–49] Furthermore, several other 4-D flow-derived hemodynamic parameters have been explored for the quantitative analysis of PH flow characteristics (see **Table 2**). Wall shear stress (WSS) plays a role in physiologic endothelial function and may contribute to pathophysiologic vascular remodeling in PH.[50] In a 2-center study with 17 PH patients, 4-D flow MRI-derived flow parameters, such as peak systolic velocity, peak flow, and stroke volume, all were significantly lower in PH patients than controls.[41] Furthermore, WSS parameters were lower in the main, left, and right pulmonary arteries of PH patients compared with healthy controls.[41,48]

A critical consequence of PH is RV dysfunction. Vortical flow duration has been suggested as a promising hemodynamic marker of RV function, measured by RV ejection fraction and end-systolic volume.[48] In addition to RV vortical flow assessment, the ventricular-vascular coupling ratio[51] showed a strong correlation with quantitative helicity in the pulmonary arteries, highlighting the interplay between RV mechanical function and alterations in pulmonary arterial flow characteristics.[52]

CHALLENGES AND FUTURE PERSPECTIVE

Over the past decade, 4-D flow MRI has emerged as a novel imaging tool for the comprehensive visualization and quantification of 3-D intracardiac and intravascular flow. Conventional and advanced 4-D flow imaging parameters characterize different 3-D blood flow details throughout the heart. In the context of HF, myocardial and vascular dysfunction lead to critical shifts in flow volumes, efficiency, and energetics. These flow-based markers may provide incremental value for assessment of HF severity and detection of subclinical cardiac dysfunction preceding global function decline.

Nevertheless, several crucial hurdles must be addressed before 4-D flow MRI and its derived hemodynamic parameters can be translated into routine clinical evaluation of HF patients. First, long scan times may be prohibitive, particularly in symptomatic HF patients who struggle to lay flat for long periods. Although current 4-D flow MRI acquisitions range from 10 minutes to 15 minutes in scan time, various acceleration techniques like compressed sensing[53] and radial acquisition[54] may offer significant reductions in 4-D flow MRI scan time. These techniques still require, however, further validation, especially for intracardiac applications. Second, an important consideration is the reproducibility and effect of age and gender on 4-D flow markers. Recent studies have worked on understanding how LV KE, hemodynamic forces, WSS, and pulmonary arterial blood flow measurements change as a function of age.[55–58] Nevertheless, these studies generally are conducted in small populations and larger comprehensive studies still are needed. In addition to interobserver and intraobserver reproducibility, more scan-rescan reproducibility studies of these 4-D hemodynamic markers are imperative to bolster their clinical applicability for serial follow-up.[59–61] Additionally, reproducibility across multiple centers has yet to be assessed because most studies are single center. Third, although many novel and potentially useful clinical applications of 4-D flow in HF patients have been reviewed, longitudinal data are crucial to risk-stratify HF patients and provide prognostic information. These longitudinal data would be essential in translating such potential hemodynamic biomarkers into clinical decision making but remain lacking.

Future applications of intracardiac and intravascular hemodynamics in HF patients should focus on developing large prospective multicenter trials to validate and build on current findings. Such trials could play an essential role in understanding how 4-D flow hemodynamic parameters tie into patient functional capacity, rate of cardiac remodeling, response to therapy, and risk of HF exacerbations. Furthermore, the diagnosis of HF with preserved ejection fraction (HFpEF) is challenging because echocardiographic measures and natriuretic peptide levels have demonstrated poor sensitivity.[62] There may be a role for 4-D flow biomarkers, especially diastolic markers, such as vortex flow, to clarify the diagnosis of HFpEF and identify patients with subclinical LV dysfunction. The majority of work has focused attention on the LV, but a few studies have investigated flow components, vorticity, and E/A ratios in RV HF pathologies.[63–66] Although the studies presented in this review focused on the most common etiologies of HF, future studies may investigate less common pathologies, such as cardiac amyloidosis, hemochromatosis, sarcoidosis, and collagen diseases.

In summary, 4-D flow MRI has emerged as a powerful imaging modality that enables, previously unattainable, 3-D cardiac blood flow evaluation in HF with intuitive flow visualization and comprehensive quantitative flow-based metrics. Current challenges in HF range from making accurate diagnoses to measuring response to therapy and to risk-stratifying patients. The use of 4-D flow MRI provides an array of intracardiac and intravascular hemodynamic markers that have

the potential to effectively complement existing techniques and biomarkers for evaluation of HF and various pathologies at risk of advancing to HF.

DISCLOSURE

M. Markl declares research support from Siemens Healthineers; a research grant from, and consulting for, Circle Cardiovascular Imaging; and a research grant from Cryolife Inc. The other authors have nothing to disclose.

REFERENCES

1. Richter Y, Edelman ER. Cardiology is flow. Circulation 2006;113(23):2679–82.
2. Carlhall CJ, Bolger A. Passing strange: flow in the failing ventricle. Circ Heart Fail 2010;3(2):326–31.
3. Yancy CW, Jessup M, Bozkurt B, et al. 2013 ACCF/AHA guideline for the management of heart failure: a report of the American college of cardiology foundation/American heart association task force on practice guidelines. J Am Coll Cardiol 2013;62(16): e147–239.
4. Markl M, Chan FP, Alley MT, et al. Time-resolved three-dimensional phase-contrast MRI. J Magn Reson Imaging 2003;17(4):499–506.
5. Markl M, Kilner PJ, Ebbers T. Comprehensive 4D velocity mapping of the heart and great vessels by cardiovascular magnetic resonance. J Cardiovasc Magn Reson 2011;13:7.
6. Pelc NJ, Herfkens RJ, Shimakawa A, et al. Phase contrast cine magnetic resonance imaging. Magn Reson Q 1991;7(4):229–54.
7. Markl M, Frydrychowicz A, Kozerke S, et al. 4D flow MRI. J Magn Reson Imaging 2012;36(5):1015–36.
8. Buonocore MH. Visualizing blood flow patterns using streamlines, arrows, and particle paths. Magn Reson Med 1998;40(2):210–26.
9. Roes SD, Hammer S, van der Geest RJ, et al. Flow assessment through four heart valves simultaneously using 3-dimensional 3-directional velocity-encoded magnetic resonance imaging with retrospective valve tracking in healthy volunteers and patients with valvular regurgitation. Invest Radiol 2009; 44(10):669–75.
10. Crandon S, Elbaz MSM, Westenberg JJM, et al. Clinical applications of intra-cardiac four-dimensional flow cardiovascular magnetic resonance: a systematic review. Int J Cardiol 2017;249:486–93.
11. Dyverfeldt P, Bissell M, Barker AJ, et al. 4D flow cardiovascular magnetic resonance consensus statement. J Cardiovasc Magn Reson 2015;17:72.
12. Kanski M, Arvidsson PM, Toger J, et al. Left ventricular fluid kinetic energy time curves in heart failure from cardiovascular magnetic resonance 4D flow data. J Cardiovasc Magn Reson 2015;17:111.

13. Eriksson J, Bolger AF, Ebbers T, et al. Four-dimensional blood flow-specific markers of LV dysfunction in dilated cardiomyopathy. Eur Heart J Cardiovasc Imaging 2013;14(5):417–24.

14. Stoll VM, Hess AT, Rodgers CT, et al. Left ventricular flow analysis. Circ Cardiovasc Imaging 2019;12(5):e008130.

15. Elbaz MS, Calkoen EE, Westenberg JJ, et al. Vortex flow during early and late left ventricular filling in normal subjects: quantitative characterization using retrospectively-gated 4D flow cardiovascular magnetic resonance and three-dimensional vortex core analysis. J Cardiovasc Magn Reson 2014;16:78.

16. Suwa K, Saitoh T, Takehara Y, et al. Intra-left ventricular flow dynamics in patients with preserved and impaired left ventricular function: analysis with 3D cine phase contrast MRI (4D-Flow). J Magn Reson Imaging 2016;44(6):1493–503.

17. Eriksson J, Zajac J, Alehagen U, et al. Left ventricular hemodynamic forces as a marker of mechanical dyssynchrony in heart failure patients with left bundle branch block. Sci Rep 2017;7(1):2971.

18. Arvidsson PM, Toger J, Pedrizzetti G, et al. Hemodynamic forces using four-dimensional flow MRI: an independent biomarker of cardiac function in heart failure with left ventricular dyssynchrony? Am J Physiol Heart Circ Physiol 2018;315(6):H1627–39.

19. Ponikowski P, Voors AA, Anker SD, et al. 2016 ESC Guidelines for the diagnosis and treatment of acute and chronic heart failure: the task force for the diagnosis and treatment of acute and chronic heart failure of the European society of cardiology (ESC) developed with the special contribution of the heart failure association (HFA) of the ESC. Eur Heart J 2016;37(27):2129–200.

20. Garg P, Crandon S, Swoboda PP, et al. Left ventricular blood flow kinetic energy after myocardial infarction - insights from 4D flow cardiovascular magnetic resonance. J Cardiovasc Magn Reson 2018;20(1):61.

21. Garg P, van der Geest RJ, Swoboda PP, et al. Left ventricular thrombus formation in myocardial infarction is associated with altered left ventricular blood flow energetics. Eur Heart J Cardiovasc Imaging 2019;20(1):108–17.

22. Svalbring E, Fredriksson A, Eriksson J, et al. Altered diastolic flow patterns and kinetic energy in subtle left ventricular remodeling and dysfunction detected by 4D flow MRI. PLoS One 2016;11(8):e0161391.

23. Brandts A, Bertini M, van Dijk EJ, et al. Left ventricular diastolic function assessment from three-dimensional three-directional velocity-encoded MRI with retrospective valve tracking. J Magn Reson Imaging 2011;33(2):312–9.

24. Bozkurt B, Colvin M, Cook J, et al. Current diagnostic and treatment strategies for specific dilated cardiomyopathies: a scientific statement from the American heart association. Circulation 2016; 134(23):e579–646.

25. Zajac J, Eriksson J, Dyverfeldt P, et al. Turbulent kinetic energy in normal and myopathic left ventricles. J Magn Reson Imaging 2015;41(4):1021–9.

26. Eriksson J, Bolger AF, Ebbers T, et al. Assessment of left ventricular hemodynamic forces in healthy subjects and patients with dilated cardiomyopathy using 4D flow MRI. Phys Rep 2016;4(3):e12685.

27. Maron BJ, Maron MS. Hypertrophic cardiomyopathy. Lancet 2013;381(9862):242–55.

28. Allen BD, Choudhury L, Barker AJ, et al. Three-dimensional haemodynamics in patients with obstructive and non-obstructive hypertrophic cardiomyopathy assessed by cardiac magnetic resonance. Eur Heart J Cardiovasc Imaging 2015; 16(1):29–36.

29. van Ooij P, Allen BD, Contaldi C, et al. 4D flow MRI and T1 -mapping: assessment of altered cardiac hemodynamics and extracellular volume fraction in hypertrophic cardiomyopathy. J Magn Reson Imaging 2016;43(1):107–14.

30. Tyszka JM, Laidlaw DH, Asa JW, et al. Three-dimensional, time-resolved (4D) relative pressure mapping using magnetic resonance imaging. J Magn Reson Imaging 2000;12(2):321–9.

31. Ebbers T, Wigstrom L, Bolger AF, et al. Estimation of relative cardiovascular pressures using time-resolved three-dimensional phase contrast MRI. Magn Reson Med 2001;45(5):872–9.

32. Ha H, Kvitting JP, Dyverfeldt P, et al. Validation of pressure drop assessment using 4D flow MRI-based turbulence production in various shapes of aortic stenoses. Magn Reson Med 2019;81(2):893–906.

33. Nishimura RA, Otto CM, Bonow RO, et al. 2014 AHA/ACC guideline for the management of patients with valvular heart disease: executive summary: a report of the american college of cardiology/American heart association task force on practice guidelines. Circulation 2014;129(23):2440–92.

34. Uretsky S, Argulian E, Narula J, et al. Use of cardiac magnetic resonance imaging in assessing mitral regurgitation: current evidence. J Am Coll Cardiol 2018;71(5):547–63.

35. Garg P, Swift AJ, Zhong L, et al. Assessment of mitral valve regurgitation by cardiovascular magnetic resonance imaging. Nat Rev Cardiol 2019; 17(5):298–312.

36. Westenberg JJ, Roes SD, Ajmone Marsan N, et al. Mitral valve and tricuspid valve blood flow: accurate quantification with 3D velocity-encoded MR imaging with retrospective valve tracking. Radiology 2008; 249(3):792–800.

37. Marsan NA, Westenberg JJ, Ypenburg C, et al. Quantification of functional mitral regurgitation by real-time 3D echocardiography: comparison with

3D velocity-encoded cardiac magnetic resonance. JACC Cardiovasc Imaging 2009;2(11):1245–52.

38. Calkoen EE, Westenberg JJ, Kroft LJ, et al. Characterization and quantification of dynamic eccentric regurgitation of the left atrioventricular valve after atrioventricular septal defect correction with 4D Flow cardiovascular magnetic resonance and retrospective valve tracking. J Cardiovasc Magn Reson 2015;17:18.

39. Feneis JF, Kyubwa E, Atianzar K, et al. 4D flow MRI quantification of mitral and tricuspid regurgitation: reproducibility and consistency relative to conventional MRI. J Magn Reson Imaging 2018;48(4): 1147–58.

40. Kamphuis VP, Roest AAW, Ajmone Marsan N, et al. Automated cardiac valve tracking for flow quantification with four-dimensional flow MRI. Radiology 2019;290(1):70–8.

41. Barker AJ, Roldan-Alzate A, Entezari P, et al. Four-dimensional flow assessment of pulmonary artery flow and wall shear stress in adult pulmonary arterial hypertension: results from two institutions. Magn Reson Med 2015;73(5):1904–13.

42. Dyverfeldt P, Kvitting JP, Carlhall CJ, et al. Hemodynamic aspects of mitral regurgitation assessed by generalized phase-contrast MRI. J Magn Reson Imaging 2011;33(3):582–8.

43. Al-Wakeel N, Fernandes JF, Amiri A, et al. Hemodynamic and energetic aspects of the left ventricle in patients with mitral regurgitation before and after mitral valve surgery. J Magn Reson Imaging 2015; 42(6):1705–12.

44. Galie N, Humbert M, Vachiery JL, et al. 2015 ESC/ERS Guidelines for the diagnosis and treatment of pulmonary hypertension: the joint task force for the diagnosis and treatment of pulmonary hypertension of the European society of cardiology (ESC) and the European respiratory society (ERS): endorsed by: association for European paediatric and congenital cardiology (AEPC), international society for heart and lung transplantation (ISHLT). Eur Heart J 2016; 37(1):67–119.

45. Reiter U, Reiter G, Kovacs G, et al. Evaluation of elevated mean pulmonary arterial pressure based on magnetic resonance 4D velocity mapping: comparison of visualization techniques. PLoS One 2013;8(12):e82212.

46. Reiter G, Reiter U, Kovacs G, et al. Magnetic resonance-derived 3-dimensional blood flow patterns in the main pulmonary artery as a marker of pulmonary hypertension and a measure of elevated mean pulmonary arterial pressure. Circ Cardiovasc Imaging 2008;1(1):23–30.

47. Reiter G, Reiter U, Kovacs G, et al. Blood flow vortices along the main pulmonary artery measured with MR imaging for diagnosis of pulmonary hypertension. Radiology 2015;275(1):71–9.

48. Odagiri K, Inui N, Hakamata A, et al. Non-invasive evaluation of pulmonary arterial blood flow and wall shear stress in pulmonary arterial hypertension with 3D phase contrast magnetic resonance imaging. Springerplus 2016;5(1):1071.

49. Sieren MM, Berlin C, Oechtering TH, et al. Comparison of 4D flow MRI to 2D Flow MRI in the pulmonary arteries in healthy volunteers and patients with pulmonary hypertension. PLoS One 2019;14(10): e0224121.

50. Ben Driss A, Devaux C, Henrion D, et al. Hemodynamic stresses induce endothelial dysfunction and remodeling of pulmonary artery in experimental compensated heart failure. Circulation 2000; 101(23):2764–70.

51. Sanz J, Garcia-Alvarez A, Fernandez-Friera L, et al. Right ventriculo-arterial coupling in pulmonary hypertension: a magnetic resonance study. Heart 2012;98(3):238–43.

52. Schafer M, Barker AJ, Kheyfets V, et al. Helicity and vorticity of pulmonary arterial flow in patients with pulmonary hypertension: quantitative analysis of flow formations. J Am Heart Assoc 2017;6(12): e007010.

53. Lustig M, Donoho D, Pauly JM. Sparse MRI: the application of compressed sensing for rapid MR imaging. Magn Reson Med 2007;58(6):1182–95.

54. Johnson KM, Lum DP, Turski PA, et al. Improved 3D phase contrast MRI with off-resonance corrected dual echo VIPR. Magn Reson Med 2008;60(6): 1329–36.

55. Wong J, Chabiniok R, deVecchi A, et al. Age-related changes in intraventricular kinetic energy: a physiological or pathological adaptation? Am J Physiol Heart Circ Physiol 2016;310(6):H747–55.

56. Wehrum T, Hagenlocher P, Lodemann T, et al. Age dependence of pulmonary artery blood flow measured by 4D flow cardiovascular magnetic resonance: results of a population-based study. J Cardiovasc Magn Reson 2016;18(1):31.

57. Crandon S, Westenberg JJM, Swoboda PP, et al. Impact of age and diastolic function on novel, 4D flow CMR biomarkers of left ventricular blood flow kinetic energy. Sci Rep 2018;8(1):14436.

58. Arvidsson PM, Toger J, Carlsson M, et al. Left and right ventricular hemodynamic forces in healthy volunteers and elite athletes assessed with 4D flow magnetic resonance imaging. Am J Physiol Heart Circ Physiol 2017;312(2):H314–28.

59. Kamphuis VP, van der Palen RLF, de Koning PJH, et al. In-scan and scan-rescan assessment of LV in- and outflow volumes by 4D flow MRI versus 2D planimetry. J Magn Reson Imaging 2018;47(2): 511–22.

60. Kamphuis VP, Westenberg JJM, van der Palen RLF, et al. Scan-rescan reproducibility of diastolic left ventricular kinetic energy, viscous energy loss and

vorticity assessment using 4D flow MRI: analysis in healthy subjects. Int J Cardiovasc Imaging 2018; 34(6):905–20.

61. Markl M, Wallis W, Harloff A. Reproducibility of flow and wall shear stress analysis using flow-sensitive four-dimensional MRI. J Magn Reson Imaging 2011;33(4):988–94.

62. Pieske B, Tschöpe C, de Boer RA, et al. How to diagnose heart failure with preserved ejection fraction: the HFA–PEFF diagnostic algorithm: a consensus recommendation from the heart failure association (HFA) of the European society of cardiology (ESC). Eur Heart J 2019;40(40):3297–317.

63. Fenster BE, Browning J, Schroeder JD, et al. Vorticity is a marker of right ventricular diastolic dysfunction. Am J Physiol Heart Circ Physiol 2015; 309(6):H1087–93.

64. Fredriksson AG, Svalbring E, Eriksson J, et al. 4D flow MRI can detect subtle right ventricular dysfunction in primary left ventricular disease. J Magn Reson Imaging 2016;43(3):558–65.

65. Browning JR, Hertzberg JR, Schroeder JD, et al. 4D flow assessment of vorticity in right ventricular diastolic dysfunction. Bioengineering (Basel) 2017; 4(2):30.

66. Barker N, Fidock B, Johns CS, et al. A systematic review of right ventricular diastolic assessment by 4D flow CMR. Biomed Res Int 2019;2019:6074984.

67. Allen BD, Barker AJ, Carr JC, et al. Time-resolved three-dimensional phase contrast MRI evaluation of bicuspid aortic valve and coarctation of the aorta. Eur Heart J Cardiovasc Imaging 2013; 14(4):399.

68. Elbaz MS, van der Geest RJ, Calkoen EE, et al. Assessment of viscous energy loss and the association with three-dimensional vortex ring formation in left ventricular inflow: in vivo evaluation using four-dimensional flow MRI. Magn Reson Med 2017; 77(2):794–805.

69. Stalder AF, Russe MF, Frydrychowicz A, et al. Quantitative 2D and 3D phase contrast MRI: optimized analysis of blood flow and vessel wall parameters. Magn Reson Med 2008;60(5):1218–31.

70. Bolger AF, Heiberg E, Karlsson M, et al. Transit of blood flow through the human left ventricle mapped by cardiovascular magnetic resonance. J Cardiovasc Magn Reson 2007;9(5):741–7.

71. Eriksson J, Carlhall CJ, Dyverfeldt P, et al. Semiautomatic quantification of 4D left ventricular blood flow. J Cardiovasc Magn Reson 2010;12:9.

Measuring Myocardial Energetics with Cardiovascular Magnetic Resonance Spectroscopy

Joevin Sourdon, PhD[a,b], Sabra C. Lewsey, MD MPH[b], Michael Schär, PhD[c], Robert G. Weiss, MD[b,*]

KEYWORDS

- Metabolism • Energetics • Cardiomyopathies • Heart failure • Cardiac magnetic resonance
- Spectroscopy

KEY POINTS

- Dysfunction of multiple important myocardial metabolic pathways and energetics occurs with several common cardiovascular diseases.
- Because myocardial metabolism fuels ongoing cardiac contractile function, metabolic and energetic abnormalities in the failing heart may contribute to contractile dysfunction, disease development, and progression.
- Cardiac magnetic resonance spectroscopy allows the noninvasive, nondestructive exploration of metabolism in the beating heart.

INTRODUCTION

This review summarizes the cardiac metabolic remodeling that occurs in major cardiac diseases and the advantage of quantifying metabolism non-invasively in the beating heart with cardiac magnetic resonance spectroscopy (CMRS).

PRIMER ON MYOCARDIAL METABOLISM

Most myocardial chemical energy is derived from the oxidation of the three main substrates: free fatty acids (FFAs), glucose, and ketone bodies.[1] Glucose and FFAs are catabolized into acetyl co-enzyme A to enter the mitochondrial tricarboxylic acid (Krebs) cycle. Adenosine triphosphate (ATP) formation then is completed by mitochondrial oxidative phosphorylation. The creatine kinase (CK) reaction is the main cardiac energy reserve reaction, which reversibly transfers the high-energy phosphate (HEP) of ATP to creatine (Cr) to form Cr phosphate (PCr):

$$PCr + ADP + H^+ \overset{kf}{\underset{kr}{\rightleftharpoons}} ATP + Cr,$$

where k_r is the reverse rate constant, k_f is the forward rate constant of CK activity, ADP is adenosine diphosphate and H is hydrogen.

Myocardial bioenergetics have been defined by HEP levels and their turnover in tissue. Thus, the CK reaction by producing PCr, may enhance intracellular delivery of HEP from mitochondrial sites of ATP production to cytoplasmic sites of ATP

[a] Aix-Marseille Université, CNRS, CRMBM, Faculté de Médecine, 27 BVD Jean Moulin, Marseille 13005, France; [b] Division of Cardiology, Department of Medicine, Johns Hopkins University School of Medicine, Baltimore, MD, USA; [c] Division of Magnetic Resonance Research, Department of Radiology, Johns Hopkins University School of Medicine, Johns Hopkins Hospital, Park 330, 600 North Wolfe Street, Baltimore, MD 21287, USA
* Corresponding author. Johns Hopkins Hospital, Blalock 544, 600 North Wolfe Street, Baltimore, MD 21287-6568.
E-mail address: rweiss@jhmi.edu

utilization. However, CK also is thought to act as a temporal HEP buffer tightly maintaining high ATP and low ADP concentrations during changes in energy demand (**Fig. 1**).[2]

Remodeling of certain metabolic pathways, substrate preferences, and PCr:ATP energy balance occurs with several common cardiovascular diseases, including heart failure (HF), and may contribute to disease development and progression.[3] Myocardial ATP turnover depends in large part on energy demand and thus *in vitro* studies may not always faithfully recapitulate the energetic profile of the *in vivo* contracting heart. Therefore, the nondestructive exploration and quantification of metabolism in the beating heart with cardiac MRS offers unique and potentially powerful means to better understand the role of altered metabolism in cardiac diseases and develop novel diagnostic and therapeutic targets.

CARDIAC MAGNETIC RESONANCE SPECTROSCOPY PRINCIPLES

CMRS allows the noninvasive measurement of proton (^1H)-containing metabolites, such as Cr; carbon (^{13}C)-containing metabolites from glucose and lipid metabolism; and phosphorus (^{31}P)-containing metabolites, such as PCr and ATP. Those nuclei have an intrinsic nuclear magnetic moment, which is called nuclear spin. These nuclear spins are aligned with or against an applied magnetic field (B_0), leading to a macroscopic equilibrium magnetization (M_0) along B_0. Radiofrequency pulses can be used to perturb the alignment of M_0, so-called excitation. The excited magnetization then precesses around B_0 and induces a measurable voltage in receiver coils tuned to the specific nucleus. The precession frequency depends on B_0, the nucleus, and its chemical environment, enabling the identification of different metabolites. The detected signal is transformed to a spectrum using the Fourier transformation to identify the different frequency components of the signal. In the spectrum, different metabolites then are identified by the frequency of their signal peaks, and the area under the peak reflects the concentration of that metabolite (**Fig. 2**). Today, CMRS typically is performed using scanners with B_0 of 4.7 Tesla (T)[4] or 11.7T[5] in cardiac preclinical applications and 1.5T,[6] 3T,[7] or 7T[8] in clinical studies.

^{31}P–Magnetic Resonance Spectroscopy

^{31}P-magnetic resonance spectroscopy (MRS) is used most commonly in studies of myocardial energy metabolism and the techniques for spatial localization often include either 1-dimensional, 2-dimensional, or 3-dimensional chemical shift imaging (CSI) or image-selected *in vivo*

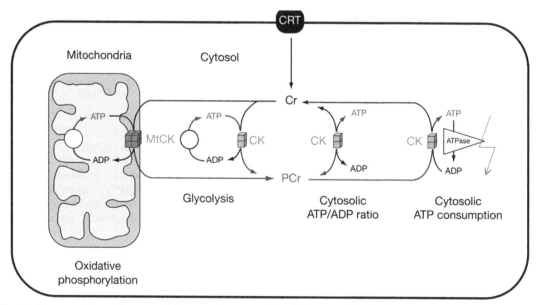

Fig. 1. Representation of myocardial energy transport. The CK energy shuttle theoretically provides ATP from mitochondria to the sites of consumption. This includes 2 main isoforms of CK, mitochondrial (MtCK) and cytoplasmic. Cr is taken up from blood through Cr transporter (CRT). (*Adapted from* Schlattner U., Tokarska-Schlattner M., Wallimann T. Metabolite channeling: creatine kinase microcompartments. In: Lennarz WJ, Lane MD, editors. Encyclopedia of Biological Chemistry (2nd edition). Waltham, MA: Academic Press; 2013. p. 80–5; with permission.)

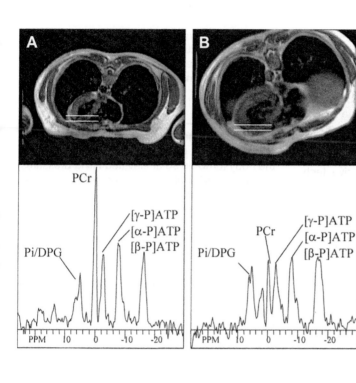

Fig. 2. Comparison of spatially localized ^{31}P-MRS of a healthy volunteer (*A*) and a patient with DCM with significant reduction of PCr (*B*). Upper images show the 1-dimensional CSI localization of ^{31}P-MRS (anterior left ventricular wall). The peaks of the spectra (*bottom panel*) show the combination of Pi and DPG, phosphodiesters, PCr, the gamma-phosphate of ATP ([γ-P]ATP), the beta-phosphate of ATP ([β-P]ATP, and the alpha-phosphate of ATP ([α-P]ATP). ppm, parts per million. (*From* Ingwall JS., Weiss RG. Is the failing heart energy starved? On using chemical energy to support cardiac function. Circulation Research 2004;95(2):137; with permission.)

spectroscopy. ^{31}P-MRS is the only technique able to nondestructively measure HEP in the *in vivo* human heart (see **Fig. 2**).

The cardiac PCr/ATP ratio was the first myocardial energetic parameter measured with spatially localized ^{31}P-MRS,[6,9,10] and PCr is approximately twice as abundant as ATP in the healthy human heart. Absolute quantification of PCr and ATP concentrations can be accomplished by comparison to an external standard and the results do not assume that ATP is constant.[11–13] A summary of major ^{31}P-MRS absolute phosphate metabolites render concentrations of PCr = 9.9 ± 0.7 μmol/g and ATP = 6.0 ± 0.5 μmol/g wet weight in the healthy human heart.[7,11–20]

Furthermore, measurement of unidirectional ATP synthesis through the CK reaction (CK flux) with ^{31}P saturation transfer MRS offers critical insight into energy turnover in cardiomyocytes. The conventional saturation transfer approach consists of saturating the magnetization of the gamma-phosphate of ATP ([γ-P]ATP) involved in the chemical exchange with PCr, which leads to a decrease of the PCr magnetization (M_0') proportional to pseudo first-order rate constant, k_f, and calculated as follows:

$$k_f = \frac{1}{T_1'}\left(1 - \frac{M_0'}{M_0}\right),$$

with T_1' the longitudinal relaxation time and M_0' and M_0 the equilibrium magnetizations of PCr

while γ-ATP is saturated or unsaturated, respectively. With conventional saturation techniques, the determination of T_1' is very time consuming, but approximately 15 years ago accelerated approaches were developed and enabled the first measurements of ATP synthesis in the human heart.[17] Multiple techniques since have been used to calculate k_f (approximately 0.33 s[−1]),[17,21–24] and subsequently CK flux that equals k_f × [PCr] (approximately 3.4 μmol/g/s) in the healthy human heart.[17,23,24] ^{31}P-MRS also can be used to noninvasively measure inorganic phosphate (Pi), to quantify cytosolic ADP (from the CK equilibrium reaction), intracellular pH (from the chemical shift of Pi relative to PCr), and the free-energy change of ATP hydrolysis (-ΔG_{ATP} [kJ/mol]).[17,25] Although these approaches have been used extensively in isolated, perfused hearts, they have been less successful and less commonly implemented in the human heart, due to overlap of blood 2,3-diacylglycerol (DPG) resonances, with the Pi resonance used for most calculations. The peak overlap may be overcome by the increased chemical shift dispersion at 7 T.[8,26]

[1]H–Magnetic Resonance Spectroscopy

Spatially localized ^{1}H-MRS has been used to measure several metabolites[27] but *in vivo* human studies are limited primarily to measuring myocardial triglycerides[28,29] and total Cr.[30] Unlike ^{13}C-MRS and ^{31}P-MRS, which require specially tuned excitation and detection coils, conventional imaging surface coils can be used for ^{1}H-MRS.

[13]C–Magnetic Resonance Spectroscopy

Although ^{13}C-MRS is a powerful technique used to study carbon substrate metabolism in animal hearts, it rarely is used in human hearts due to the low sensitivity of the ^{13}C nucleus and the expense of ^{13}C-labeled substrates. Dynamic nuclear polarization, however, an innovative technique, theoretically improves sensitivity 10,000-fold.[31] Metabolites labeled with ^{13}C are hyperpolarized in a polarizer and then injected into a living system.[32,33] Although the entire process is complex in practice and the hyperpolarization is short-lived, this technique allows real-time assessment of the Krebs cycle[34] and soon may be applicable in people.[35]

APPLICATIONS
Heart Failure Risk Factors: Ischemia, Infarction, and Diabetes

Early ^{31}P-MRS studies in isolated animal hearts during acute, severe ischemia demonstrated rapid and significant decreases in PCr and increases in Pi with initially preserved ATP.[36–38] ATP decline appears after prolonged ischemia and PCr depletion, but the PCr signal recovers rapidly during reperfusion in viable tissue.[39]

^{31}P-MRS also has been utilized *in vivo* to detect energetic changes during myocardial ischemia in humans.[40] During isometric handgrip exercise (IHE) stress, spatially localized ^{31}P-MRS detected significant stress-induced reductions in cardiac PCr/ATP in patients with significant coronary artery disease but not in healthy subjects or those with nonischemic disease. Furthermore, stress-induced myocardial PCr/ATP decline resolved after successful revascularization.[40] These observations of IHE stress-induced declines in cardiac PCr/ATP in CAD patients were reproduced by others.[41,42]

The chronic disruption of myocardial metabolism following infarction has been identified with ^{31}P-MRS, whereby viable myocardium (more PCr and ATP),[12,43] ischemic without infarction (intermediate PCr and ATP),[12] and scarred postinfarct (less PCr and ATP)[12,43] myocardium can be distinguished.[43] ^{1}H-MRS can detect lower CR in infarcted areas in canine[44] and human hearts[30] and ^{31}P-MRS saturation transfer techniques identified reduced CK flux in infarcted myocardial regions.[19]

^{31}P-MRS has identified reduced PCr/ATP in myocardium of patients with risk factors for HF, such as those with hypertension with diastolic dysfunction,[45] type 2 diabetes mellitus,[46,47] type 1 diabetes mellitus,[48] and/or obesity.[49] Moreover, ^{1}H-MRS assessed decreased Cr in the myocardium of various nonischemic heart diseases.[50]

Heart Failure

HF often is defined as the inability of the heart to pump sufficient blood to meet the demands of the body (or to do so at elevated filling pressures) and the decades-old energy-deprivation hypothesis of HF[51] posits that the failing heart has insufficient metabolic energy to fuel normal contraction. The emergence of MRS measures of energy metabolism in the beating heart have addressed several gaps in this theory.

Early animal and human tissue studies[52] supported the energy-starvation hypothesis whereby progressive and insidious loss of ATP with a loss of the total purine pool, most evident when HF is severe, were reported as well as an early reduction in the Cr pool.[53] Isolated human myocardial tissues are difficult to obtain rapidly, especially in patients with early, mild disease, but seminal studies demonstrated significant reductions in ATP, total adenine nucleotides, and nicotinamide adenine dinucleotide[54] in Cr content[55] and in CK activity[56] in patients with HF. Given the invasive nature of tissue biopsies, ^{31}P-MRS and ^{1}H-MRS have been the primary methodologies to better understand cardiac metabolism in HF under physiologic conditions. Several early groups reported a 20% to 30% reduction in cardiac PCr/ATP at rest in systolic HF and dilated cardiomyopathy (DCM) patients.[57–61] The subsequent ability to noninvasively quantify HEP concentrations[11,13] revealed that the PCr/ATP ratio, in fact, may underestimate the reductions observed in absolute concentration of PCr, especially in end-stage HF. Cardiac ATP flux through CK is reduced by approximately 50% in patients with HF and nonischemic DCM[17] and by approximately 70% in patients with left ventricular hypertrophy and HF.[18] Cardiac CK flux declines before ATP loss in human HF and the reduction is greater than changes in absolute metabolite concentrations or PCr/ATP. In addition, extensive energetic abnormalities, including derangements in HEP metabolism,[6,62] reduced CK flux,[17,18,56,63,64] and lipid accumulation,[65,66] have been reported in human HF.

An early study[58] demonstrated lower PCr/ATP in aortic valve disease patients with symptomatic HF than in those without. Cardiac PCr/ATP was shown to correlate with New York Heart Association functional class of symptom severity in DCM patients, and reported to improve or even normalize with implementation of conventional medical therapy over 3 months (angiotensin-converting enzyme inhibitors; β-blockers).[59] In the late 1990s, low cardiac PCr/ATP was found to predict all-cause and cardiovascular mortality in DCM patients.[67] More recently, rates of ATP synthesis through CK, rather than PCr/ATP, independently predicted HF related events, including transplant and cardiovascular mortality in HF patients on contemporary therapy.[63] More recently CK flux in HF patients was shown to correlate with myocardial mechanical power and mechanical efficiency, suggesting that CK energy deprivation is associated closely with cardiac dysfunction.[64] Thus, myocardial energetic abnormalities not only occur in HF and are related to symptom and functional severity but also predict subsequent adverse cardiovascular outcomes.

Eighty years of cardiac metabolic research has collectively improved understanding of energetic dysfunction and its contribution to the failing human heart; however, many questions remain. Pathways of future investigation of energetics in HF include (1) understanding metabolic differences in HF with reduced versus preserved ejection fraction, (2) defining biochemical remodeling and myocardial mitochondrial function in a new age of conventional therapy, and (3) developing novel metabolic drug targets.

LIMITATIONS AND PERSPECTIVES

Spatial resolution and depth of detection can limit the application of ^{31}P-MRS for heterogenous diseases, such as myocardial infarction. Higher magnetic field strength in clinical applications (7T) will improve signal-to-noise ratio, accelerate acquisitions, and may allow the exploration of Pi and energetics in small myocardial regions. In addition, the development of chemical exchange saturation transfer and hyperpolarized ^{13}C-MRS techniques are promising techniques to map *in vivo* free CR and PCr and assess pyruvate dehydrogenase flux. A current gap in the understanding of bioenergetics in HF is the evaluation of individuals with HF with preserved ejection fraction.

SUMMARY

Myocardial energetics are impaired in systolic HF and acute ischemia. Metabolic remodeling has been demonstrated in progressive HF stages, chronic infarction, and even in conditions associated with increased HF risk, including hypertension, diabetes, and obesity. Some energetic abnormalities have been shown to correlate with symptom severity and significant HF outcomes, including mortality. CMRS has been fundamental in building understanding of energy deprivation in the failing heart and likely will continue to be a pioneering technology in the development and evaluation of new era HF therapeutics with focused metabolic targets.

DISCLOSURE

The authors acknowledge support from the National Institutes of Health (HL61912, HL63030, HL149742, AG063661) and from the Clarence Doodeman Endowment in Cardiology at Johns Hopkins.

REFERENCES

1. Stanley WC, Recchia FA, Lopaschuk GD. Myocardial substrate metabolism in the normal and failing heart. Physiol Rev 2005;85(3):1093–129.
2. Saks V, Dzeja P, Schlattner U, et al. Cardiac system bioenergetics: metabolic basis of the Frank-Starling law. J Physiol 2006;571(Pt 2):253–73.
3. Neubauer S. The failing heart - an engine out of fuel. N Engl J Med 2007;356(11):1140–51.
4. Chacko VP, Aresta F, Chacko SM, et al. MRI/MRS assessment of in vivo murine cardiac metabolism, morphology, and function at physiological heart rates. Am J Physiol Heart Circ Physiol 2000;279(5): H2218–24.
5. Perrine SA, Michaels MS, Ghoddoussi F, et al. Cardiac effects of MDMA on the metabolic profile determined with 1H-magnetic resonance spectroscopy in the rat. NMR Biomed 2009;22(4):419–25.
6. Bottomley PA. Noninvasive study of high-energy phosphate metabolism in human heart by depth-resolved 31P NMR spectroscopy. Science 1985; 229(4715):769–72.
7. El-Sharkawy A-MM, Gabr RE, Schär M, et al. Quantification of human high-energy phosphate metabolite concentrations at 3 T with partial volume and sensitivity corrections. NMR Biomed 2013;26(11): 1363–71.
8. Rodgers CT, Clarke WT, Snyder C, et al. Human cardiac 31P magnetic resonance spectroscopy at 7 Tesla. Magn Reson Med 2014;72(2):304–15.
9. Bottomley PA, Herfkens RJ, Smith LS, et al. Noninvasive detection and monitoring of regional myocardial ischemia in situ using depth-resolved 31P NMR spectroscopy. Proc Natl Acad Sci U S A 1985; 82(24):8747–51.
10. Blackledge MJ, Rajagopalan B, Oberhaensli RD, et al. Quantitative studies of human cardiac metabolism by 31P rotating-frame NMR. Proc Natl Acad Sci U S A 1987;84(12):4283–7.
11. Bottomley PA, Hardy CJ, Roemer PB. Phosphate metabolite imaging and concentration

measurements in human heart by nuclear magnetic resonance. Magn Reson Med 1990;14(3):425–34.

12. Yabe T, Mitsunami K, Inubushi T, et al. Quantitative measurements of cardiac phosphorus metabolites in coronary artery disease by 31P magnetic resonance spectroscopy. Circulation 1995;92(1):15–23.

13. Bottomley PA, Atalar E, Weiss RG. Human cardiac high-energy phosphate metabolite concentrations by 1D-resolved NMR spectroscopy. Magn Reson Med 1996;35(5):664–70.

14. Okada M, Mitsunami K, Inubushi T, et al. Influence of aging or left ventricular hypertrophy on the human heart: Contents of phosphorus metabolites measured by 31P MRS. Magn Reson Med 1998; 39(5):772–82.

15. Meininger M, Landschütz W, Beer M, et al. Concentrations of human cardiac phosphorus metabolites determined by SLOOP 31P NMR spectroscopy. Magn Reson Med 1999;41(4):657–63.

16. Schneider-Gold C, Beer M, Köstler H, et al. Cardiac and skeletal muscle involvement in myotonic dystrophy type 2 (DM2): a quantitative 31P-MRS and MRI study. Muscle Nerve 2004;30(5):636–44.

17. Weiss RG, Gerstenblith G, Bottomley PA. ATP flux through creatine kinase in the normal, stressed, and failing human heart. Proc Natl Acad Sci U S A 2005;102(3):808–13.

18. Smith CS, Bottomley PA, Schulman SP, et al. Altered creatine kinase adenosine triphosphate kinetics in failing hypertrophied human myocardium. Circulation 2006;114(11):1151–8.

19. Bottomley PA, Wu KC, Gerstenblith Gy, et al. Reduced myocardial creatine kinase flux in human myocardial infarction. Circulation 2009;119(14): 1918–24.

20. Abraham MR, Bottomley PA, Dimaano VL, et al. Creatine kinase adenosine triphosphate and phosphocreatine energy supply in a single kindred of patients with hypertrophic cardiomyopathy. Am J Cardiol 2013;112(6):861–6. https://doi.org/10.1016/j.amjcard.2013.05.017.

21. Schär M, El-Sharkawy A-MM, Weiss RG, et al. Triple repetition time saturation transfer (TRiST) 31P spectroscopy for measuring human creatine kinase reaction kinetics. Magn Reson Med 2010;63(6): 1493–501.

22. Schär M, Gabr RE, El-Sharkawy A-MM, et al. Two repetition time saturation transfer (TwiST) with spill-over correction to measure creatine kinase reaction rates in human hearts. J Cardiovasc Magn Reson 2015; 17(1). https://doi.org/10.1186/s12968-015-0175-4.

23. Bashir A, Gropler R. Reproducibility of creatine kinase reaction kinetics in human heart: a 31P time-dependent saturation transfer spectroscopy study. NMR Biomed 2014;27(6):663–71.

24. Clarke WT, Robson MD, Neubauer S, et al. Creatine kinase rate constant in the human heart measured with 3D-localization at 7 tesla. Magn Reson Med 2017;78(1):20–32.

25. Hirsch GA, Bottomley PA, Gerstenblith G, et al. Allopurinol acutely increases adenosine triphospate energy delivery in failing human hearts. J Am Coll Cardiol 2012;59(9):802–8.

26. Valkovič L, Clarke WT, Schmid AI, et al. Measuring inorganic phosphate and intracellular pH in the healthy and hypertrophic cardiomyopathy hearts by in vivo 7T 31P-cardiovascular magnetic resonance spectroscopy. J Cardiovasc Magn Reson 2019;21(1):19.

27. Keller AM, Sorce DJ, Sciacca RR, et al. Very rapid lactate measurement in ischemic perfused hearts using 1H MRS continuous negative echo acquisition during steady-state frequency selective excitation. Magn Reson Med 1988;7(1):65–78.

28. Reingold JS, McGavock JM, Kaka S, et al. Determination of triglyceride in the human myocardium by magnetic resonance spectroscopy: reproducibility and sensitivity of the method. Am J Physiol Endocrinol Metab 2005;289(5):E935–9.

29. Hammer S, van der Meer RW, Lamb HJ, et al. Progressive caloric restriction induces dose-dependent changes in myocardial triglyceride content and diastolic function in healthy men. J Clin Endocrinol Metab 2008;93(2):497–503.

30. Bottomley PA, Weiss RG. Non-invasive magnetic-resonance detection of creatine depletion in nonviable infarcted myocardium. Lancet 1998; 351(9104):714–8.

31. Ardenkjaer-Larsen JH, Fridlund B, Gram A, et al. Increase in signal-to-noise ratio of > 10,000 times in liquid-state NMR. Proc Natl Acad Sci U S A 2003; 100(18):10158–63.

32. Golman K, Petersson JS, Magnusson P, et al. Cardiac metabolism measured noninvasively by hyperpolarized 13C MRI. Magn Reson Med 2008;59(5):1005–13.

33. Schroeder MA, Clarke K, Neubauer S, et al. Hyperpolarized magnetic resonance: a novel technique for the in vivo assessment of cardiovascular disease. Circulation 2011;124(14):1580–94.

34. Schroeder MA, Atherton HJ, Ball DR, et al. Real-time assessment of Krebs cycle metabolism using hyperpolarized 13C magnetic resonance spectroscopy. FASEB J 2009;23(8):2529–38.

35. Rider OJ, Tyler DJ. Clinical implications of cardiac hyperpolarized magnetic resonance imaging. J Cardiovasc Magn Reson 2013;15:93.

36. Hollis DP, Nunnally RL, Taylor GJ, et al. Phosphorus nuclear magnetic resonance studies of heart physiology. J Magn Reson (1969) 1978;29(2):319–30.

37. Jacobus WE, Taylor GJ, Hollis DP, et al. Phosphorus nuclear magnetic resonance of perfused working rat hearts. Nature 1977;265(5596):756–8.

38. Garlick PB, Radda GK, Seeley PJ. Studies of acidosis in the ischaemic heart by phosphorus

nuclear magnetic resonance. Biochem J 1979; 184(3):547–54.

39. Wolfe CL, Moseley ME, Wikstrom MG, et al. Assessment of myocardial salvage after ischemia and reperfusion using magnetic resonance imaging and spectroscopy. Circulation 1989;80(4): 969–82.

40. Weiss RG, Bottomley PA, Hardy CJ, et al. Regional Myocardial Metabolism of High-Energy Phosphates during Isometric Exercise in Patients with Coronary Artery Disease. N Engl J Med 1990;323(23): 1593–600.

41. Buchthal SD, den Hollander JA, Merz CN, et al. Abnormal myocardial phosphorus-31 nuclear magnetic resonance spectroscopy in women with chest pain but normal coronary angiograms. N Engl J Med 2000;342(12):829–35.

42. Yabe T, Mitsunami K, Okada M, et al. Detection of myocardial ischemia by 31P magnetic resonance spectroscopy during handgrip exercise. Circulation 1994;89(4):1709–16.

43. Friedrich J, Apstein CS, Ingwall JS. 31P nuclear magnetic resonance spectroscopic imaging of regions of remodeled myocardium in the infarcted rat heart. Circulation 1995;92(12): 3527–38.

44. Bottomley PA, Weiss RG. Noninvasive localized MR quantification of creatine kinase metabolites in normal and infarcted canine myocardium. Radiology 2001;219(2):411–8.

45. Lamb HJ, Beyerbacht HP, van der Laarse A, et al. Diastolic dysfunction in hypertensive heart disease is associated with altered myocardial metabolism. Circulation 1999;99(17):2261–7.

46. Scheuermann-Freestone M, Madsen PL, Manners D, et al. Abnormal cardiac and skeletal muscle energy metabolism in patients with type 2 diabetes. Circulation 2003;107(24):3040–6.

47. Diamant M, Lamb HJ, Groeneveld Y, et al. Diastolic dysfunction is associated with altered myocardial metabolism in asymptomatic normotensive patients with well-controlled type 2 diabetes mellitus. J Am Coll Cardiol 2003;42(2):328–35.

48. Shivu GN, Phan TT, Abozguia K, et al. Relationship between coronary microvascular dysfunction and cardiac energetics impairment in type 1 diabetes mellitus. Circulation 2010;121(10):1209–15.

49. Rider OJ, Francis JM, Ali MK, et al. Effects of catecholamine stress on diastolic function and myocardial energetics in obesity. Circulation 2012;125(12): 1511–9.

50. Nakae I, Mitsunami K, Matsuo S, et al. Myocardial creatine concentration in various nonischemic heart diseases assessed by 1H magnetic resonance spectroscopy. Circ J 2005;69(6):711–6.

51. Herrmann G, Decherd GM. The chemical nature of heart failure. Ann Intern Med 1939;12(8):1233.

52. Olson RE, Schwartz WB. Myocardial metabolism in congestive heart failure. Medicine (Baltimore) 1951;30(1):21–41.

53. Shen W, Asai K, Uechi M, et al. Progressive loss of myocardial ATP due to a loss of total purines during the development of heart failure in dogs: a compensatory role for the parallel loss of creatine. Circulation 1999;100(20):2113–8.

54. Starling RC, Hammer DF, Altschuld RA. Human myocardial ATP content and in vivo contractile function. Mol Cell Biochem 1998;180(1): 171–7.

55. Ingwall JS, Kramer MF, Fifer MA, et al. The creatine kinase system in normal and diseased human myocardium. N Engl J Med 1985;313(17): 1050–4.

56. Nascimben L, Ingwall JS, Pauletto P, et al. Creatine kinase system in failing and nonfailing human myocardium. Circulation 1996;94(8): 1894–901.

57. Hardy CJ, Weiss RG, Bottomley PA, et al. Altered myocardial high-energy phosphate metabolites in patients with dilated cardiomyopathy. Am Heart J 1991;122(3 Pt 1):795–801.

58. Conway MA, Allis J, Ouwerkerk R, et al. Detection of low phosphocreatine to ATP ratio in failing hypertrophied human myocardium by 31P magnetic resonance spectroscopy. Lancet 1991;338(8773): 973–6.

59. Neubauer S, Krahe T, Schindler R, et al. 31P magnetic resonance spectroscopy in dilated cardiomyopathy and coronary artery disease. Altered cardiac high-energy phosphate metabolism in heart failure. Circulation 1992;86(6):1810–8.

60. Masuda Y, Tateno Y, Ikehira H, et al. High-energy phosphate metabolism of the myocardium in normal subjects and patients with various cardiomyopathies–the study using ECG gated MR spectroscopy with a localization technique. Jpn Circ J 1992;56(6): 620–6.

61. de Roos A, Doornbos J, Luyten PR, et al. Cardiac metabolism in patients with dilated and hypertrophic cardiomyopathy: assessment with proton-decoupled P-31 MR spectroscopy. J Magn Reson Imaging 1992;2(6):711–9.

62. Buser PT, Camacho SA, Wu ST, et al. The effect of dobutamine on myocardial performance and high-energy phosphate metabolism at different stages of heart failure in cardiomyopathic hamsters: a 31P MRS study. Am Heart J 1989;118(1):86–91.

63. Bottomley PA, Panjrath GS, Lai S, et al. Metabolic rates of ATP transfer through creatine kinase (CK Flux) predict clinical heart failure events and death. Sci Transl Med 2013;5(215):215re3.

64. Gabr RE, El-Sharkawy A-MM, Schär M, et al. Cardiac work is related to creatine kinase energy supply in human heart failure: a cardiovascular magnetic

resonance spectroscopy study. J Cardiovasc Magn Reson 2018;20(1):81.

65. Sharma S, Adrogue JV, Golfman L, et al. Intramyocardial lipid accumulation in the failing human heart resembles the lipotoxic rat heart. FASEB J 2004; 18(14):1692–700.

66. Nakae I, Mitsunami K, Yoshino T, et al. Clinical features of myocardial triglyceride in different types of cardiomyopathy assessed by proton magnetic resonance spectroscopy: comparison with myocardial creatine. J Card Fail 2010; 16(10):812–22.

67. Neubauer S, Horn M, Cramer M, et al. Myocardial phosphocreatine-to-ATP ratio is a predictor of mortality in patients with dilated cardiomyopathy. Circulation 1997;96(7):2190–6.

Cardiovascular Magnetic Resonance in Congenital Heart Disease: Focus on Heart Failure

Vivek Muthurangu, MD(res)

KEYWORDS

- Congenital heart disease • Ventricular dysfunction • Cardiovascular magnetic resonance

KEY POINTS

- In the present era, heart failure is most commonly seen in patients with repaired congenital heart disease.
- The main roles of Cardiovascular Magnetic Resonance in congenital heart disease with heart failure are to quantify ventricular volume and function and identify possible causes of dysfunction.
- The most common types of congenital heart disease patients with ventricular dysfunction are those with unrepaired Atrial Septal Defects, repaired Tetralogy of Fallot, Transposition of the Great arteries repaired with an intra-atrial baffle, and functionally single ventricles.

INTRODUCTION

Congenital heart disease (CHD) has an incidence of 6 to 8 per 1000 in neonates.[1] Life expectancy of individuals with CHD has increased significantly due to improvements in diagnosis and treatment (both surgical and interventional). In the current era, a majority of children born in developed countries with CHD survive into adulthood. This has led to an increasing prevalence of patients with CHD in the general population, most of whom require ongoing evaluation.

Imaging is fundamental to the follow-up of CHD patients, helping to guide management decisions, evaluate interventions, and guide prognosis. Echocardiography still is considered the first-line imaging modality for pediatric and adult CHD assessment. This is because it is available in all institutions, is portable, and provides immediate anatomic and physiologic information. For cooperative patients with good acoustic windows, echocardiography alone can guide the diagnosis and management of many conditions. This is true particularly in the neonatal period and early childhood. Echocardiography, however, is highly user-dependent, can be limited by acoustic windows, and provides poor visualization of the distal

vasculature. Thus, historically, echocardiographic assessment has been augmented with cardiac catheterization. Cardiac catheterization not only allows high-resolution delineation of vascular and intracardiac anatomy but also provides reference standard hemodynamic information. Unfortunately, cardiac catheterization is limited by its invasive nature and exposure to ionizing radiation. In addition, conventional x-ray fluoroscopy provides only a projection image and has limited 3-dimensional (3-D) capabilities.

In the past 20 years, cardiovascular magnetic resonance (CMR) has become a vital part of the imaging follow-up in CHD. It provides comprehensive noninvasive evaluation of anatomy and physiology but without exposure to ionizing radiation. One of the major advantages of CMR over other imaging modalities is that it provides both 3-D and unrestricted 2-dimensional (2-D) visualization of the cardiovascular anatomy. Thus, CMR is able to accurately delineate complex intracardiac and vascular abnormalities, irrespective of body habitus. This makes CMR useful particularly in adults with CHD, because they often have poor acoustic windows. For this reason, CMR is recommended in recent guidelines regarding multimodality imaging and the management of adults with

Institute of Cardiovascular Science, University College London, 30 Guilford Street, London WC1N 1EH, UK
E-mail address: v.muthurangu@ucl.ac.uk

Heart Failure Clin 17 (2021) 157–165
https://doi.org/10.1016/j.hfc.2020.08.012

CHD.[2-4] Another advantage of CMR in CHD is reference standard assessment of ventricular volumes, mass, and function. This is due to the easier delineation of endocardial and epicardial borders in high-contrast CMR images as well as the ability to quantify without geometric assumptions.[5-7] The advantages of CMR are particularly valuable for right ventricular (RV) assessment, because its position and complex shape often make it difficult to fully evaluate with echocardiography. For this reason, CMR is vital in the assessment of patients who have CHD with ventricular dysfunction. A final important general indication for CMR is assessment of blood flow. Multiple studies have shown that it provides accurate measurement of cardiac output, regurgitation fraction, and the pulmonary–to–systemic flow ratio (Qp:Qs).[8-11]

CARDIAC FUNCTION

Many CHDs result in ventricular dysfunction and much of the morbidity and mortality experienced by these patients is due to cardiac failure. Thus, measuring ventricular function is a vital aspect of continuing assessment and management of these patients. Cardiac failure often is defined as an inability to produce sufficient cardiac output to supply the bodies metabolic needs. Thus, measuring cardiac output can provide important clinical information regarding cardiac failure. Most CHD patients have normal cardiac output at baseline due to cardiac compensation (eg, ventricular dilation, hypertrophy, and increased filling pressures). In these patients, evaluation of the ventricles may provide a better correlate of symptoms.

One common ventricular manifestation of CHD is dilation, whether this be due to volume loading (eg, valvar regurgitation or shunts) or ventricular failure. Dilation is known to increase the risk of arrhythmia, as well as causing increased wall stress and consequent contractile failure. Thus, measuring ventricular volumes is an important part of the evaluation of CHD. Measuring ventricular volumes also is necessary for precise measurement of ejection fraction. Ejection fraction is the percentage of blood ejected from the heart with every heartbeat. It is a well-recognized measure of cardiac function and ventricular arterial coupling and an important prognostic marker in many forms of CHD.[12,13] Ventricular volumes can be estimated by 2-D echocardiography, but most methods rely on significant geometric assumptions. Although these may hold true for the left ventricle (LV), they are inadequate to describe the crescentic RV.[14] New 3-D echocardiographic techniques do enable volumetric assessment but still suffer from operator dependence and inadequate echocardiographic windows. As discussed previously, CMR has some important advantages over echocardiography, including not being limited by body habitus and unrestricted 2-D imaging. Thus, CMR can image contiguous slices covering the both ventricles, enabling true 3-D assessment of biventricular volumes.[15] Finally, modern steady-state free precession techniques provide high blood pool myocardial contrast, aiding segmentation and further postprocessing.[16] Several studies have shown that CMR provides highly accurate and reproducible measurement of ventricular volumes and ejection fraction data in CHD.[17-19] For these reasons, CMR now should be considered the reference standard method of measuring left volumetric and right volumetric data.

Although assessment of ventricular volumes is a vital element of the CMR protocol for CHD, it does not provide a full picture of cardiac dysfunction. Increasingly, it has been recognized that local myocardial motion may be a more sensitive marker of both early systolic and diastolic ventricular dysfunction. Local myocardial motion can be evaluated by several metrics, such as longitudinal/radial contraction, twisting/torsion, and wall thickening. Some or all of these metrics can be measured with echocardiography using tissue Doppler or strain imaging. Like all echocardiographic techniques, however, they suffer from inadequate windows and operator dependence. Thus, CMR also plays an important role in the evaluation of local myocardial motion. Several CMR techniques can be used for this purpose and these include tissue tagging, tissue phase mapping, and strain/displacement encoding.[20,21] Over the past decade, these techniques have been used to better understand pathophysiology in CHD. Significant clinical utility has not been demonstrated, however, and most sequences still are considered research technologies. More recently, strain (and strain rate) data have been derived from conventional CMR cine data. This has allowed retrospective analysis of historical cine data and demonstration of clinical utility. Several studies have now shown that strain metrics can independently predict outcome (eg, death or major cardiac event) and exercise tolerance in patients with CHD.[22-24] No large studies, however, have demonstrated that CMR strain measures outperform conventional ventricular volumes or ejection fraction data.

There are some limitations in using CMR to measure ventricular volumes and ejection fraction in patients with CHD. In some patients, in particular children, breath holding is difficult and free breathing approaches are required. These include signal averaged gated cine acquisitions and real-time acquisitions. Real-time sequences increasingly are becoming used in pediatric imaging, with new accelerated techniques now reaching the quality of conventional breath hold cines.[25] Several studies have validated real-time CMR for measurement of ventricular volumes and they are a useful alternative in patients who cannot breath hold.

BLOOD FLOW

Assessing ventricular volumes and ejection fraction remains the prime CMR method of evaluating heart failure in CHD patients. Quantification of blood flow, however, also plays an important role. This is because flow-related lesions (eg, shunts or valvar regurgitation) are one of the main causes of ventricular dysfunction in CHD. The reference standard method of measuring shunts in CHD is invasive oximetry with measurement of oxygen saturations (or content) in the pulmonary and systemic arterial and venous systems. From these data, the Qp:Qs can be calculated, which is a measure of both the magnitude and direction of a shunt. This approach is invasive in nature, however, and can be associated with morbidity. In addition, there are some technical problems with invasive oximetry. These include the requirement for multiple blood samples that can result in error propagation[26] and shunt quantification only being possible if sampling can be performed distal to the shunt, which is not possible in some extracardiac lesions (ie, systemic-pulmonary arterial collaterals).

Valvar regurgitation usually is assessed using Doppler echocardiography. The main benefit of this approach is that echocardiography already is the first-line method of evaluating anatomy and cardiac function in CHD. Unfortunately, echocardiographic evaluation of regurgitation either is qualitative or at best semiquantitative. Thus, it is prone to inaccuracy and cannot provide accurate measures of regurgitation fraction or volumes.

CMR can be used to accurately assess blood flow using the velocity-encoded phase-contrast magnetic resonance (PCMR) technique.[8–11,27] In PCMR, the average velocity of blood in each pixel is encoded and thus blood flow in a region of interest (eg, a vessel) can be calculated. As PCMR is a cine acquisition the resulting flow curve can be integrated to calculate metrics, such as stroke volume and cardiac output. There are a significant number of studies that have demonstrated good agreement between PCMR and both direct measurement of flow in phantom studies[11,28] and invasive oximetry in patient studies.[8,11,27] As well as being noninvasive, PCMR has a distinct advantage over invasive oximetry because measurement of

Qp:Qs is not limited to measurement of flow in the pulmonary trunk and aorta. This can be useful particularly in situations where invasive oximetry fails, such as patients with systemic to pulmonary arterial collaterals. The ability to accurately evaluate flow throughout the cardiac cycle also means that PCMR is able to provide truly quantitative measures or pulmonary or aortic valve regurgitation. Furthermore, combining great arterial flow with ventricular volume data also can allow calculation of atrioventricular (AV) valve regurgitation. Thus, CMR can be used to better evaluate the important primary causes of heart failure in CHD, aiding clinical decision making in these patients.

Another area PCMR can be used is assessment of diastolic function. Diastolic dysfunction often is overlooked as a cause of symptoms in CHD. The traditional method of assessing diastolic function is echocardiographic assessment of AV valve inflow. Specifically, the ratio of early to late inflow velocities (E/A ratio) is an important indicator of ventricular diastolic dysfunction. The E/A ratio also can be measured using PCMR and some studies have demonstrated clinical utility.[29]

SPECIFIC LESIONS

Not all CHDs result in heart failure, and many patients have minimal symptoms after successful repair in the infant period. There are 4 instances, however, in which ventricular dysfunction and accompanying symptoms are common and these are discussed in more detail.

Shunt Lesions

Many shunt lesions are identified in early life, in particular ventricular septal defects (VSDs) and patent ductus arteriosus (PDA). In younger children, both VSDs and PDAs can be identified easily and assessed using echocardiography. Children with complex or multiple VSDs[30] or difficult-to-visualize ducts, however, may benefit from CMR for full 3-D evaluation. In addition, CMR measurement of the Qp:Qs and LV volume may be important in determining management in older children and adults.[2]

Consequently, the most common indication for CMR in patients with shunts is assessment of older children and adults with unrepaired atrial septal defects (ASDs). ADSs are an anatomically heterogeneous group of lesions, and the natural history and management of this disease depend on the specific type. Ostium secundum defects are the most common lesions and are located in the fossa ovalis. Ostium primum defects, on the other hand, are a type atrioventricular septal defect and associated with some degree of atrioventricular valve abnormality. Sinus venosus defects are found at the junction of the right atrium and either of the caval veins and often are associated with partial anomalous pulmonary venous drainage. The final type of ASD is an unroofed coronary sinus, which is not strictly a defect in the atrial septum but is associated with similar physiology. A majority of isolated ASDs result in left-to-right shunts and right volume overload due to the fact that the shunt occurs before the atrioventricular valves.

The use of CMR in patients with ASDs falls into 2 main categories: (1) comprehensive assessment of anatomy and (2) evaluation of physiology. In terms of anatomic assessment, definitive diagnosis and evaluation of possible sinus venosus defects and anomalous pulmonary venous connection are among the most important CMR indications.[31,32] This is because these lesions often are difficult to image with echocardiography, particularly in adults, where they easily can be missed. This also is true for patients with unroofed coronary sinus, which often are difficult to visualize with transthoracic echocardiography. Although secundum defects usually can be identified with transthoracic echocardiography, CMR can be used determine suitability for transcatheter or surgical closure,[33–35] providing a noninvasive alternative to transesophageal echocardiography with better sensitivity for anomalous pulmonary venous connections.

The other aspect of CMR assessment in these patients is quantification of the magnitude of the shunt through calculation of Qp:Qs and measurement of RV volumes and function. This provides important information for clinical decision making, particularly in borderline lesions.

Tetralogy of Fallot

Another group of patients with RV volume overload are those with repaired tetralogy of Fallot (ToF) and pulmonary regurgitation. ToF is the most common cyanotic congenital heart defect, with an incidence of approximately 420 per million live births.[1] It is caused by malalignment of the infundibular septum, which leads to RV outflow (RVOT) obstruction, a subaortic VSD with aortic override, and RV hypertrophy. Current management consists of early single-stage reconstructive surgery,[36] although staged procedures are necessary in more complex cases. This procedure has the benefit of leaving the patient acyanotic and has good survival rates.[37] Because symptoms appear in early life in most patients, echocardiography usually is sufficient for initial diagnosis and assessment.[38] Prior to the initial repair, CMR rarely is needed but it may have a role in

assessing the pulmonary arteries in more complex cases.[39–41]

The main role of magnetic resonance (MR) in patients with ToF is assessment of postoperative complications. Operative repair of ToF consists of VSD closure and relief of RVOT obstruction, often with placement of a transannular patch. This compromises pulmonary valve integrity, resulting in pulmonary regurgitation. Pulmonary regurgitation results in RV volume overload and ultimately RV dysfunction. In some patients, either as part of the initial repair or subsequent pulmonary valve replacement (PVR), an RV to pulmonary artery conduit is placed. In conduits, the main mode of failure is mixed dysfunction with some degree of both RVOT obstruction and pulmonary regurgitation. Due to this RVOT dysfunction, a majority of patients require PVR. CMR is useful in these patients for determining both the timing of PVR and the type of PVR performed (eg, surgical or catheter based).

Accurate quantification of regurgitation and/or stenosis is important in deciding the type and timing of procedures. PCMR has been shown to quantify pulmonary regurgitation accurately and has been validated internally against MR ventricular volumetry in patients with ToF.[42] PCMR also can assess differential regurgitation in the branch pulmonary arteries accurately. This is important in patients with PVR with metallic components (eg, Hancock valve), because artifact may prevent accurate flow mapping in the pulmonary trunk. Although regurgitation can be qualitatively assessed using transthoracic or transesophageal echocardiography, the ability of MR to quantify regurgitant fraction and volume accurately makes it a superior technique. PCMR also can be used to measure peak velocities at the level RVOT obstruction. Conventional PCMR, however, underestimates peak velocity[43] and Doppler echocardiography still should be considered the reference standard method of measuring peak velocities. CMR also is useful in delineating anatomic abnormalities of RVOT, which is important for planning surgical or interventional valve replacement.

The result of RVOT dysfunction is volume and/or pressure loading, which results in RV failure as well as LV dysfunction due to ventricular interdependence. Because morbidity and mortality in these patients ultimately are related to ventricular dysfunction, volumetric evaluation is a vital aspect of the follow-up in ToF patients. Measuring ventricular volumes function also is important when evaluating the effect of any invasive procedure.[44–46] It has been shown that when using a combination of MR ventricular volumetry and tricuspid and pulmonary flow maps, precise information about global and diastolic ventricular function can be assessed in patients with repaired ToF.[47] Importantly, CMR-derived parameters inform risk-stratification[13,48–50] and referral for PVR,[44,51,52] and figure prominently in published clinical management guidelines.[2–4,53] The presence of localized ventricular scarring or fibrosis also has been associated with arrhythmia and ventricular dysfunction in patients after repair of ToF.[48] Thus, late gadolinium enhancement is an important component of assessing older patients with repaired ToF.

Systemic Right Ventricle

Ventricular dysfunction due to volume overload (eg, shunts or valvar regurgitation) is common in CHD. Pressure overload, however, also is an important cause of ventricular dysfunction in some CHD patients. This is true particularly in patients with systemic RVs. This group includes patients born with transposition of the great arteries (TGA) who have undergone an atrial switch procedure and congenitally corrected TGA (CCTGA). TGA is the second most common cyanotic CHD[1] and is defined as ventriculoarterial discordance with an anterior aorta arising from the RV and the pulmonary artery arising from the LV. Surgical therapy for this condition was revolutionized with the introduction of the Senning procedure in which an intra-atrial baffle was used to divert blood from the right atrium to the LV and the left atrium to the RV.[54] A further variation was the Mustard procedure in which a pericardial patch was used to construct the intra-atrial baffle.[55] Both procedures produced a physiologically normal but an anatomically abnormal circulation (systemic venous return to the left atrium, LV, and then pulmonary artery; pulmonary venous return to the right atrium, RV, and then aorta). Although the intra-atrial repair has been superseded by the arterial switch operation, there is a sizable population of adults who have undergone either a Senning or Mustard operation. The most common complications of intra-atrial repair are baffle obstruction or leak, arrhythmias, and RV dysfunction. Baffle obstruction is more common in the Mustard operation,[56] probably due to calcification and poor growth of the pericardial tissue used to construct the baffle. The venous pathways have a complex 3-D structure and are difficult to assess accurately with transthoracic echocardiography. Thus, 3-D MR imaging is extremely useful in demonstrating the anatomy of the Senning/Mustard anatomy and has been

shown to be able to detect baffle narrowing.[57] Obstruction of either the superior venocaval or inferior venocaval limb of the intra-atrial baffles can be corroborated from MR angiographic by identifying venous collaterals, which divert blood from the obstructed venous system. PCMR also can be useful in identifying baffle obstruction, with in-plane PCMR visualizing flow turbulence at the site of baffle narrowing and through-plane PCMR confirming loss of the typical, phasic, venous flow profile. Baffle leaks can be difficult to visualize even with CMR cine imaging. They result, however, in a shunt and easily can be detected measuring Qp:Qs using PCMR.

The etiology of RV dysfunction in patients with intra-atrial baffles is complex. Deranged atrioventricular coupling as a result of the baffles may be important.[58] Studies have shown that atrial baffle function limits RV filling rates during exercise or pharmacologic stress, despite appropriate responses in load-independent indices of RV contraction and relaxation.[59] RV dysfunction may be present, however, without abnormal coupling and it is likely that the RV also is inherently unprepared to pump against systemic afterload. RV systolic function has been assessed in patients with intra-atrial repair of TGA using CMR and has been shown to be lower than in matched controls.[58] Studies also have demonstrated areas of focal myocardial fibrosis using late gadolinium enhancement techniques in adults late after atrial baffle repair of TGA.[60,61] These studies demonstrated that the presence of fibrosis was associated with RV systolic dysfunction, poor exercise tolerance, arrhythmia, and progressive clinical deterioration.

CCTGA is a rare disorder characterized by atrioventricular and ventricle-arterial discordance (right atrium to LV to pulmonary artery and left atrium to RV to aorta). Thus, these patients also have a systemic RV. CCTGA may be asymptomatic and, in some patients, an incidental finding. A majority of patients with CCTGA, however, have associated cardiac lesions, which often are the source of cardiac problems. The most common associated lesions are VSDs, pulmonary stenosis, and tricuspid valve abnormalities (ie, Ebstein abnormality).[62] Even without associated abnormalities, a majority of patients with CCTGA develop systemic ventricular failure over time. The main roles of MR are in evaluation of associated lesions, quantification of ventricular function, and assessment of postoperative complications. RV function has been assessed in patients with CCTGA using CMR[58] and has been shown to be reduced both at baseline and in response to dobutamine stress.[58]

Single Ventricle

The final example of patients with CHD and ventricular dysfunction is those born with a functionally single ventricle. Because most patients present in the newborn period, echocardiography is the primary imaging tool during initial evaluation. In some cases, however, CMR may be used to determine whether a 1-ventricle versus 2-ventricle repair should be pursued.[63,64] CMR also can be useful in more complex forms of heterotaxy syndrome,[65,66] because it provides reliable 3-D visualization of intracardiac and vascular anatomy. Nevertheless, the common use of CMR in these in infants and younger children is as a noninvasive alternative to cardiac catheterization during staged palliation toward a Fontan circulation. Multiple studies have shown CMR outperforms echocardiography and can substitute routine diagnostic catheterization in selected patients prior to the bidirectional cavopulmonary connection (Glenn shunt or a hemi-Fontan procedure)[67–70] and total cavopulmonary connection (Fontan procedure).[71–73] In addition, CMR measurements of systemic–to–pulmonary artery collateral flow predict postoperative outcomes, such as hospital length of stay,[74–76] and can be used for optimization of hospital resources. After the Fontan procedure, patients remain at risk for numerous complications, including ventricular and valve dysfunction, Fontan baffle obstruction, pulmonary artery stenosis, aortic coarctation, systemic–to–pulmonary venous collateral formation, and intracardiac thrombus formation. CMR has a key role in surveillance for these complications because echocardiography alone often is inadequate.[77,78] Finally, CMR-derived parameters, such as ventricular volume and myocardial fibrosis, have been shown to be associated with adverse outcomes.[79,80]

SUMMARY

Over the past decade, CMR has become a mainstream noninvasive imaging tool for assessment of adult and pediatric patients with CHD. It provides comprehensive anatomic and hemodynamic information that echocardiography and catheterization alone do not provide. Extracardiac anatomy can be delineated with high spatial resolution, intracardiac anatomy can be imaged in multiple planes, and functional assessment can be made accurately and with high reproducibility. In patients with heart failure, CMR provides not only reference standard evaluation of ventricular volumes and function but also information about the possible causes of dysfunction (eg, shunts and valvar regurgitation). It, therefore, should be considered a vital part of the follow-up in this group of patients.

CLINICS CARE POINTS

- Cardiovascular Magnetic Resonance provides accurate and reproducible measures of ventricular volume and function.
- Cardiovascular Magnetic Resonance provides enables accurate quantification of shunts and valvar regurgitation.

DISCLOSURE

The author has nothing to disclose.

REFERENCES

1. Hoffman JI, Kaplan S. The incidence of congenital heart disease. J Am Coll Cardiol 2002;39(12): 1890–900.
2. Baumgartner H, Bonhoeffer P, De Groot NM, et al. ESC Guidelines for the management of grown-up congenital heart disease (new version 2010). Eur Heart J 2010;31(23):2915–57.
3. Kilner PJ, Geva T, Kaemmerer H, et al. Recommendations for cardiovascular magnetic resonance in adults with congenital heart disease from the respective working groups of the European Society of Cardiology. Eur Heart J 2010; 31(7):794–805.
4. Stout KK, Daniels CJ, Aboulhosn JA, et al. 2018 AHA/ACC Guideline for the Management of Adults With Congenital Heart Disease: Executive Summary: A Report of the American College of Cardiology/ American Heart Association Task Force on Clinical Practice Guidelines. J Am Coll Cardiol 2018; 73(12):1494–563.
5. Buechel EV, Kaiser T, Jackson C, et al. Normal right- and left ventricular volumes and myocardial mass in children measured by steady state free precession cardiovascular magnetic resonance. J Cardiovasc Magn Reson 2009;11:19.
6. Robbers-Visser D, Boersma E, Helbing WA. Normal biventricular function, volumes, and mass in children aged 8 to 17 years. J Magn Reson Imaging 2009; 29(3):552–9.
7. Sarikouch S, Peters B, Gutberlet M, et al. Sex-specific pediatric percentiles for ventricular size and mass as reference values for cardiac MRI: assessment by steady-state free-precession and phase-contrast MRI flow. Circ Cardiovasc Imaging 2010; 3(1):65–76.
8. Beerbaum P, Korperich H, Barth P, et al. Noninvasive quantification of left-to-right shunt in pediatric patients: phase-contrast cine magnetic resonance imaging compared with invasive oximetry. Circulation 2001;103(20):2476–82.

9. Beerbaum P, Korperich H, Gieseke J, et al. Rapid left-to-right shunt quantification in children by phase-contrast magnetic resonance imaging combined with sensitivity encoding (SENSE). Circulation 2003;108(11):1355–61.

10. Hundley WG, Li HF, Hillis LD, et al. Quantitation of cardiac output with velocity-encoded, phase-difference magnetic resonance imaging. Am J Cardiol 1995;75(17):1250–5.

11. Muthurangu V, Taylor A, Andriantsimiavona R, et al. Novel method of quantifying pulmonary vascular resistance by use of simultaneous invasive pressure monitoring and phase-contrast magnetic resonance flow. Circulation 2004;110(7):826–34.

12. Bokma JP, de Wilde KC, Vliegen HW, et al. Value of Cardiovascular Magnetic Resonance Imaging in Noninvasive Risk Stratification in Tetralogy of Fallot. JAMA Cardiol 2017;2(6):678–83.

13. Valente AM, Gauvreau K, Assenza GE, et al. Contemporary predictors of death and sustained ventricular tachycardia in patients with repaired tetralogy of Fallot enrolled in the INDICATOR cohort. Heart 2014;100(3):247–53.

14. Greutmann M, Tobler D, Biaggi P, et al. Echocardiography for assessment of right ventricular volumes revisited: a cardiac magnetic resonance comparison study in adults with repaired tetralogy of Fallot. J Am Soc Echocardiogr 2010;23(9):905–11.

15. Geva T. Is MRI the preferred method for evaluating right ventricular size and function in patients with congenital heart disease?: MRI is the preferred method for evaluating right ventricular size and function in patients with congenital heart disease. Circ Cardiovasc Imaging 2014;7(1):190–7.

16. Hudsmith LE, Petersen SE, Francis JM, et al. Normal human left and right ventricular and left atrial dimensions using steady state free precession magnetic resonance imaging. J Cardiovasc Magn Reson 2005;7(5):775–82.

17. Beygui F, Furber A, Delepine S, et al. Routine breath-hold gradient echo MRI-derived right ventricular mass, volumes and function: accuracy, reproducibility and coherence study. Int J Cardiovasc Imaging 2004;20(6):509–16.

18. Clarke CJ, Gurka MJ, Norton PT, et al. Assessment of the accuracy and reproducibility of RV volume measurements by CMR in congenital heart disease. JACC Cardiovasc Imaging 2012;5(1):28–37.

19. Mooij CF, de Wit CJ, Graham DA, et al. Reproducibility of MRI measurements of right ventricular size and function in patients with normal and dilated ventricles. J Magn Reson Imaging 2008;28(1): 67–73.

20. Khalaf A, Tani D, Tadros S, et al. Right- and left-ventricular strain evaluation in repaired pediatric Tetralogy of Fallot patients using magnetic resonance tagging. Pediatr Cardiol 2013;34(5):1206–11.

21. Fogel MA, Gupta KB, Weinberg PM, et al. Regional wall motion and strain analysis across stages of Fontan reconstruction by magnetic resonance tagging. Am J Physiol 1995;269(3 Pt 2):H1132–52.

22. Menting ME, van den Bosch AE, McGhie JS, et al. Assessment of ventricular function in adults with repaired Tetralogy of Fallot using myocardial deformation imaging. Eur Heart J Cardiovasc Imaging 2015; 16(12):1347–57.

23. Kalaitzidis P, Orwat S, Kempny A, et al. Biventricular dyssynchrony on cardiac magnetic resonance imaging and its correlation with myocardial deformation, ventricular function and objective exercise capacity in patients with repaired tetralogy of Fallot. Int J Cardiol 2018;264:53–7.

24. Schmidt R, Orwat S, Kempny A, et al. Value of speckle-tracking echocardiography and MRI-based feature tracking analysis in adult patients after Fontan-type palliation. Congenit Heart Dis 2014; 9(5):397–406.

25. Steeden JA, Kowalik GT, Tann O, et al. Real-time assessment of right and left ventricular volumes and function in children using high spatiotemporal resolution spiral bSSFP with compressed sensing. J Cardiovasc Magn Reson 2018;20(1):79.

26. Antman EM, Marsh JD, Green LH, et al. Blood oxygen measurements in the assessment of intracardiac left to right shunts: a critical appraisal of methodology. Am J Cardiol 1980;46(2):265–71.

27. Hundley WG, Li HF, Lange RA, et al. Assessment of left-to-right intracardiac shunting by velocity-encoded, phase-difference magnetic resonance imaging. A comparison with oximetric and indicator dilution techniques. Circulation 1995;91(12): 2955–60.

28. Greil G, Geva T, Maier SE, et al. Effect of acquisition parameters on the accuracy of velocity encoded cine magnetic resonance imaging blood flow measurements. J Magn Reson Imaging 2002;15(1):47–54.

29. Paelinck BP, Lamb HJ, Bax JJ, et al. MR flow mapping of dobutamine-induced changes in diastolic heart function. J Magn Reson Imaging 2004;19(2): 176–81.

30. Bhatla P, Tretter JT, Ludomirsky A, et al. Utility and Scope of Rapid Prototyping in Patients with Complex Muscular Ventricular Septal Defects or Double-Outlet Right Ventricle: Does it Alter Management Decisions? Pediatr Cardiol 2017;38(1):103–14.

31. Prompona M, Muehling O, Naebauer M, et al. MRI for detection of anomalous pulmonary venous drainage in patients with sinus venosus atrial septal defects. Int J Cardiovasc Imaging 2011;27(3): 403–12.

32. Valente AM, Sena L, Powell AJ, et al. Cardiac magnetic resonance imaging evaluation of sinus venosus defects: comparison to surgical findings. Pediatr Cardiol 2007;28(1):51–6.

33. Beerbaum P, Korperich H, Esdorn H, et al. Atrial septal defects in pediatric patients: noninvasive sizing with cardiovascular MR imaging. Radiology 2003;228(2):361–9.

34. Teo KS, Disney PJ, Dundon BK, et al. Assessment of atrial septal defects in adults comparing cardiovascular magnetic resonance with transoesophageal echocardiography. J Cardiovasc Magn Reson 2010;12:44.

35. Thomson LE, Crowley AL, Heitner JF, et al. Direct en face imaging of secundum atrial septal defects by velocity-encoded cardiovascular magnetic resonance in patients evaluated for possible transcatheter closure. Circ Cardiovasc Imaging 2008;1(1):31–40.

36. Lillehei CW, Varco RL, Cohen M, et al. The first open heart corrections of tetralogy of Fallot. A 26-31 year follow-up of 106 patients. Ann Surg 1986;204(4): 490–502.

37. Nollert G, Fischlein T, Bouterwek S, et al. Long-term survival in patients with repair of tetralogy of Fallot: 36-year follow-up of 490 survivors of the first year after surgical repair. J Am Coll Cardiol 1997;30(5):1374–83.

38. Tworetzky W, McElhinney DB, Brook MM, et al. Echocardiographic diagnosis alone for the complete repair of major congenital heart defects. J Am Coll Cardiol 1999;33(1):228–33.

39. Beekman RP, Beek FJ, Meijboom EJ. Usefulness of MRI for the pre-operative evaluation of the pulmonary arteries in Tetralogy of Fallot. Magn Reson Imaging 1997;15(9):1005–15.

40. Geva T, Greil GF, Marshall AC, et al. Gadolinium-enhanced 3-dimensional magnetic resonance angiography of pulmonary blood supply in patients with complex pulmonary stenosis or atresia: comparison with x-ray angiography. Circulation 2002; 106(4):473–8.

41. Holmqvist C, Hochbergs P, Bjorkhem G, et al. Pre-operative evaluation with MR in tetralogy of fallot and pulmonary atresia with ventricular septal defect. Acta Radiol 2001;42(1):63–9.

42. Rebergen SA, Chin JG, Ottenkamp J, et al. Pulmonary regurgitation in the late postoperative follow-up of tetralogy of Fallot. Volumetric quantitation by nuclear magnetic resonance velocity mapping. Circulation 1993;88(5 Pt 1):2257–66.

43. Steeden JA, Jones A, Pandya B, et al. High-resolution slice-selective Fourier velocity encoding in congenital heart disease using spiral SENSE with velocity unwrap. Magn Reson Med 2012;67(6): 1538–46.

44. Frigiola A, Tsang V, Bull C, et al. Biventricular response after pulmonary valve replacement for right ventricular outflow tract dysfunction: is age a predictor of outcome? Circulation 2008;118(14 Suppl):S182–90.

45. Heng EL, Gatzoulis MA, Uebing A, et al. Immediate and Midterm Cardiac Remodeling After Surgical Pulmonary Valve Replacement in Adults With Repaired Tetralogy of Fallot: A Prospective Cardiovascular Magnetic Resonance and Clinical Study. Circulation 2017;136(18):1703–13.

46. Vliegen HW, van Straten A, de Roos A, et al. Magnetic resonance imaging to assess the hemodynamic effects of pulmonary valve replacement in adults late after repair of tetralogy of fallot. Circulation 2002;106(13):1703–7.

47. Helbing WA, Niezen RA, Le Cessie S, et al. Right ventricular diastolic function in children with pulmonary regurgitation after repair of tetralogy of Fallot: volumetric evaluation by magnetic resonance velocity mapping. J Am Coll Cardiol 1996;28(7): 1827–35.

48. Babu-Narayan SV, Kilner PJ, Li W, et al. Ventricular fibrosis suggested by cardiovascular magnetic resonance in adults with repaired tetralogy of fallot and its relationship to adverse markers of clinical outcome. Circulation 2006;113(3):405–13.

49. Knauth AL, Gauvreau K, Powell AJ, et al. Ventricular size and function assessed by cardiac MRI predict major adverse clinical outcomes late after tetralogy of Fallot repair. Heart 2008;94(2):211–6.

50. Orwat S, Diller GP, Kempny A, et al. Myocardial deformation parameters predict outcome in patients with repaired tetralogy of Fallot. Heart 2016;102(3): 209–15.

51. Lee C, Kim YM, Lee CH, et al. Outcomes of pulmonary valve replacement in 170 patients with chronic pulmonary regurgitation after relief of right ventricular outflow tract obstruction: implications for optimal timing of pulmonary valve replacement. J Am Coll Cardiol 2012;60(11):1005–14.

52. Oosterhof T, van Straten A, Vliegen HW, et al. Preoperative thresholds for pulmonary valve replacement in patients with corrected tetralogy of Fallot using cardiovascular magnetic resonance. Circulation 2007;116(5):545–51.

53. Geva T. Repaired tetralogy of Fallot: the roles of cardiovascular magnetic resonance in evaluating pathophysiology and for pulmonary valve replacement decision support. J Cardiovasc Magn Reson 2011;13:9.

54. Senning A. Correction of the transposition of the great arteries. Ann Surg 1975;182(3):287–92.

55. Mustard WT. Recent experiences with surgical management of transposition of the great arteries. J Cardiovasc Surg (Torino) 1968;9(6):532–6.

56. Sarkar D, Bull C, Yates R, et al. Comparison of long-term outcomes of atrial repair of simple transposition with implications for a late arterial switch strategy. Circulation 1999;100(19 Suppl):176–81.

57. Fogel MA, Hubbard A, Weinberg PM. Mid-term follow-up of patients with transposition of the great arteries after atrial inversion operation using two- and three-dimensional magnetic resonance imaging. Pediatr Radiol 2002;32(6):440–6.

58. Tulevski II, van der Wall EE, Groenink M, et al. Usefulness of magnetic resonance imaging dobutamine stress in asymptomatic and minimally symptomatic patients with decreased cardiac reserve from congenital heart disease (complete and corrected transposition of the great arteries and subpulmonic obstruction). Am J Cardiol 2002;89(9):1077–81.

59. Derrick GP, Josen M, Vogel M, et al. Abnormalities of right ventricular long axis function after atrial repair of transposition of the great arteries. Heart 2001; 86(2):203–6.

60. Giardini A, Lovato L, Donti A, et al. Relation between right ventricular structural alterations and markers of adverse clinical outcome in adults with systemic right ventricle and either congenital complete (after Senning operation) or congenitally corrected transposition of the great arteries. Am J Cardiol 2006;98:1277–82.

61. Babu-Narayan SV, Goktekin O, Moon JC, et al. Late gadolinium enhancement cardiovascular magnetic resonance of the systemic right ventricle in adults with previous atrial redirection surgery for transposition of the great arteries. Circulation 2005;111: 2091–8.

62. Bjarke BB, Kidd BS. Congenitally corrected transposition of the great arteries. A clinical study of 101 cases. Acta Paediatr Scand 1976;65(2):153–60.

63. Banka P, Schaetzle B, Komarlu R, et al. Cardiovascular magnetic resonance parameters associated with early transplant-free survival in children with small left hearts following conversion from a univentricular to biventricular circulation. J Cardiovasc Magn Reson 2014;16:73.

64. Grosse-Wortmann L, Yun TJ, Al-Radi O, et al. Borderline hypoplasia of the left ventricle in neonates: insights for decision-making from functional assessment with magnetic resonance imaging. J Thorac Cardiovasc Surg 2008;136(6):1429–36.

65. Hong YK, Park YW, Ryu SJ, et al. Efficacy of MRI in complicated congenital heart disease with visceral heterotaxy syndrome. J Comput Assist Tomogr 2000;24(5):671–82.

66. Yim D, Nagata H, Lam CZ, et al. Disharmonious Patterns of Heterotaxy and Isomerism: How Often Are the Classic Patterns Breached? Circ Cardiovasc Imaging 2018;11(2):e006917.

67. Brown DW, Gauvreau K, Powell AJ, et al. Cardiac magnetic resonance versus routine cardiac catheterization before bidirectional glenn anastomosis in infants with functional single ventricle: a prospective randomized trial. Circulation 2007;116(23):2718–25.

68. Brown DW, Gauvreau K, Powell AJ, et al. Cardiac magnetic resonance versus routine cardiac catheterization before bidirectional Glenn anastomosis: long-term follow-up of a prospective randomized trial. J Thorac Cardiovasc Surg 2013;146(5):1172–8.

69. Krupickova S, Muthurangu V, Hughes M, et al. Echocardiographic arterial measurements in complex congenital diseases before bidirectional Glenn: comparison with cardiovascular magnetic resonance imaging. Eur Heart J Cardiovasc Imaging 2017;18(3):332–41.

70. Muthurangu V, Taylor AM, Hegde SR, et al. Cardiac magnetic resonance imaging after stage I Norwood operation for hypoplastic left heart syndrome. Circulation 2005;112(21):3256–63.

71. Ait-Ali L, De Marchi D, Lombardi M, et al. The role of cardiovascular magnetic resonance in candidates for Fontan operation: proposal of a new algorithm. J Cardiovasc Magn Reson 2011;13:69.

72. Fogel MA. Is routine cardiac catheterization necessary in the management of patients with single ventricles across staged Fontan reconstruction? No! Pediatr Cardiol 2005;26(2):154–8.

73. Prakash A, Khan MA, Hardy R, et al. A new diagnostic algorithm for assessment of patients with single ventricle before a Fontan operation. J Thorac Cardiovasc Surg 2009;138(4):917–23.

74. Glatz AC, Rome JJ, Small AJ, et al. Systemic-to-pulmonary collateral flow, as measured by cardiac magnetic resonance imaging, is associated with acute post-Fontan clinical outcomes. Circ Cardiovasc Imaging 2012;5(2):218–25.

75. Grosse-Wortmann L, Drolet C, Dragulescu A, et al. Aortopulmonary collateral flow volume affects early postoperative outcome after Fontan completion: a multimodality study. J Thorac Cardiovasc Surg 2012;144(6):1329–36.

76. Odenwald T, Quail MA, Giardini A, et al. Systemic to pulmonary collateral blood flow influences early outcomes following the total cavopulmonary connection. Heart 2012;98(12):934–40.

77. Margossian R, Schwartz ML, Prakash A, et al. Comparison of echocardiographic and cardiac magnetic resonance imaging measurements of functional single ventricular volumes, mass, and ejection fraction (from the Pediatric Heart Network Fontan Cross-Sectional Study). Am J Cardiol 2009;104(3):419–28.

78. Williams RV, Margossian R, Lu M, et al. Factors impacting echocardiographic imaging after the Fontan procedure: a report from the pediatric heart network fontan cross-sectional study. Echocardiography 2013;30(9):1098–106.

79. Rathod RH, Prakash A, Kim YY, et al. Cardiac magnetic resonance parameters predict transplantation-free survival in patients with fontan circulation. Circ Cardiovasc Imaging 2014;7(3):502–9.

80. Rathod RH, Prakash A, Powell AJ, et al. Myocardial fibrosis identified by cardiac magnetic resonance late gadolinium enhancement is associated with adverse ventricular mechanics and ventricular tachycardia late after Fontan operation. J Am Coll Cardiol 2010;55:1721–8.

Moving?

Make sure your subscription moves with you!

To notify us of your new address, find your **Clinics Account Number** (located on your mailing label above your name), and contact customer service at:

Email: journalscustomerservice-usa@elsevier.com

800-654-2452 (subscribers in the U.S. & Canada)
314-447-8871 (subscribers outside of the U.S. & Canada)

Fax number: 314-447-8029

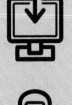

Elsevier Health Sciences Division
Subscription Customer Service
3251 Riverport Lane
Maryland Heights, MO 63043

Printed and bound by CPI Group (UK) Ltd, Croydon, CR0 4YY

03/10/2024

01040372-0016